Child Growth and Nutrition
in Developing Countries

Food Systems and Agrarian Change

Edited by Frederick H. Buttel, Billie R. DeWalt, and
Per Pinstrup-Andersen

CHILD GROWTH AND NUTRITION IN DEVELOPING COUNTRIES

Priorities for Action

EDITED BY

Per Pinstrup-Andersen

David Pelletier

Harold Alderman

Cornell University Press

ITHACA AND LONDON

First published 1995 by Cornell University Press.

Printed in the United States of America

⊗ The paper in this book meets the minimum requirements of the American National Standard for Information Sciences—Permanence of Paper for Printed Library Materials, ANSI Z39.48-1984.

Library of Congress Cataloging-in-Publication Data

Child growth and nutrition in developing countries : priorities for
    action / [edited by] Per Pinstrup-Andersen, David Pelletier, Harold
    Alderman.
        p.   cm. — (Food systems and agrarian change)
    "Revised August 1993"—CIP t.p.
    Includes bibliographical references and index.
    ISBN 0-8014-8189-9 (alk. paper)
        1. Nutrition policy—Developing countries. 2. Children—
Developing countries—Nutrition. 3. Women—Developing countries—
Nutrition. 4. Children—Developing countries—Growth.
I. Pinstrup-Andersen, Per. II. Pelletier, David L. III. Alderman, Harold, 1948–   .
IV. Series.
TX360.5.C49   1994
363.8'8'083—dc20   94-31497

Contents

Preface

Improved nutritional status for young children is one of the most highly desired results of a science-based development effort in poor nations emphasizing agriculture, health, population, and the environment. Food deficiency, of course, leads to poor nutrition, but so do infections and other illnesses; and food deficiencies and poor health are in turn related to ineffective family planning and child spacing. An unsafe and deteriorating ecological environment threatens nutritional sustainability. Our best statistical efforts reveal that about 40 percent of the world's children under age five, 141 million, are chronically undernourished. Studies around the world have shown the dramatic increased risk of death among these children, many of whom die from minor diseases that become fatal in the dangerous milieu of malnutrition. Those who live may suffer long-term reductions in their capacity to learn and to work. Yet a high proportion of this waste of human potential, with its toll on national development, can be avoided by implementing simple nutrition and growth-promoting strategies that are financially and technically feasible. The international community knows more about what to do technically than about how to do it. Operationally useful information on cost-effective ways to reach, hear, and respond to needs of vast numbers of impoverished families, especially mothers, with diverse cultural values and practices is woefully scarce.

This volume grows out of an effort led by Per Pinstrup-Andersen and sponsored by the Rockefeller Foundation to take stock of existing knowledge of nutritional improvement and attempt to analyze the web of constraints that have slowed the translation of technical information into effective ongoing action on the ground. The book builds from the analytical and conceptual to an understanding of how and why things do or do not work in practice. By attempting to examine both the behavior of high-risk households and past intervention experience, the authors have directed their research toward evaluative and operational ends. There is particular emphasis on the role of information as it affects the design and implementation of nutritional interventions from the household level through to community action and on to national policies that influence the socioeconomic environment within which community action takes place. Despite the tremendous gains in scientific knowledge about nutritional deficiencies and their technical relief, real payoffs must ultimately come through the effectiveness of locally tailored approaches to the specifics of community circumstances. This, in turn, suggests greater emphasis on applied behavioral studies and community involvement in identifying their own nutritional solutions. Future nutritional research and operational interventions, as the volume demonstrates, can be brought closer together in the continuing global effort to promote the health and well-being of our children now at risk.

JOYCE LEWINGER MOOCK
ASSOCIATE VICE PRESIDENT
THE ROCKEFELLER FOUNDATION
New York, New York

*Child Growth and Nutrition
in Developing Countries*

I

Beyond Child Survival:
An Overview of the Issues

Per Pinstrup-Andersen, David Pelletier,
and Harold Alderman

In 1990 over 1.1 billion people in developing countries were living in poverty, nearly half of them in extreme poverty. About half of the developing world's poor—more than 500 million people—live in South Asia. East Asia is home to another 15 percent, Sub-Saharan Africa to 19 percent, and Latin America and the Caribbean to 10. In both South Asia and Sub-Saharan Africa about 50 percent of the population is poor.

Projections indicate that if significant efforts are made along various avenues, both the depth and the breadth of poverty can be reduced. Gains are looked for particularly in East and South Asia. In Sub-Saharan Africa, on the other hand, for a variety of reasons, the number of poor people is expected to increase by almost 50 percent by the year 2000.

Poverty and hunger work hand in hand against the children of the developing world. Even those who escape serious disease are likely to be significantly underweight, a condition that spirals back on itself to retard growth in other areas. Moreover, the number of underweight children under five years of age is rising, from some 164 million in 1980 to 184 million in 1990, with a projection of 200 million by the turn of the century. Again, a major increase is expected in Sub-Saharan Africa, but the situation in South Asia is also bleak; almost half the children there are projected to be significantly underweight by 2000.

Micronutrient deficiencies are also widespread. About 14 million preschool children have eye damage as a result of vitamin A deficiency. Between a quarter and a half a million such children go blind each year from lack of vitamin A, and two thirds of these die within months of

I

going blind. Iron deficiency—leading to anemia, which diminishes learning capacity as well as lowering physical health—also affects about a billion people in the world, particularly children and women of childbearing age.

The immediate causes of growth faltering among preschool children—insufficient intake of energy, nutrients, or both, and prevalence of infectious diseases—are known and their effects generally understood. They are outcomes of a complex web of biological, social, and economic factors and relationships, which are location-specific and often poorly understood for a particular population group, location, and time period.

Efforts to alleviate malnutrition often fail to reflect both complexity and location-specificity. In some cases, comprehensive attempts have been made to deal with all major factors as, for example, multisectoral nutrition planning efforts. Other attempts have focused on one or more factors believed to be the major causes of existing malnutrition. The impact on nutrition of either of the two types of efforts, although not uniformly small, has not been impressive. Recent attempts have been made to tailor integrated health and nutrition programs to particular geographic areas, taking location-specific factors and relationships into account, with varying degrees of participation by the intended beneficiaries. These attempts have shown considerable promise, although there have been some disappointments.

To enhance the probability of success, future efforts to alleviate malnutrition and growth faltering among preschool children should be based on the experience of past efforts and current knowledge. This book provides the results of syntheses of such experience and related research results. The syntheses are based on the relevant theory and conceptual relationships, and the authors attempt to separate evidence founded on solid research and evaluation from that which is more speculative. Claims based on simplistic reasoning and without solid support, a not uncommon phenomenon in the nutrition literature, are ignored or identified as such. As a reflection of the multidisciplinary nature of the problem, the book covers research from several disciplines, and we have tried to keep jargon to a minimum to facilitate access to the material. To the fullest extent possible, we have provided references for the reader to pursue issues raised.

The syntheses presented in this book cover the following issues and interventions:

1. Household Behavior
   a. Demand for food
   b. Demand for health care

    c. Child care
    d. Breastfeeding
    e. Family planning
    f. Women's time allocation
2. Interventions Influencing Behavior
    a. Nutrition education
    b. Growth monitoring
    c. Women's education and employment
3. Interventions Influencing Health
    a. Child survival interventions
    b. Integrated health and nutrition programs
    c. Water and sanitation projects
    d. Family planning
4. Interventions Influencing Access to Food
    a. Food and income transfers
    b. Agricultural programs and policies
5. Organization, Information, and Action
    a. Community participation
    b. Multisectoral nutrition planning
    c. Information
    d. Lessons for action

Although referred to in several chapters, the magnitudes of malnutrition and growth faltering and associated functional and economic consequences are not explicitly dealt with in this volume. The reader is referred to Pinstrup-Andersen, Burger, Habicht, and Peterson (1993) for a recent treatment of these issues. Micronutrients are not explicitly treated either, because two initiatives on micronutrients, one by the World Bank and the other by the Commission on International Health, began at the time the present work was initiated.

This chapter provides an overview of the issues covered in the book and some of the major findings. No overview can do justice to the richness of each chapter, but some highlighting will be useful to readers.

In Chapter 2, Reynaldo Martorell examines the rationale for emphasizing normal child growth and avoiding growth faltering. In addition to the epidemiology, prevalence, and measurement of growth faltering in developing countries, Martorell identifies the functional consequences and potential benefits of alleviating growth faltering and suggests related research needs.

Martorell emphasizes the importance of growth, rather than small size per se, as an indicator of health and nutrition stress. Growth faltering is often associated with weaning and usually occurs before children are three years old. Little catch-up growth seems to occur subsequently. Therefore, nutrition interventions should give priority to children under three years old with emphasis on the weaning period. Children's growth rates reflect their general health and nutritional status, but they do not identify the contribution of specific factors to growth. Therefore, growth monitoring must be accompanied by the search for other information to identify the reasons for growth faltering.

External assistance may be essential, but the actions of households in general and mothers in particular are the most critical component of overall efforts to assure good nutrition for preschool children. Household behavior determines how household resources—including those resulting from external nutrition intervention programs—are allocated, given the constraints within which the household must operate. Therefore, an understanding of how households with members at risk of malnutrition behave is paramount in understanding how best to alleviate such risk.

Chapters 3 to 7 deal with household behavior and action aimed at changing such behavior, including nutrition education, growth monitoring, and improved child care.

In Chapter 3, Jere Behrman presents a conceptual framework for the consideration of household behavior regarding health and nutrition of preschool children, summarizes the related empirical evidence, and identifies the implications for information needs for households, communities, and governments. Using a health production function as the base, Behrman identifies issues important for the design and implementation of nutrition intervention, including understanding the interactions among inputs, that is, whether they are substitutes or complements. Identification of possible substitutions may greatly improve cost-effectiveness of individual interventions, while complementarity would argue for more integrated programs. For example, under what conditions are formal education and nutrition education complements or substitutes? Do more educated women make better use of specialized nutrition information, or is such information likely to have a greater impact among uneducated women? Should more emphasis be placed on the alleviation of community-level constraints, such as sanitation and clean drinking water, than on enhancing household resources? Answers to these and many related questions require sound understanding of the behavior of the target households.

A more general question raised by Behrman is whether nutrition education can change household behavior by changing preferences or by enhancing household awareness of options and consequences. The author argues that the latter aim is likely to be more justifiable in consequences for individual welfare. Finally, the chapter provides a review of common methodological fallacies in studies of household behavior that have resulted in misinterpretation of findings.

Nutrition education is the most common approach used to alleviate malnutrition by changing household and individual behavior. In Chapter 4, Maria Teresa Cerqueira and Christine M. Olson examine the education components of selected recent successful nutrition projects. Most past nutrition education efforts have failed in part because they have used the medical model as a guide. Such efforts were often implicitly or explicitly of a prescriptive and curative nature, as illustrated by use of the term "compliance" to assess whether the prescribed behavioral changes occurred. In this model households were merely passive recipients, and the active participation of intended beneficiaries in the design and implementation of nutrition education projects was not deemed necessary. Similarly, the need to understand the socioeconomic environment within which nutrition education was to work was not fully appreciated. Although this model is still the basis for much ongoing nutrition education, it has been rejected by most experts.

Chapter 4 draws from experience to demonstrate the importance of a thorough understanding of the nutrition problem, household behavior, and the reasons for prevailing behavior as well as the environment constraining the intended beneficiaries. Community participation is considered an important strategy to ensure that nutrition education activities address the issues of concern to the beneficiaries, although surprisingly few of the programs reviewed explicitly facilitated community involvement. Some of the successful projects examined show very little community participation, but all are based on a clear understanding of the target group and their behavior. Receiver-oriented, rather than sender-oriented, messages should be sent, and interactive, multichannel approaches appear to be particularly promising. The question of substitution versus complementarity between nutrition education and other interventions arises in this chapter as well, particularly regarding the interaction between nutrition education and income transfers and formal education.

Growth monitoring is a key component in many recent nutrition education projects, including those reviewed in Chapter 4. In Chapter 5, Marie T. Ruel argues that the controversy over growth monitoring results partly from a lack of clarity and consensus about what growth monitoring really is, what it can potentially achieve, and how it should be evaluated. The chapter attempts to clarify these issues and compares, for each form of growth monitoring, the theoretical objectives and expectations with actual achievements in various programs and projects.

Ruel divides growth-monitoring activities into three broad categories, according to purpose: an educational and promotional tool, an integrating strategy, and a source of information for mothers and professionals. Whatever the purpose, growth monitoring is intended to lead to action to improve nutrition; it is not itself a nutrition intervention. Ruel concludes that growth monitoring has great potential but that poor implementation and ineffective use in nutrition education have often prevented the potential from materializing. Growth monitoring has achieved more success in community activities than in clinics. Its effectiveness for screening and surveillance appears limited. Use of growth monitoring to educate mothers may be incompatible with its use for nutritional surveillance because of the competition for the health worker's time and the different needs for reporting and processing data. The author suggests that a decision should be made as to which purpose to pursue.

As in previous chapters, the question of substitution and complementarity is discussed. In particular, it is important to identify conditions and programs that are likely to deter or enhance the usefulness of growth monitoring for a given purpose.

The synthesis of behavioral issues related to nutrition is continued in Chapter 6, in which Patrice L. Engle stresses the importance of the interaction between mothers or other caregivers and children in efforts to assure good nutrition. She proposes a transactional model that takes into account the interaction between the child and its environment. Engle argues that such a model will result in more relevant and cost-effective interventions. Several examples of programs inappropriate to address an existing problem and behavior are given. These include nutrition education to convince mothers to feed children during periods of diarrhea, when mothers already do so, and food supplementation program directed toward children who do not consume all the food they are served.

Engle concludes that the amount of food available in the home is not a good proxy for the quantity consumed by the child. Other variables must be considered, including frequency of feeding, the child's appetite, amount refused, energy density, the caregiver's feeding behavior, and beliefs about feeding children. Mothers' time devoted to activities other than child care often reduces the quality of interaction with the child, and Engle concludes that mothers' work may have negative effects on the nutritional status of young infants. Maternal work for earnings has been seen to have positive effects for older children, however.

Three groups of interventions are identified on the basis of the transactional model. These are aimed to (a) increase the responsiveness of the child, (b) increase the resources of the caregiver, and (c) enhance interactions within the household. Engle stresses that technological solutions such as the perfect weaning food are less likely to be effective than interventions tailored to specific circumstances.

As illustrated in Chapter 6, women generally play the central role in assuring adequate nutrition for children. One way they do so is by assuring adequate nutrition for themselves during pregnancy and lactation. As Joanne Leslie discusses in Chapter 7, however, adequate nutrition for women is also a goal in itself, independent of its effect on children. The extent and major types of malnutrition among women and some of the main determinants of these are discussed, and the author synthesizes information on how household and community practices, and nutrition interventions themselves, influence women's nutrition. Finally, she makes recommendations for improving their nutrition and enhancing the role of information.

Leslie suggests that a clear distinction be made between women as a target for behavioral change and women as intended beneficiaries of nutrition intervention. The former is much more common than the latter. A number of factors Behrman identified as influencing child nutrition, such as women's education, time allocation, and self-esteem, also influence the nutritional status of women. Furthermore, because women's nutritional status during pregnancy, lactation, and other periods affects children's nutritional status, there is clearly a considerable commonality between efforts to improve women's nutrition and efforts to improve children's. For example, the small size of women resulting from previous nutritional insults is associated with low birth weight and high infant mortality. Thus the goal of improving the nutritional status of premenopausal women appears compatible with improving the nutritional status of preschool children.

Although this book is about nutritional deficiencies, Leslie reminds us that obesity is becoming a significant nutrition problem among women in certain countries, including low-income women in some developing countries. Thus, although most low-income women would benefit from reduced energy expenditures, behavioral changes may be needed to accompany changes in life-styles. Education may also be needed to counter what appears to be a widespread "eating down" during pregnancy aimed at keeping the birth weight low among women who are already at risk of having low-birth-weight babies.

Leslie recommends a series of actions likely to improve women's nutrition and suggests that gender-specific information is needed, including community-level information design future interventions correctly.

The book then turns to syntheses of program experiences and research related to health interventions and immediate causes of infectious diseases, including assessments of the impact of child survival interventions on child growth and nutrition, recent integrated health and nutrition programs, water and sanitation projects, and the interaction between family planning and health and nutrition.

Action to assure child survival has received considerable support from national governments and funding agencies. In Chapter 8, Sandra L. Huffman and Adwoa Steel examine the impact of this action on child growth and nutrition. Growth faltering and poor nutrition among children below two years of age are generally associated with high rates of mortality. The authors ask whether and to what extent action to promote child survival has been successful in reducing mortality without reducing the prevalence of malnutrition and poor growth—the "dark side" of child survival.

The chapter discusses the following child survival interventions: improved infant and child feeding (including breastfeeding and improved weaning practices), oral rehydration therapy, measles immunization, and control of acute respiratory infections. Efforts to promote breastfeeding have been successful, and breastfeeding has proven to be extremely effective in assuring adequate nutrition in infants. Conforming to findings in other chapters, Huffman and Steel identify the weaning period as the most critical period for nutrition and suggest that interventions related to child feeding should play a major role in future action to improve nutrition. Immunization against measles affects mortality but appears to have little or no impact on nutrition, although improved nutrition has been shown to reduce the prevalence and severity of some childhood diseases.

Huffman and Steel present cost estimates for health interventions for child survival as well as nutrition interventions and conclude that current expenditures on nutrition are too low relative to expenditures on health. They further conclude that community participation and more extensive use of nongovernmental organizations (NGOs) are likely to enhance the cost-effectiveness of nutrition intervention.

In Chapter 9, Susan E. Burger and Steven A. Esrey address two principal causes of infectious diseases: poor sanitation and contaminated water. The chapter is divided into two parts. The influence of improved water and sanitation in reducing exposure to pathogens and disease is reviewed first, followed by the influence of improved water supplies on time savings and improved child health. The issue of substitution and complementarity or, to use the authors' terms, compensation and complementation, between interventions and between interventions and environmental factors mentioned in several chapters is tackled head-on in this chapter.

Burger and Esrey state that "people live over a film of contamination," which implies that removing one pathway for pathogen exposure leaving others intact may do little to reduce infections. A case in point is the finding that improving the quality of water in a very contaminated environment generally does little to reduce infections whereas providing access to larger quantities of water often is more effective.

Many examples support the conclusion that water and sanitation interventions can either complement existing efforts, such as health education, or compensate for undesirable conditions, such as a lack of breastfeeding, to reduce pathogen transmission. Single interventions will be effective only if they break the transmission of pathogens not dealt with by other means. Alternatively, a package of interventions to prevent transmission from all existing major routes would be needed.

Burger and Esrey also conclude on the basis of available evidence that improvements in water supply frequently result in major savings in women's time. Such time may be spent on nutrition-related activities, including child care and income generation. The evidence suggests that the nutritional status of children improves where water supplies have been improved even though diarrhea was affected little or not at all. This may be a result of changes in time allocation, but existing information does not support a definitive conclusion. Information is also insufficient on other related issues, and the authors suggest areas where additional research would contribute to better interventions for the future.

In Chapter 10, John S. Haaga reviews two bodies of evidence concerning the relationship between demographic factors and child health, survival, and growth. The first concerns the extent to which demographic risk factors are consistently associated with infant and child mortality, low birth weight, and postnatal growth across populations, including consideration of the possible mechanisms and confounding factors underlying these relationships. The review finds that short birth interval, young and old maternal age, and high parity are consistently associated with low birth weight, infant mortality, and child mortality. Although fewer studies are available, there is evidence of similar relationships with postnatal growth. The possible mechanisms of action for various risk factors include the maternal depletion syndrome, increased transmission of disease from older siblings to infants, competition among siblings for scarce household resources (food, maternal care, and health care), and health conditions that differentially affect young versus old mothers (e.g., pregnancy-induced hypertension, urogenital tract infections).

The second body of evidence concerns the impact of family planning programs on child health outcomes. The review finds that well-managed programs have reduced the incidence of births to mothers in some high-risk groups, notably those at the extremes of the age distribution and at high parity. On this basis and building on the first body of evidence, Haaga concludes that these programs have improved child health outcomes as well. The review also highlights the unexpected result that birth intervals are shorter in countries where contraceptive use is greatest, probably because of interference with breastfeeding, and puts forth hypotheses for why this may be a real (i.e., not spurious) result that represents an urgent area for further research. Finally, the review notes that, despite the health rationale for family planning programs often stated by donors and governments, the setting of program targets, choice of target groups of women, and choice of evaluation indicators all suggest that health improvement is viewed as a potentially fortuitous by-product of the real objective of these programs (fertility reduction). These problems and other information gaps, notably in sub-Saharan Africa, are discussed in the final section of the chapter.

Moving to the food side of the nutrition problem, Beatrice Rogers, in Chapter 11, reviews past experience and research results regarding feeding programs and food-related transfers. She identifies five factors to be considered in efforts to enhance the effects of these programs. First, the programs must be effectively targeted. Second, coverage of the most vulnerable population must be assured. Third, the size of the benefit should be sufficient. Fourth, barriers to participation, especially time and monetary constraints, should be removed; and fifth, the programs should be based on local information about the nature of the problem and the feasibility of alternative solutions. Rogers argues strongly for programs that are tailored to specific communities and environments rather than generalized programs aimed at many communities and environments.

Further probing for solutions on the food side of the nutrition equation, Saba Mebrahtu, David Pelletier, and Per Pinstrup-Andersen examine in Chapter 12 the nutritional effects of changes in agriculture, with emphasis on agricultural research and technological change, commercialization of semisubsistence farming, rural development projects, land tenure changes, and agricultural pricing and marketing policies.

In the past, simplistic reasoning about the links between agriculture and nutrition resulted in erroneous conclusions about likely nutrition effects of agricultural changes. Although agriculture and nutrition are closely linked, the links are less direct than previously assumed. For example, changes in national food production are usually a poor proxy for changes in the nutritional status of children. The authors identify six pathways through which changes in agriculture may affect nutrition: (1) incomes of households with at-risk members, including level, fluctuations, control, and sources; (2) food prices; (3) time allocation of household members, particularly women; (4) energy and nutrient expenditures; (5) infectious diseases; and (6) changing nutrient composition of individual commodities.

Technological change and commercialization have helped raise incomes of farmers and landless laborers in regions suited for these changes. In these regions the smaller and larger farmers have adopted technological change and participated in commercialization equally except in cases where existing institutions were biased against small farmers, and employment has usually increased. Furthermore, multiplier effects associated with increased income have further amplified regional incomes and employment. As a result of higher incomes from commercialization, food consumption by food-deficit households and individuals has increased and the nutritional status of preschool children has improved, although very slightly. The nutrition effect may be constrained by infectious diseases, lack of knowledge, or other factors that hinder nutrition improvements despite increased food consumption. Only short-run effects have been estimated, however. In the longer run enhanced incomes will likely influence constraints other than insufficient food, including community sanitation. The studies reviewed also identify groups of households that appear to have lost from the above changes, including some farmers who lost land to commercialization schemes. No short-run negative nutrition effects were detected among any of these groups.

Authors of several chapters have identified community participation as a critical element of successful nutrition intervention programs. In Chapter 13, Roger Shrimpton examines the record of community participation in government-promoted food and nutrition programs in four countries. He develops an analytical framework for measuring community participation and assesses the importance of information.

Shrimpton concludes that community participation has contributed to the success of all the programs analyzed, although the degree and type of such participation varied. In three of the four programs studied, participation was limited to achieving efficiency objectives and only one program—the Iringa program in Tanzania—pursued both efficiency and empowerment goals. Furthermore, only Iringa used community participation in needs assessment and strategy formulation. Community-based growth monitoring was common to all programs, but the usage of the generated information varied.

The author suggests that the real barrier to achieving community participation is a lack of organization. He argues that efficiency goals are insufficient if we are pursuing long-term sustained improvements. Empowerment is essential. To promote real community participation we initially need simple interventions to produce visible and desirable effects. Growth monitoring may be an effective component of such initial efforts. A clearer understanding of how to use nutrition information at the community level, including that generated by growth monitoring, would strengthen efforts to improve nutrition. In particular, the sustainability of such efforts would be enhanced if information could be more effectively used in the community empowerment process, creating more autonomy and self-sufficiency at the community level.

Continuing the review of organizational issues in Chapter 14, F. James Levinson focuses on the national level. As opposed to agriculture and health, nutrition is usually not considered a sector and does not have a natural home in government bureaucracies. In view of the multisectoral nature of nutrition and in response to the poor performance of past supply-oriented nutrition interventions, the idea of multisectoral nutrition planning gained considerable momentum during the early 1970s. Levinson reviews the experience gained and the lessons learned.

The author concludes that although multisectoral nutrition planning did not become a widespread organizational tool, it has had a very significant impact on subsequent nutrition-related action by conditioning thinking and analysis of causality, by stressing disaggregation of households and targeting, and by raising sensitivity of agricultural and health professionals to the nutrition effects of their work. Although most nutrition programs may be sectoral, the lessons from multisectoral nutrition planning may help us avoid certain pitfalls. Levinson identifies a return to the supply-oriented "magic bullet" interventions as one such pitfall.

Levinson identifies food policy analysis as one legacy of multisectoral nutrition planning. In Chapter 15, Harold Alderman examines whether and how information generated by such analyses influences food and nutrition policy. He recognizes a range of roles for information generated from research, from its use in creating awareness among the general public and recruiting support within a political arena to redefining both conventional wisdom and research priorities among professionals. These are long-run processes and differ greatly from an idealized process in which decision makers act directly on a study initiated by those individuals to address a felt information gap. It is noteworthy that when such cases can be found, they can usually be linked to the promotion of findings by a few committed insiders or to a long-term interaction between the researchers and policy makers. Usable knowledge implies a user; a scientist does not necessarily abandon scientific objectivity by identifying such actors and including them in discussions to facilitate the dissemination of information.

Alderman feels that the political nature of competing information is not necessarily antithetical to good science. Indeed, controversy attracts scrutiny and, therefore, reinforces methodological rigor. Underlying this view is an assumption that science is self-correcting. Policies and technology, however, are generally path dependent, hence, there are often appreciable costs to misguided policies that persist long after researchers have modified the perspectives on which the policies were based. This observation stresses the importance of communication between scientists and the individuals who make and implement policies.

The last two chapters provide syntheses across the subjects covered in the previous chapters and attempt to draw general lessons for future action. In Chapter 16, David Pelletier synthesizes the findings presented in previous chapters with respect to the role of information. The previous chapters clearly show that information needs are much greater than can be provided by nutritional surveillance. This chapter attempts to integrate the various categories of required information into a generalized framework for use at national, community, or household levels, indicating in broad terms how it might be operationalized at each level. Nutritional surveillance, whether conceived in a broad or a narrow sense, is an implicit part of this framework along with a variety of other information strategies not generally recognized as part of nutritional surveillance.

The resulting framework, if fully operationalized at the national level, is acknowledged to be too resource-demanding to be feasible. It nonetheless provides the basis for rationalizing the use of existing resources such that priority information needs can be identified and pursued in keeping with national conditions. When operationalized at community or district levels, the framework provides a mechanism for harmonizing the need to achieve some degree of community participation for efficiency or empowerment purposes with the realistic need for governments to maintain some degree of control over many programmatic aspects. At that level the purpose is to better inform the decisions and actions of government agencies concerning location-specific needs, constraints, and opportunities during the process of planning and implementation.

Finally, in Chapter 17 we attempt to identify the most important lessons for future action to assure healthy growth and adequate nutrition for preschool children. The nature and determinants of child nutrition, as well as the constraints to adequate nutrition and the opportunities for their removal, vary among households, communities, and countries, and so must approaches for sustainable nutrition improvement. Efforts to alleviate child malnutrition across countries or across all high-risk household groups within a given country by means of a prepackaged general solution have failed in the past and will fail if tried again. Because of the high degree of location-specificity, the content of the interventions is seldom generalizable across communities. The process, on the other hand, appears to be more generalizable.

Past experience has shown that a high degree of participation by intended beneficiaries in the diagnosis of problems and the design and implementation of intervention greatly enhances the probability of success.

Instead of prepackaged interventions for widespread application, external agencies, such as government agencies, should offer an array or menu of intervention components from which each community could choose. A change from prepackaged interventions for widespread application to a menu of options will require stronger institutional, administrative, and logistical frameworks, particularly those related to the delivery of goods and services, including health care, food or food entitlements, and information. It will also require attitudinal changes at all levels.

Government agencies also should make available information about technical and economic feasibility of various options, and they should provide technical assistance to communities to initiate and strengthen their capabilities to diagnose and solve their nutrition problems. In other words, government participation in community action might be more appropriate than community participation in action designed and implemented by external agencies. The policy environment is critical for the success of community-level efforts. The often ignored nutrition effects of government policies not explicitly aimed at nutrition may be very important indeed.

2

Promoting Healthy Growth:
Rationale and Benefits

Reynaldo Martorell

As the end of the century approaches, governments and agencies in developing countries which deal with child welfare are becoming more concerned with quality of life than with mere survival. Quality of life can be broadly defined as physical and mental well-being. Health-related indicators of physical well-being include adequate nutritional status, as measured by anthropometric, biochemical, and clinical indicators and freedom from disease.

Anthropometric measures are generally the best global indicators of physical well-being in children because inadequate food intake, poor nutritional quality of the diet, and various infections affect growth. Poor growth is also a predictor of other undesirable outcomes such as increased morbidity and mortality in early childhood. Finally, the end result of poor growth in early childhood, small adult body size, has functional consequences such as diminished work capacity and increased obstetric risk for women.

The emerging view emphasizing quality of life has been clearly articulated by Rhode (1988). This book is another example of the changing perception. Both stress the need for adequate growth in children on the premise that if adequate growth is achieved, the probability is high that children will be healthy and well-nourished.

This view is supported in this chapter, but it is emphasized that in enhancing or promoting growth one should advocate that *growing bigger is better* rather than *big is better*. This distinction is extremely important from a programmatic point of view. As Beaton (1989) notes, identifying children who are failing to grow is more likely to lead to effective and timely intervention than focusing on small body size as the problem. Older children who may be small because of past growth retardation may be growing at the expected rate, and younger children whose body sizes are not yet markedly small may be growing poorly (i.e., in the process of becoming small). Only a focus on growth retardation rather than on its outcome, small body size, would identify the latter group as being in poorer health. The notion that adequacy of growth rates is to be emphasized over achieved size is, of course, the raison d'être for growth-monitoring programs.

This chapter is meant as a general introduction to others that follow on specific policies and programs. Its chief goal is to examine the rationale for the proposition that enhancing child growth is the key to improving child health and nutrition in developing countries. The chapter also reviews the measurement of growth faltering, discusses the choice of reference population, describes the epidemiology of growth faltering in developing countries, briefly reviews data about the prevalence of growth retardation in poor countries, identifies the functional correlates and outcomes of growth retardation, considers research needs, and, finally, discusses the potential benefits of alleviating growth faltering.

This chapter is focused on the rationale for promoting growth and is not a review of experiences with growth-monitoring programs in developing countries. Though it is now widely recognized that such programs often fail to trigger actions to improve growth for a variety of technical, logistic, and other reasons, the goal of growth promotion continues to be advocated (UNICEF, 1992b; Latham, 1991).

Measurement of Poor Growth

Poor growth is ultimately a response to limited nutrient availability or utilization—or both—at the cellular level. Little is known about the nature and sequencing of responses to varying types and levels of nutrient deficiencies. At severe levels of protein-energy deficiency, linear growth probably ceases altogether and tissue reserves (e.g., fat, lean body mass) are likely used as energy and protein sources to maintain vital functions. At less severe stages, however, little or no wasting may occur because it may be possible to cope with deficiencies simply by slowing the rate of linear growth and perhaps through other compensatory mechanisms as well. Almost nothing is known about the role of diminished physical activity in coping with energy deficiency in children.

Two basic types of growth responses can be monitored: linear growth and wasting. Further, these responses may be measured either in dynamic fashion as changes over time or statically at any one time.

The most common measure of linear growth used is total body length (or height in older children), and the most widely used measure of wasting is weight-for-length (or weight-for height), though other measures of localized tissue reserves are often used (e.g., arm circumference, skinfold measurements). Weight, the single most common measure taken in developing countries, reflects the degree of adequacy of both linear growth and mass-to-length status.

By tracking changes through time, as in growth monitoring, one can assess whether a child is growing adequately. "Adequate growth" or the converse, "growth faltering," are frequently used but poorly defined terms. Loss of weight or failure to gain any weight between consecutive measures (i.e., over a specified span of time, often monthly) are the usual definitions followed in growth-monitoring approaches and have the virtue of simplicity. The inadequate weight gain method is also used in some programs. This is failure to gain a specified amount of weight per unit of time at certain ages.

There are problems with these definitions. For example, at some ages, the absolute rate of growth per month (e.g., the second year of life) is small in comparison to instrument precision and intraindividual, nonnutritional causes of variation (e.g., weight fluctuations caused by sweat losses, intake of food and water, micturition, and defecation). Though incremental growth charts are available (Roche and Himes, 1980; Roche et al., 1989), they are difficult for untrained personnel to interpret and, therefore, cannot be used easily to guide growth-monitoring programs. Ideally, internationally accepted reference data should be available about weight gain and its variability at various ages (by every month of age) and for various intervals (as short as one month and as long as six months). This information would permit one to estimate the rate of false positives (i.e., healthy children identified as faltering) for various criteria. Also, data are needed on how children grow in rich and poor countries to estimate the proportion expected to falter using various definitions (Martorell and Shekar, forthcoming). The criterion for triggering action might conceivably be adjusted to make sure that the proportion of children identified at risk, and therefore deserving of focused attention, is in keeping with program resources.

Onetime anthropometric assessments relate measures of body size (e.g., length/height, weight) obtained to age-sex specific values in the reference population or evaluate wasting by comparing the weight measured to that of the median weight of children of similar lengths/heights and sex in the reference population. A variety of ways of expressing the data, including percentile rankings, percent of median values, and standard deviation or z-scores, are used (Waterlow et al., 1977). The criterion of less than two standard deviations below the reference median ($z = -2$) is widely accepted as a definition of small body size (i.e., stunting) or wasting.

Choice of Reference Population

The issue of which reference population to use in assessing the extent of growth faltering has been a cause of much controversy (Goldstein and Tanner, 1980; Graitcer and Gentry, 1981). The emerging consensus appears to be that healthy preschool children of diverse ethnic groups have surprisingly similar growth patterns (Martorell, 1985). Population differences of "genetic" origin are evident for some comparisons, but these differences are apparently quite small. Differences that can be attributed to environmental factors, however, are remarkably large. For example, in the United States blacks are taller than whites before puberty, leading Garn and Clark (1976) to propose separate reference curves for blacks, a suggestion that has been ignored because the differences in stature are small (Himes, 1984). For some groups, for example Japanese and Koreans, differences compared to children of European ancestry may be somewhat greater, but it is not clear whether the secular trend in growth has reached a plateau in these Asian populations (Martorell, 1985). Yip and colleagues (1992) have documented remarkable improvement in the growth status of successive cohorts of young children born to Asian refugees in the United States; over time, differences with respect to U.S. whites are being reduced significantly.

The World Health Organization (WHO) has adopted the reference curves of the National Center of Health Statistics (NCHS) for worldwide use (Waterlow et al., 1977). These curves are based on several sources of data from the United States (Hamill et al., 1979). For children under two years of age the data used are from the Fels Research Institute in Yellow Springs, Ohio, and come from studies of a white, middle-class population. For older children the data come from nationally representative surveys of children in the United States and include all ethnic groups and social classes. In addition to the reference curves, the Centers for Disease Control (CDC) have made available computer subroutines, which allow for comparisons of anthropometric data to the reference curves (i.e., the programs yield percentile rankings, percent of median values, and z-scores) upon specification of length/height, weight, age, and sex information for all subjects (Dibley et al., 1987a). These curves and the CDC program have a number of technical problems because two distinct data sets were used to construct the reference curves (Dibley et al., 1987b; Yip and Trowbridge, 1989). The implications of these problems for the analyses and interpretation of anthropometric data in developing countries are not fully known but are thought to be minor.

Concern has also been expressed that the NCHS curves are inappropriate for healthy, breastfed infants. Some authors believe that these infants tend to be lighter, nearly as long, but similar in head circumference when compared to the NCHS reference curves (Butte et al., 1984; Neville and Oliva-Rashbach, 1989; Dewey et al., 1992). Some researchers, by contrast, have concluded that there are no significant differences in growth between breast- and bottle-fed infants (Roche et al., 1989). This issue deserves further investigation.

The difficulties in perfecting reference curves for the United States illustrate those inherent in generating statistically sound and appropriate growth curves. Large, representative sample sizes and sophisticated statistical expertise are required in constructing the curves. Not all developing countries have these resources.

The Timing of Growth Faltering and Its Causes

Adults and children from disadvantaged areas of developing countries are considerably smaller than upper-class adults and children from the same countries or those from industrialized nations (Martorell, 1985). Considerable information has accumulated to show that almost all of the growth retardation observed in developing countries has its origins in the first 2 or 3 years of life. Data from Egypt, Kenya, and Mexico from the Nutrition Collaborative Research Support Program (CRSP) indicate that most of the deceleration in growth occurs before age 2 (Calloway et al., 1992). A study of poor Indian boys found that stunting at 5 years of age was the key factor determining small adult stature (Satyanarayana et al., 1980). Shorter children did not catch up relative to taller children; specifically, the gain in height from 5 to approximately 18 years was independent of the degree of stunting at 5 years of age. In fact, the gain in height was of similar magnitude in poor Indians as in well-to-do Indians and only 2 to 3 cm less than reported for samples of European origin. A later study by the same authors found a somewhat different situation in Indian girls (Satyanarayana et al., 1981). Indian girls grew from 5 to 18 years of age by an amount equal or greater than that recorded for European girls. In contrast to boys, catch-up growth occurred, but not enough to eliminate the deficit incurred in early childhood. For example, the tallest and shortest groups of girls differed by 14.2 cm at 5 years but by only 7.7 cm at 18 years. Long-term prospective studies from rural Guatemala also indicate that growth retardation is largely confined to the first few years of life. No catch-up growth occurred in either boys or girls over 5 years of age. Also, the gain in height from 5 years to adulthood for rural Guatemalans was similar to that observed for children of Mexican origin growing up in the United States and only slightly less than the gain predicted by the NCHS reference curves (Martorell et al., 1990).

A study from Nigeria found that boys and girls classified into groups according to stature at 5 years of age maintained parallel growth curves to 17 years of age (Hussain, Nwaka, and Omololu, 1985). This finding implies that increments were independent of stature at 5 years. A study from The Gambia showed that the gain in height from 3 years to adulthood was the same in local boys and girls as in British subjects (Billewicz and McGregor, 1982). The authors of this study concluded that the losses caused by growth faltering in early life in developing countries are never regained. Finally, a study of a middle-class Indian group showed that adult deficits in height were almost entirely a product of prepubertal growth (Hauspie et al., 1980).

It seems that growth lost during the early years is not often regained during later childhood and adolescence (Martorell, et al., 1994). The reasons are not entirely clear. It may be that a poor environment limits the potential for compensatory growth. This is probably not the case in Guatemala during the preschool period; food supplementation improved growth rates in younger children (under 3 years) but not in older children (3 to 7 years), who were already growing as well as healthy children (Schroeder et al., forthcoming). Perhaps failure to catch up is largely a matter of lost opportunity. The rate at which children grow is a function of biological age; for example, the astonishing rates of growth during early infancy are never again matched, even at peak height velocity during adolescence. Thus the capacity for catch-up growth in children[1] may be largely limited to the degree of developmental delay, which predicts how much growing time is left. Malnutrition is known to affect the biological clock, but its effects are less than those on growth velocity (Martorell et al., 1979; Bogin et al., 1989; Martorell et al., 1994). Consequently, the possibilities for catch-up growth after early childhood may be limited unless maturation is delayed markedly.

Growth faltering is clearly a phenomenon intimately associated with the perils of weaning (in traditional societies, the transition from total dependence on mother's milk to complete reliance on the local diet). The

---

[1] Severely malnourished children experience rates of weight gain up to fifteen times faster than those observed in well-nourished children (Ashworth, 1969). This rapid rate of weight gain occurs until adequate weight-for-length is achieved.

evidence from numerous studies unequivocally indicates that the *immediate* causes of growth faltering are poor diets and infection (principally gastrointestinal) and that these are interactive (Chen, 1983; NAS, 1989a). Recent information from the CRSP studies indicates that dietary factors constraining growth include energy as well as micronutrients; a small amount of animal protein may be desirable, not necessarily because of protein but because of the vitamins and minerals it contains (Calloway et al., 1992). Numerous factors determine nutrient intake and disease patterns, including infant feeding practices, the nature of the local diet and the foods offered to children, the child's appetite, environmental sanitation, and the degree of contamination of foods and liquids. The web of causality, although similar across regions, is sufficiently different to caution against a simple list of risk factors.

Why are children most affected in the first 2 or 3 years of life? Among the possible reasons are the following:

(1) Growth rates are highest in infancy, and adverse factors have a greater potential for causing retardation at this time.
(2) Younger children have higher nutritional requirements per kilogram of body weight.
(3) Young children are immunologically naive and, consequently, more susceptible to infections.
(4) Young children are less able to make their needs known and are more vulnerable to the effects of poor parenting.

Growth is of lower priority than the maintenance of vital functions. Thus growth retardation is a nonspecific response to many adverse factors and situations. Nevertheless, children who are growing poorly will respond quickly to improvements (Schroeder et al., forthcoming; Rivera, 1988). These two qualities, poor specificity and high responsiveness, characterize anthropometric indicators and have important programmatic implications.

Arising from its nonspecificity, growth retardation clearly can indicate only that a problem exists; it provides no information about its nature. Thus the measurement of growth alone is not enough for action programs. The causes of growth faltering are extremely complex, and the relative mix of causes varies greatly by region of the country and even by locality. Therefore, to mount effective actions at the individual or population level, one needs to know the probable causes of growth faltering and have at one's disposal interventions that work effectively in the local context. Once actions are taken, the measurement of growth provides sensitive indicators to assess effectiveness.

Prevalence of Growth Retardation in the Third World

The *Second Report on the World Nutrition Situation* (ACC/SCN, 1992), issued by the Administrative Committee on Coordination/Subcommittee on Nutrition (ACC/SCN) of the United Nations, compiled available weight-for-age data from around the world in order to assess levels and trends in the prevalence of low weight-for-age, defined as less than two standard deviations below the reference median and termed "underweight" in the report. Prevalence estimates for 1990 for various regions of the world were as follows: sub-Saharan Africa, 30 percent; Near East and North Africa, 13 percent; South Asia, 59 percent; Southeast Asia, 31 percent; China, 22 percent; Middle America and the Caribbean, 15 percent; and South America, 8 percent. The prevalence expected in a population similar in distribution to the reference population is 2.5 percent. Trends from 1980 through 1990 indicate increased prevalence or lack of change in most of sub-Saharan Africa and decrements in the other regions. Overall, the proportion of underweight children fell from 38 percent in 1980 to 34 percent in 1990.

Low weight-for-age can reflect both stunting and wasting. In most of the developing countries, except in Asia, low weight-for-age is primarily related to stunting. In Asia, low weight-for-age also results from a higher prevalence of wasting (Victora, 1992).

These contrasting patterns may reflect a greater severity of problems in Asia than in Latin America. In Latin America children may be confronted with chronic but moderate deficiencies of nutrients; they may respond by growing less in height without altering weight-for-height ratios. In Asia the severity of adverse factors may be increased, and, in addition to much wasting, even greater retardation in height may result. A greater incidence of infections, which can quickly lead to wasting in poorly nourished children, may be a critical factor explaining the high levels of wasting found in Asia. Dietary patterns may also play a role; for example, energy intakes may be lower than required in Asia, compared with Latin America. Nonetheless, as noted by Haaga et al. (1985), regional differences in the pattern of low weight-for-age should be interpreted with caution (e.g., the much lower prevalence of low weight-for-age in sub-Saharan Africa compared with South Asian nations, such as India) because the causes of the differences, as well as their functional implications, are not clearly understood (Victora, 1992).

Immediate Functional Correlates of Growth Retardation

Seckler (1982) has advanced the "small but healthy" hypothesis, which regards stunting as an effective adaptation to poor nutrition; that is, it carries no functional implications. In his view, most nutritional scientists believe in the "deprivation theory," which holds that an individual is healthy and well nourished if he grows along his genetically determined growth curve. Growth significantly below this curve indicates that the individual is malnourished and in poor health. Seckler believes that this view is incorrect and proposes instead the "homeostatic theory of growth" in which the single potential growth curve is replaced by the concept of a broad array of potential growth curves. Within the bounds of this potential growth space, the child may move through various paths of size and shape without suffering any functional implications. Seckler states that although the deprivation theory of nutritionists postulates a continuous functional relationship between small body size and impairments, his homeostatic theory postulates a threshold relationship. Seckler goes on to tell us that "smallness may not be associated with functional impairments over a rather large range of variation; but the system explodes into a high incidence of functional impairments at the lower bound of size" (p. 129). The stunted but not the wasted child is within this safe zone or "small but healthy." The truly malnourished, according to Seckler, are children showing clinical signs of malnutrition or wasting. This controversial view has been criticized by several authors, including Gopalan (1983), Latham (1984), and Martorell (1989). Reference to this debate is appropriate here because, if the "small but healthy" hypothesis is true, the emerging strategy of growth promotion has little basis.

Seckler's views may arise partly because he focuses on the outcome, small body size, rather than on the process of becoming small, growth faltering. A focus on the process would lead one to note that factors which markedly affect growth also have other functional effects. Although it may be true that minor differences in growth patterns with respect to genetic potential may carry no adverse functional implications or may even be beneficial, such as the slightly shorter lengths and lower levels of fatness of breastfed infants in parts of the United States (Butte et al., 1984; Dewey et al., 1992), the situation in developing countries is usually one of marked deviations in growth leading to massive and widespread "nutritional dwarfism." These levels of growth retardation are risky; marasmus is, in fact, nothing more than the end of a continuum of responses to nutritional deficits.

A serious correlate of growth faltering and wasting is depressed immunocompetence, leading to increased risk of morbidity and mortality. Several authors have reviewed this rapidly growing body of literature (Martorell and Ho, 1984; Tomkins and Watson, 1989). The nature of these relationships is poorly understood, but they are probably not linear. Some studies have detected magnified effects, or even threshold levels, at more marked stages of stunting and wasting. Not all studies have controlled for socioeconomic status in examining these relationships. This would provide important information about the possible reasons for the relationship because growth retardation is probably a proxy of environmental sanitation and the resources available for preventive and curative care, as well as of immunodepression.

Although growth retardation does not *cause* depressed immunocompetence, the factors that cause growth faltering, such as infection and inadequate intakes of specific nutrients, also result in immunodepression. All components of immunocompetence, particularly cellular immunity, are affected. Once socioeconomic status is taken into account, poor growth generally predicts severity of infection (e.g., duration, symptomatology, complications, and fatality rates) to a greater extent than incidence. In other words, children may get infected for reasons largely determined by their environment, but, once they are infected, the course of the infection will be influenced strongly by nutritional status, reflected by the degree of growth retardation.

Poor growth is consistently associated with health risks, yet the predictive power of indicators (e.g., weight-for-age, height-for-age, arm circumference, and weight-for-height) varies widely in different settings. Many factors, including differences among populations in the causes of growth retardation, variability in the length at follow-up in the study, and differences in the ages of study subjects, probably account for this variability. Variability in the mix of causes of growth retardation is probably very important.

Pelletier (1991a) reanalyzed data from six prospective studies in order to clarify the nature of the relationship between weight-for-age and mortality. He found that mortality increased exponentially with declining weight-for-age but had no apparent threshold in the relationship. The primary difference across studies was in baseline levels of mortality which determined the intercept of the line but not its slope, which was similar across studies.

Choice of outcome variable and length of follow-up affect the predictive power of anthropometric indicators. Short-term risk (i.e., 1 to 3 months following assessment) appears to be better predicted by measures of wasting than of stunting, particularly in the case of morbidity. On the other hand, measures of achieved status, such as height-for-age and weight-for-age, are better predictors of longer-term risk (e.g., 18 to 24 months) than measures of wasting (Martorell and Ho, 1984; Pelletier, 1991a; Tomkins and Watson, 1989).

Age at assessment is another important factor to consider when studying the health risks associated with anthropometric indicators because it is related to both mortality and growth retardation patterns. Mortality is related negatively to age in young children: rates are highest in infancy, remain high in the second year of life, and decrease rapidly thereafter. Relationships with age vary greatly by anthropometric indicator. Cumulative indicators of growth retardation, such as height-for-age and weight-for-age, are positively related to age, with the lowest values achieved by 2 to 3 years of age. Wasting is more common among 2-year-olds than among infants and older children. Hence investigations that involve wide age ranges (e.g., 0 to 60 months) should control for age in assessing the relative merits of anthropometric indicators. For example, in very young children height-for-age is a strong predictor of mortality (Chen et al., 1980), but in studies that also include older children, predictive power is less (Smedman et al., 1987; Kasongo Project Team, 1983; Katz et al., 1989; Alam et al., 1989c; Bågenholm and Nasher, 1989). In Guinea-Bissau, height-for-age was predictive of mortality but only before 36 months of age (Smedman et al., 1987). Katz et al. (1989) also found the same result in a study in West Java. Odds ratios for mortality over 18 months are expressed in Figure 2.1 relative to rates for the group with least retardation, above 95 percent height-for-age. A relationship is evident for all but the oldest group (i.e., 3 to 5 years). These authors also found that the mortality risk associated with mild wasting (80–90 percent of the reference median) declined with increasing age; however, for moderate to severe wasting (less than 80 percent of the reference median), the risk of dying was actually greater in older children.

In explaining their findings, Katz et al. (1989) state that "the lack of association between attained height and mortality among older children may reflect their selective adaptation to chronic nutritional and morbid stress, in contrast with younger children" (p. 1225). A different explanation is that stunting may be more important in young children because this is when they are in the process of becoming small or failing to grow. Many children older than 3 years are stunted but grow adequately, which implies reduced risk. Wasting, however, is a risk indicator at all ages and

Figure 2.1. Age-specific 18-month mortality odds ratios in West Java (reference category is > 95 height-for-age)

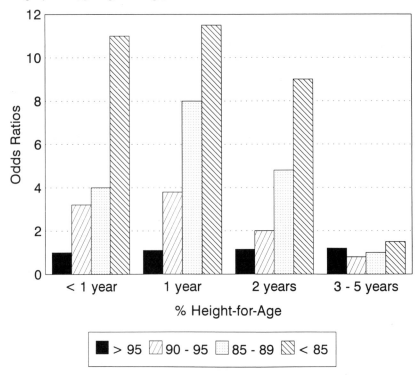

Source: Katz et al., 1989.

may be particularly revealing in older children, in whom it is rarer than in toddlers.

The above findings suggest that growth rates should be useful indexes to predict mortality. The few such studies that have been carried out consistently show growth rates to be predictive of increased mortality risk (Bairagi et al., 1985; Kasongo Project Team, 1986; Briend and Bari, 1989). In Zaire cross-sectional measures did not predict mortality, whereas growth velocities did (Kasongo Project Team, 1986). In Bangladesh weight-for-age and height-for-age performed better than weight and height velocities in predicting mortality during a 1-year period in children 1 to 4 years of age (Bairagi et al., 1985). Using a multivariate approach, Briend and Bari (1989) showed that weight-for-age was a stronger predictor of mortality than weight velocity in another study from Bangladesh. Briend and Bari (1989) also showed that changes in weight were associated with risk of death, even after controlling for weight-for-age and selected diseases, suggesting that combining weight-for-age and weight loss improves the assessment of risk of death.

Briend and Bari (1989) suggest that the poor performance of weight velocity as a risk indicator of mortality may be a result of measurement errors. When changes over a few months are assessed, errors due to measurement techniques or to nonnutritional variation may overwhelm the assessment of weight or height gain and attenuate relationships with mortality. Obviously, further work in this area is necessary. Although the theoretical prediction that growth rates provide dynamic information not contained in cross-sectional measures of attained size (weight-for-age, height-for-age) has not been invalidated, concerns have been raised about the practicality of velocities as routine screening indicators.

Finally, physical activity is also likely to be affected concurrently with growth rates as part of the complex of responses to cope with energy limitations. The data to confirm this statement are limited. This is an important area of research because decreased physical activity may mean listlessness and apathy and limited interaction with peers, adults, and the environment, which would adversely influence cognitive development.

Long-Term Functional Correlates of Stunting

Measures of growth retardation, such as stunting, are strongly associated with poor psychological test performance and low school achievement (Pollitt, 1990). These complex relationships are probably a result of third factors, such as those related to poverty, which cause both physical and developmental retardation. According to Ricciuti (1981), animal and human studies suggest that nutrition improvements alone (which would allow for adequate growth) or environmental stimulation programs alone produce modest effects in populations at risk of developmental retardation, but combined interventions interact to produce more dramatic results. Pollitt (1990) proposes that satisfactory school performance cannot be achieved without a multifaceted approach, including appropriate health and nutrition interventions in early childhood. These interventions would also lead to improved growth.

Work capacity, as measured by maximal oxygen consumption, is highly related to body size (Spurr, 1983). Growth retardation in early childhood results in small adult body size and reduced lean body mass (Satyanarayana et al., 1979; Martorell et al., 1992). For example Martorell et al. (1992) have shown that Guatemalan boys who were severely stunted (i.e., less than -3 standard deviations below the reference median) at 3 years of age had 6.4 kg less in fat-free mass as adults compared to subjects who were not stunted at 3 years of age (i.e., above -2 standard deviations). A study of Indian boys has related stunting at 5 years of age with reduced work capacity as measured by maximal oxygen consumption (Satyanarayana et al., 1979).

From a social point of view, the key question is whether reduced work capacities result in lower labor effort or productivity. According to Spurr (1983), work capacity probably limits productivity in moderate to heavy work, a situation that he considers common to developing countries. Research shows that up to 35–40 percent of maximal oxygen consumption can be sustained for an eight-hour day by individuals in good physical condition. Any task can be measured by its oxygen cost and expressed as a percentage of maximal oxygen consumption. According to Spurr (1983), the effort required to complete a moderate to heavy task might be such that individuals with reduced work capacities would need to work at unsustainable levels of maximal oxygen consumption. Individuals so limited would be forced to work a shorter day or increase periods of rest, with important reductions in total work effort.

The available literature offers confirmation that body size, a proxy of work capacity, is related to labor effort or productivity, particularly for demanding tasks such as sugarcane cutting (Spurr, 1983; Martorell and Arroyave, 1988). Economists view most of the biological literature on what they term the efficiency wage hypothesis, the notion that "there is a technically determined relationship between nutritional status and labor effort or productivity," as being methodologically flawed in that the analyses have tended to ignore the potential bidirectional nature of the nutrition-productivity effect (Behrman and Deolalikar, 1988, p. 683). Simply stated, work capacity may determine work output and, hence, income; but income may also affect dietary intakes and, ultimately, work capacity. This is a serious concern because it is clear from observational and experimental evidence that energy intakes, anemia, and deficiencies in thiamine, riboflavin, vitamin B_6, and vitamin C affect work capacity (Martorell and Arroyave, 1988; Bates et al., 1989). Therefore, to the extent that nutritional deficiencies among study subjects exist and that dietary intakes are constrained by incomes, increased productivity might lead to improved diets through increased incomes. If this is the case, studies need to control for the bidirectional nature of nutrition-productivity relationships. This can be done through statistical or econometric approaches or by experimental manipulation of diet in appropriately controlled studies.

For purposes of the present discussion, there is a need to distinguish between current nutritional status (e.g., dietary intakes, nutritional bio-chemistry, weight-for-height) and long-term measures (e.g., height). Of the studies that have considered bidirectional relationships, those by Strauss (1986), Sahn and Alderman (1988), and Deolalikar (1988) do not provide information about the long-term consequences of growth retardation in early childhood. Strauss (1986) and Sahn and Alderman (1988) used household energy intakes expressed on a per capita basis as their only measure of nutrition, while Deolalikar (1988) used two measures: individual energy intakes and weight-for-height. Height was not included in these investigations. A study of agricultural productivity in the Philippines considered three measures of nutrition: energy dietary intakes, weight-for-height, and stature (Haddad and Bouis, 1990). They found that higher wages appear to result from greater heights and not from increased energy intakes or greater weight-for-heights. In this setting stunting matters, but current nutritional status does not (in which case bidirectionality is not an issue). Different results might be expected in other areas, depending upon the level of physical and economic well-being of workers as children and as adults and the nature of the tasks examined. For example, in India, Deolalikar (1988) found that weight-for-height, but not energy intakes, was associated with agricultural productivity.

Maternal size and reproductive success are clearly related. One of the most frequently cited risk factors of low birth weight in developing countries is maternal stature (Kramer, 1987). This relationship might be a result of nutritional mechanisms (e.g., maternal size may be a proxy for nutritional reserves, or size may be important for birth weight, simply because it partly determines how much women eat), mechanical considerations (e.g., the growth potential of the fetus may be constrained in a small woman, or the fetus may crowd maternal organs to a greater degree in stunted women and thus limit maternal gastric capacity), or yet other mechanisms. Whatever the reason, the relationship between maternal size and birth weight is strong and consistent. Maternal size is similarly related to infant mortality, probably mediated through birth weight (Martorell et al., 1981). Short maternal stature is also a risk factor for prolonged labor and cesarean section because of cephalopelvic disproportion (Adadevoh et al., 1989; Mahmood et al., 1988), perhaps indicating a relationship between stunting and reduced pelvic inlet diameter. Finally, stunting has been hypothesized to be related to increased maternal mortality because of increased risk of obstructed labor (Royston and Armstrong, 1989).

Guatemalan studies provide clear evidence linking stunting in early childhood with a wide range of adverse outcomes in the adult, including reduced fat-free mass, short adult stature, and constrained intellectual achievement as measured through tests of intelligence, numeracy, literacy, and school attainments (Martorell et al., 1992). Also, nutrition interventions in early childhood substantially reduce the risk of stunting and its adverse consequences in the adult (Martorell, 1993; Pollitt et al., 1993).

Research Needs

Important research gaps that limit our understanding of the causes and implications of growth retardation and introduce significant uncertainty in program design, implementation, and evaluation have been identified in the previous sections. A summary list of needed clinical and epidemiological research about growth is given below. Operational research needs are addressed by others in this volume.

- Research about the nature and sequencing of responses to varying types and levels of nutrient deficiencies and different types of infections, with due consideration to linear growth retardation, wasting, and physical activity.
- Studies of healthy populations to generate appropriate international reference data for growth rates, particularly for weight and length/height. Also research to clarify whether separate reference data are required for breast-fed infants.
- Research about the timing of growth retardation in populations exposed to varying conditions. Investigations of the extent to which catch-up growth is possible in different populations beyond the age when growth is severely affected.
- Studies to clarify the causes of regional variability in patterns of stunting, wasting, and low weight-for-age and to shed light on the implications of these differences for program planning and allocation of resources.
- Research about the value of various patterns and levels of growth retardation as predictors of depressed immunocompetence and increased risk of morbidity and mortality in different regions of the world, with assessment of the shape of these relationships at different ages. Investigations of the value of growth velocities as predictors of risk.
- Clarification of the long-term implications of growth retardation in early childhood, not only for work capacity but for labor productivity as well.
- Elucidation of the mechanisms through which growth retardation in early childhood affects future female reproductive performance. Assessment of obstetric mortality risks associated with short maternal stature.
- Investigations to extend knowledge of the long-term functional implications of growth retardation in early childhood to other areas, such as school and occupational achievement, risk of chronic degenerative diseases, and adult life span.

Potential Benefits of Alleviating Growth Faltering

What are the potential benefits of a strategy to promote healthy growth? Because much is unknown, all answers to this question will necessarily involve speculation as well as fact. A personal view is given below.

Most benefits of achieving healthy growth are indirect and arise because the interventions necessary to improve growth also affect other functional domains. A child who is growing well will in all probability be more physically active and interact more intensely with his or her environment than one who is growing poorly. Listlessness and apathy, whether induced by energy dietary deficits or infection, place a child at risk of developmental retardation. The conditions that improve growth will also improve cognitive development, especially if emphasis is placed on interventions to promote behavioral stimulation.

A child who is growing well is likely to have healthy immunological defenses against infection. Better growth thus means decreased risk of severe infections, case fatality rates, and child mortality. In effect, a focus on the quality of life will lead to lower infant and child mortality rates and extend the gains made by child survival programs.

Over the long term, youths who grew adequately during childhood will perform better in school than those who grew poorly. Again, this is not a causal relationship but simply a reflection of the fact that altering the environment to promote healthy growth also enhances development and learning capacity.

Youths and adults will, of course, be bigger as a result of improved growth in early childhood. This implies an increased dietary maintenance cost. Roughly, every kilogram added will contribute to basal metabolic needs at the rate of one kcal per hour throughout adult life. But the work capacity will be enhanced as well, leading to increased productivity in situations of moderate to heavy work loads.

Another important benefit of larger body size in women is lower risk of delivering low-birth-weight infants and, hence, lower risk of infant mortality. Improved maternal stature will also lead to fewer delivery complications and perhaps lower maternal mortality rates.

The short answer to the question posed in this final section is that a focus on the promotion of healthy growth in early childhood will result in youths with a greater potential for being productive members of society. Good physical growth results in increased human capital.

3

Household Behavior, Preschool Child Health and Nutrition, and the Role of Information

Jere R. Behrman

The actions of household members (defined here as those who share residence, hearth, and other resources), primarily the parents and especially the mother,[1] substantially determine the health and nutrition of preschool children in developing countries. Of course, other people, such as neighbors and kin who are not coresident, and entities, such as formal and informal groups based on religion, occupation, regional origin, clan, caste, and tribe, may directly influence child health and nutrition. Beyond the proximate determinants of preschool child health and nutrition may be factors ranging from the governmental provision and regulation of local health-related services, to exchange rate policy, to conditions in world commodity markets. Nevertheless, it can fairly be said that the household probably plays the major proximate role in determining the preschool child's health and nutrition.

More and better information can affect nutrition by changing the behavior of the household, the community, the government, and any other entity that interacts on some level with the household. Household and

Helpful comments on a preliminary outline and an earlier version of this chapter were offered by Harold Alderman, Alain de Janvry, Kathleen DeWalt, Marcia Griffiths, Elena Hurtado, Sandra Huffman, Joanne Leslie, Judith McGuire, David Pelletier, Per Pinstrup-Andersen, Beatrice Rodgers, Ligia Rodriguez, Roger Shrimpton, and Judith Timyan.

[1] In some societies fairly high proportions of children do not live with their parents. Ainsworth (1991), for example, reports that about a quarter of 7- to 14-year-old children in a random sample from the Ivory Coast are fostered out to other households, apparently primarily for economic reasons. Such fostering is strongly associated with age, however. Fewer than 10 percent of preschool-age children are fostered.

community members can practice better health and nutrition if they learn how. Communities may affect preschool health and nutrition by learning to take collective action and more effectively representing their needs and claims on other resources to governments, NGOs, and other outside organizations. Appropriate information pertaining to the range of relevant options and household and community responses to the direct and indirect effects of policies can help governments make more educated policy decisions that relate to the health and nutrition of preschool children.

Although better information at the household, community, and government levels may lead to better health and nutrition for preschool children, the monetary, time, social, religious, and political costs of changing behavior in the way suggested by better information may be considered too great.

Nevertheless, improving information to improve preschool child health and nutrition and closing the current gaps in such information are attractive for two reasons. First, many people (this author included) believe that improved child health and nutrition in the developing world is desirable in itself, though there also may be some reasons to want to do so in the pursuit of other goals (e.g., increased productivity, equity).[2] Second, sufficient information is not likely to be provided by private individuals and entities because its production is unprofitable. The collection and dissemination of information requires time and other resources, but it has public good characteristics. The consumption by one person of a given quantity of most goods and services, sometimes called private goods, makes it unavailable for consumption by another. Information about a new method of improving health (e.g., oral rehydration therapy, ORT), however, *can* be made available to all without diluting its value for any particular individual. This public good characteristic of information renders its private production less desirable from the producer's standpoint because it is less likely to be profitable. The producer of the information will be unable to sell the information to every user. Information used by one person is still available to others. Thus, although the social benefits of information production far outweigh the costs, the private reward to the producer of information may be small. Therefore, the case is strong for information-oriented public policies.

This chapter will explore both the known and unknown qualities of information at the household, community, and government and its role in the household in determining preschool child health and nutrition. The

---

[2] More persuasive evidence is accumulating that improved health and nutrition can have important productivity effects for poor populations, quite possibly with higher rates of return than for other investments such as schooling (see Behrman, 1993; Behrman, Foster, and Rosenzweig, 1994).

next section outlines a conceptual framework for considering household behavior regarding preschool child health and nutrition and the implications of such a framework for empirical analysis. The following section summarizes empirical evidence regarding household behavior related to preschool child health and nutrition and its implications for information needs for households, communities, and governments.

Household Behavior regarding Preschool Health and Nutrition: Conceptual Framework and Implications for Empirical Estimates

Most preschool children live in households whose members share resources and have considerable proximate effects on the children's health and nutrition.[3] At the same time, the members are involved in other relations and organizations, generally including market relations, that determine the monetary or in-kind rate at which they can exchange a range of goods and services with one another or that affect their personal esteem, satisfaction, and options. But important nonmarket relations also shape household behavior. Moreover, household members' preferences and perceptions are conditioned by the culture of the larger community in which they live and have lived. Therefore, the household should be considered within this larger context.

Within this larger context, a given household's behavior can be systematized depending upon its members' preferences, rules about intrahousehold resource allocations, and limiting constraints to satisfaction of preferences relating to household production of outcomes such as child health, the endowments of individual household members, and the prices, services, and other relations that the household faces in the communities in which its members interact.

Preferences or tastes characterize the trade-offs an individual is willing to make among his or her consumption of various goods and services, the consumption of others, and the changes of such trade-offs with changes in resources. Preferences indicate, for example, how many additional kilograms of coarse grains an individual would consume in order to reduce consumption of good quality rice by 1 kg, what improvements in the oldest son's health a parent would be willing to trade for 10 percent improvement in another child's health, and what compositional shifts in consumption would be chosen if income increased by 10 percent. The

---

[3] Related frameworks for the analysis of nutritional issues in which household behavior is embedded are presented in Habicht and Butz (1985) and Martorell et al. (1985). For a survey of the economic literature on intrafamily allocations and references to other studies, see Behrman (1995).

nature of such preferences thus relates to the extent to which the individual would substitute among the consumption of various goods and services if their full relative costs (including monetary and time) change, as well as to how the individual would want to change consumption with a change in resources. Such preferences could be defined for many goods and services, including child health (directly or indirectly as a potential determinant of resources for the parents) and factors that directly affect child health such as different time uses. If preferences are presumed to be given and if people attempt to maximize their preferences subject to constraints such as those discussed below, then a change in behavior in response to an external change can be interpreted to improve the welfare of the individual in comparison with the situation in which the same external change occurred and the individual did not change his or her behavior. If an external change alters preferences, however, it is difficult to give meaning to the question of whether an individual is made better off by an external change because the criterion for judgment has changed.

What determines preferences? Whether adult preferences are fixed or mutable, most social scientists would agree that they arise from some combination of genetic and environmental factors. The latter reflects the immediate microenvironment in which one is raised, generally including the household and the culture and associated norms of the larger community in which the household is located. These norms, in turn, may reflect long-existing (though not necessarily still-existing) relative scarcities, as Harris (1978) has argued. Of greater concern than the question of how preferences originate is the question of whether, how, and how quickly they can be changed. For example, is it useful to think of changes in information changing tastes, perhaps by increasing awareness of options? Or is it more useful analytically to think of such information merely permitting the satisfaction of some basic underlying stable preferences by different channels?

Intrahousehold allocation rules or procedures may substantially affect preschool child health and nutrition for a given set of preferences for individual household members and constraints on their actions, particularly if the preferences of individual household members differ substantially. Though economists often model the household as if there were unified preferences, such an assumption seems strong. Instead, it is probably preferable to consider that intrahousehold allocations are the result of implicit or explicit bargaining among household members, individual bargaining positions (which may depend partly on their individual command over resources), and various cultural norms that could affect individual preferences that shape the bargaining and allocation processes. For example, it is often assumed that mothers tend to have greater concern about small children than do fathers. If so, and if bargaining power were to shift toward mothers (for example, because of increased esteem emanating from social or economic relations outside of the household or more control over economic resources resulting from higher wages for women), child health and nutrition are likely to improve because of the change in intrahousehold allocations in addition to any resource effect. In this context, information may change bargaining outcomes by changing the options outside of the households for one or more household members. For example, information about a new rural bank credit program, such as the Grameen Bank in Bangladesh or similar programs elsewhere, may significantly increase the options of women whose access to credit markets had previously been very limited or nonexistent. Information about new options might significantly increase bargaining power, even if the option is not exercised.

Household constraints limit the household's options for obtaining the goods and services that affect the preferences of individual household members. These include resource and technological constraints embedded in production relations that determine how much output can be obtained from a given set of inputs. The household directly controls some of the inputs needed to produce child health, government policy affects others, and some inputs are independent of both. This last group of factors may be important both in limiting the possible impact of policy on preschool child health and nutrition and in trying to understand empirically the impact of those factors that can be changed. Among the major inputs into the production of preschool child health are nutrients, water quality, preventive health care such as inoculations, curative health care such as drugs, the child's genetic endowments and time use, the mother's or other caregivers' time devoted to health-related activities and productivity in such activities (probably related partially to the caregiver's formal education), the general household environment regarding such characteristics as shelter and sanitation, and the larger environment surrounding the household, which includes natural features, such as climate, and human-made features, such as water control and pollution.

This chapter sets forth two important questions regarding one of the constraints, the health production function. First, how do various inputs interact? How easy is it to substitute among them? To what extent are relations complementary, that is, to what extent is one particular input dependent on another particular input? The easier it is to substitute, the easier it is to maintain or to improve preschool child health, and the stronger the complementarities, the higher the payoffs are to integrated efforts to improve child health and nutrition. Second, what is the role of information about the child health production process? Information concerning this health production function is imperfect, so the child's health depends in part on others' beliefs about it. For example, if certain foods that are rich in some relatively scarce nutrients are believed to be bad for children, the result will be less satisfactory child health than would occur with the same resources and more accurate information. Likewise, information about the nature of available inputs into the health production function can significantly affect child health.

Another important household production function is that which determines the nutrient intakes available to the child. These nutrient intakes depend on whether the child is breastfeeding and whether the child is consuming other food. If the child is breastfeeding, the mother's health status, milk production, and time to feed the infant are important. If the child is consuming other food, the range, quantity, and quality of these foods and how they are prepared (which in turn may depend on the knowledge of the food preparer as well as the availability of capital equipment such as refrigeration) may be important. The extent of substitution among foods in the production of nutrients is another important question. The more such substitution, the easier it is to make nutrients available to the child under various conditions of food availability and prices. Here, again, the role of information is important. Just as information can improve the health production function, better information about the nutrient qualities of food, food preparation, and the range of nutrient options tends to increase nutrient availability to preschool children.

Endowments are characteristics that are predetermined and not affected by choices made by the individual. For the purpose of this chapter, among the most important individual endowments are the genetic endowments of the children of interest; the predetermined ability, knowledge, and habits of the mother (particularly related to health and nutrient intake production but also to her productivity in other activities); and other human resource endowments of individual household members (such as prior schooling, time, physical and financial assets, and preferences). Household endowments include all collective assets of the household. Community endowments include the environmental, social, cultural, and economic context in which the household exists. Information about many endowments of household members is often imperfect. Information about an infant's endowments at birth, for example, is relatively limited, but more is acquired over time by observing the child's development and robustness. Nevertheless, some dimensions of the child's endowments remain unknown, though some genetic effects may become apparent later. Likewise, many dimensions of the household and community endowments are likely to be unknown, though some may be knowable through existing tests. For example, water tests can lead to better information about its quality and advisable precautions with regard to its use. This could certainly lead to better preschool child health.

Empirical Evidence on Household Behavior and Preschool Child Health and Nutrition

Relevant surveys already exist (e.g., Behrman, 1990a, 1990b; Leslie and Gupta, 1989). Rather than summarizing these surveys, relatively detailed summaries are presented of some selected studies of particular interest because of their approaches or because they are well-known and reflect other work much more broadly. A focus is maintained on studies that relate explicitly to preschool child health and nutrition, but some relevant studies that address broader populations are summarized as well. This discussion is organized with reference to the three levels of the preschool child health and nutrition–household-information nexus identified at the beginning of the chapter: information at the household level, information at the community level involving households' knowledge on related topics, and information for the design of related governmental policies.

Information at the Household Level regarding Preschool Child Health and Nutrition

This section presents three broad topics: accuracy of household information pertaining to preschool child health and nutrition, level of education and information of the household, and intrahousehold allocation processes that might indicate appropriate targeting of relevant information to particular household members.

Accuracy of Household Information Relevant to Proximate Determinants of Preschool Child Health and Nutrition. Little systematic direct analysis has been made of large populations regarding the accuracy of household information about the determinants of preschool child health and nutrition, including practices and the availability, quality, and time and money costs of health options. Misinformation about any of these topics might lead to diminished preschool child health and nutrition. A priori it is hard to know the importance of such information. In static situations with considerable interaction among individuals, information generally seems to be fairly adequate, even among the very poor (Schultz, 1975). Situations in which knowledge, prices, and quality and availability of relevant goods and services are rapidly changing have greater information inadequacies—especially in geographically isolated areas and areas where interpersonal communication is limited. Ewbank and Preston

(1990), for example, argue that government dissemination of information about the germ theory was a major factor in changing mothers' behavior and reducing infant and child mortality in the fairly dynamic 1900 to 1930 period in the United States.

Investigations into the extent of misinformation in households and a comparison between the rate of return of policies for the rapid dissemination of information and other uses of resources might be very useful in formulating effective policies. To calculate such rates of return, obviously, analysts must account for all costs and the particular social and cultural contexts of the households of interest. Very strong dietary prescriptions that preclude eating foods containing scarce nutrients, for example, must be recognized in analysis of policies directed toward increasing information about the nutritional advantages of such foods. If such prescriptions are very hard to modify, they could render impossible an information policy with a very high rate of return, even if all other circumstances were favorable to a high rate of return. Difficult questions arise, however, if such information deliberately or inadvertently changes personal preferences regarding diet or other determinants of preschool child health and nutrition. These questions are addressed below.

Education of Household Members and Information Related to Child Health and Nutrition. Although direct evidence of misinformation about the proximate determinants of preschool child health and nutrition is limited and largely anecdotal, much more systematic evidence has been found concerning the association between preschool child health and nutrition and education, particularly maternal education. In fact, the association between the two is perhaps the strongest and most positive in the relevant empirical literature. Therefore, increased schooling for females often is advocated as a major channel for improving child health and nutrition (e.g., World Bank, 1981; Colclough, 1982; Eisemon, 1988; King, 1990; King and Hill, 1993; Mensch et al., 1985; Schultz, 1993a, b).

The strong association between maternal schooling and preschool child health and nutrition raises at least five major questions. The latter two are discussed in subsequent sections on intrahousehold allocations and policy interactions.

First, if such schooling is important because it improves information-gathering capacity, might the rate of return not be higher if there were some other way of providing needed information? The gestation period for the return for schooling of current primary-school age girls is quite long in terms of their own children's health. Might it not be possible to improve relevant information of current mothers? Casual evidence of this possibility suggests that the answer is sometimes yes. The more optimistic appraisals of programs such as the GOBI (growth monitoring, oral rehydration therapy, breastfeeding, immunization) efforts, for example, depend on a positive assessment of the efforts to improve information and practices regarding growth monitoring, oral rehydration, and other factors. In other cases, however, the success appears much more limited, particularly in measuring longer-term, as opposed to isolated, episodes of child health. Systematic efforts to investigate the value of such information within a household modeling context, moreover, do not uniformly suggest high rates of return to the direct provision of health and nutrition information. In a study of a rural Philippine sample, for instance, Bouis and Haddad (1990a) found no significant association between the mothers' nutritional knowledge and their children's health once other characteristics, including mothers' schooling, were controlled for. Perhaps the capacity to use such information depends so much on the characteristics associated with formal schooling that it is difficult to separate such direct information provision from formal schooling. DaVanzo and Levy (1989, p. 42), for instance, claim that in Malaysia "decisions about breastfeeding seem to be responsive to the information that is available at the time about the effectiveness of breastfeeding in producing health and contraceptive outcomes" because they find "a greater negative effect of mother's education [on breastfeeding] in the earlier time period than in the later time period." They explain that this pattern "is consistent with [their] ... hypothesis that in the 1970s new information became available about the health benefits of breastfeeding and educated women should have been most likely to be exposed to this information and to take advantage of it" (pp. 42–43). Their interpretation depends upon their maintained hypothesis that more formally educated women are more likely to be aware of and to use new information so that it may not be sensible to provide information per se if the educational level is not sufficient to use it.

Second, might the estimated effects of parental schooling on preschool child health and nutrition be misleading because of the indicator of schooling that is used for such estimates? In estimates of the impact of adult schooling on various outcomes, schooling typically is measured by grades or years of schooling, or what might be called the "quantity" of schooling. Yet some evidence has been found in labor market outcomes in developing countries that not only the quantity but also the quality of schooling is relevant (e.g., Behrman and Birdsall, 1983, Behrman et al., 1994). Moreover, Behrman and Birdsall argue on a priori grounds, and Birdsall (1985) provides empirical evidence for Brazil, that higher-quality schools induce greater quantity of schooling. If so, the failure to control for the quality of schooling in empirical estimates of the impact of parental schooling on child outcomes biases the estimate of the impact of the quantity of schooling. There are no well-known estimates of the magnitude of such an effect in the determination of preschool child health and nutrition. But the Behrman and Sussangkarn (1989) estimates for other child outcomes in Thailand suggest that the impact of the quality as well as the quantity of parental schooling is important and the failure to control for the schooling quality biases the estimated impact of schooling quantity for those at lower schooling levels.

Third, exactly what does schooling represent in such estimates? To this point schooling is assumed to represent at least in part the capacity to acquire and use information relevant for child health and nutrition. Schooling also may represent a range of other phenomena: productivity in using a given set of inputs to produce health and nutrition; preferences that favor healthy children; and parents' abilities and motivation (or endowments) that lead to greater schooling and to better health and nutrition for their preschool children. It is essential to determine the extent to which, among these and other possibilities, schooling does in fact lead to better capacities to acquire and use knowledge, rather than substituting for other attributes. Rosenzweig and Schultz (1982a) attempt to distinguish, in a Colombian sample, the extent to which parental schooling is associated with a better set of inputs into the production of child health and to which it is associated with better use of a given set of inputs. Their results suggest that the former, not the latter, is dominating. This finding is consistent with an important information-related role for schooling, though not conclusive, because they do not control for unobserved endowments that may be correlated with schooling. Thomas, Strauss, and Henriques (1991) attempt to sort out what mothers' schooling represents in estimates of the determination of heights of 1,378 children under age six in rural northeastern Brazil in 1986 by presenting a set of estimates with varying degrees of control for the mothers' information-related activities (e.g., listening to the radio, watching TV, reading newspapers) and of community characteristics. They conclude that much of the effect of maternal education on child health in rural areas is "transmitted through . . . better information gathering or processing" (p. 17). In fact, however, their procedure allows the confident identification only of schooling being associated with these information-related activities, not that schooling works through them or that they or schooling represents only the effects of schooling per se rather than correlated unobserved endowments.

Results from recent studies are disconcerting, however, for those who interpret the effects of parental schooling on preschool child health and nutrition to represent positive effects of schooling per se, perhaps partly through increasing the capacity for acquiring and using information. These studies illustrate how the estimated impact of parental schooling in such relations changes with better control for parental background characteristics, or endowments, for which schooling in part may be proxying. Briefly summarized are results from four recent studies. First, Rosenzweig and Wolpin (1988) estimate a simple dynamic model of infant health that incorporates unobserved heterogeneity in health endowments across households and uncertainty regarding individual children's endowments before birth and also learning by the parents about such endowments subsequent to birth (even though the data do not have direct observations on such endowments). They estimate health production functions for weight-for-age at birth and at six months in Colombian households from 1968 to 1974, controlling for simultaneity and fixed effects for unobserved household and individual endowments. These estimates then are used to estimate individual child and household endowments, and the latter is correlated positively with parental schooling. That means that parental schooling partly represents the unobserved (to the social scientist) household health environment, *not* the effects of parental schooling alone. Second, Barrera (1987, 1990) estimates a reduced-form relation for age-standardized child height for 3,821 children in households in Bicol, Philippines, in 1978 with and without partial control for unobserved dimensions of maternal backgrounds by including mothers' heights. He finds that maternal schooling has a positive impact on child height and that it decreases as the child's age increases. But the estimated effects are substantially less—from 26 to 81 percent, depending on the age group—if the height control for mothers' background is included. This suggests that in the standard estimates a mother's schooling proxies substantially for other correlated dimensions of her background that in her youth affected both her nutrition (and thus her adult height) and her schooling. Third, Thomas, Strauss, and Henriques (1990) follow a similar procedure in their estimates of child height-for-age for 41,233 Brazilian households in 1974–1975 and find that the failure to control for parental height results in schooling estimates that are biased upward by 25 to 100 percent. Fourth, Behrman and Wolfe (1987a) and Wolfe and Behrman (1987) present four sets of estimates of child anthropometric outcome production functions for Nicaraguan households in 1976–1977: ordinary least squares estimates, similar estimates with control for simultaneity of nutrient intakes, fixed effects estimates for adult sisters to control for the unobserved childhood background characteristics that were shared by the sisters and that may have affected their schooling and other characteristics, and latent variable estimates to control for such characteristics. The first two sets of estimates (which follow standard procedures for most studies before their investigation) indicate a strong positive impact of maternal schooling on child health. The last two sets of estimates, with control for unobserved dimensions of mothers' endowments, indicate that the impact of mothers' schooling is insignificant. Thus these studies raise considerable doubt that, in existing cross-sectional studies, schooling in fact represents only the effects of schooling per se, including those related to information acquisition and use, rather than substantial other unobserved individual and household characteristics that have positive impact on preschool child health and nutrition and are associated with, but not necessarily caused by, parental schooling.

Intrahousehold Allocations and Focus on Providing Information for Particular Types of Individuals to Improve Preschool Health and Nutrition. Empirical studies document very widely that females provide substantially more child care, particularly for infants and small children, than do males. This pattern of specialization of tasks among household members might be related to the nature of birth and breastfeeding, in which women are much more central than men for biological reasons and possibly because of differential opportunity costs of time in economic activities, as Becker (1991) sometimes seems to argue.[4] The pattern of child care also might reflect the nature of the distribution of power within the household or differential preferences, as Folbre (1986) and others seem to suggest (see Behrman 1995 for further references). Better understanding of intrahousehold allocation processes for the purpose of targeting specific individuals helps to improve child health and nutrition. To separate such possibilities is difficult because observations on critical variables (e.g., preferences, bargaining power with controls for opportunity costs[5]) are missing. The latter point is illustrated by Thomas (1990), who studied urban Brazilian household nutrient and child anthropometric outcome demand relations for a 1974–1975 sample and distinguished among the effects of unearned income of women, men, and other sources. If women and men have different preferences regarding these outcomes and if unearned income represents purely relative bargaining power over intrahousehold allocations, then estimates that indicate differential impact of women's versus men's unearned income support an inference of differential preferences and perhaps of directing information-related policies more toward the group with the most interest in child health and nutrition. Thomas's estimates indicate that women's unearned incomes are more related than men's to the investigated outcomes. Therefore, his estimates can be interpreted to support the bargaining model of intrahousehold

[4] Gender discrimination in the labor market also has implications for time allocation within the household because of the differential opportunity costs of time in economic activities and the impact on bargaining power.

[5] Sometimes variables such as schooling and income are used to represent bargaining power. But such variables also may represent the opportunity costs of time or preferences and therefore change the allocation of household resources. See the interchange between Folbre (1984) and Rosenzweig and Schultz (1984).

allocation and the reallocation of resources (and perhaps information) from men to women to improve child health and nutrition. They also indicate that women's unearned income has a greater association with daughters' than with sons' anthropometric measures and (somewhat more weakly) the opposite for men's unearned income, thus suggesting some parental own-gender preference. But the critical maintained assumption that unearned income does not reflect the opportunity costs of time is not persuasive, especially because the major sources of unearned income are pension and social security payments and savings from past labor market earnings, which probably are highly correlated with wage rates and thus the opportunity costs of time in the labor market. Therefore, these results may reflect simply that women who are more productive in the labor market also are more productive in household activities that affect their household nutrient intakes and their children's health, given their specialization in child care, and *not* that shifting resources to women would improve health and nutrition. Thus, although this study is very provocative and more careful than its predecessors in attempting to separate the income/bargaining power effect from the opportunity cost of time/productivity effect,[6] it does not ultimately succeed. Though some experiments would permit such a separation (e.g., by randomly distributing resources to women), available data simply do not permit confident identification of the income effect from price and taste effects.

The variable that is generally included in estimates of household relations that determine child health and nutrition that is most closely related to information, once again, is parental schooling. A priori it does not seem obvious that only mothers' schooling should matter, particularly as it concerns the acquisition of information rather than because of productivity effects. Certainly mothers in most societies spend much more time in child care, including that related to health and nutrition, than do fathers. But for the purpose of obtaining better information related to child health and nutrition, it does not necessarily follow that mothers' schooling is of greater importance than that of other family or household members. The analogy that comes to mind is the work of Rosenzweig and Wolpin (1985) on the adoption of new agricultural technology. They suggest that relatively high schooling of any individual in the household, not necessarily only of those who primarily work in the fields, affects positively the adoption of new technology by the household (presumably by affecting the probability that the household is aware of the new technology). Like-

---

[6] Previous studies have used wage rates, total income (including income earned in the labor market), or schooling for estimates. Such variables are likely to be even more subject to the criticism in the text than is the unearned income variable used by Thomas (and also by Schultz, 1990, in a related study).

wise, at least for some types of information that may improve preschool health and nutrition, any household member might conceivably be the channel through which the information flows. The schooling of anyone in the household besides the mother may be important.

Many studies, however, include only the mothers' schooling in relations that determine child outcomes, a priori restricting the impact of the fathers' or other household members' schooling to zero. If the schooling of other household or family members is in fact important and schooling is correlated with the mother's schooling, the results of this restriction are misleading both by falsely forcing all of the schooling effect to be that of the mother and by biasing upward the estimated impact of the mother's schooling. For example, Behrman and Sussangkarn (1989) find for child outcomes in Thailand that the father's schooling tends to be at least as important as the mother's, that substitution between father's and mother's schooling (that is, the effect of one is less if the effect of the other is greater) does occur, and that if father's schooling in fact does have an impact on such outcomes but is constrained a priori to have no effect in the estimated relations, the estimated impact of mother's schooling is biased upward by 40 to 70 percent. These results suggest that the impact of parental schooling on child outcomes, presumably in part through improved access to and use of information, may be more complicated than is often assumed. A priori restrictions on the schooling of others, based on the conventional wisdom that only mothers' schooling counts, may bias upward the estimated impact of mothers' schooling.

Information at the Community Level That Might Result in Household Behavior That Leads to Better Preschool Child Health and Nutrition

Most household members are involved in several communities (through occupation, ethnic origin, language groups, religion, clan, relatives, castes, tribes, neighborhoods, and other characteristics) that enable them to organize collective action for better health and nutrition. Lobbying with other organizations and governments can be effective, and activities with public good characteristics, such as the dissemination of information directly related to preschool child health and nutrition, are particularly promising. Some community organizations in developing countries have been effective in working to improve preschool child health and nutrition (e.g., the sarvodaya movement in Sri Lanka), although a number of similar efforts have been abortive. More systematic information or more broadly disseminated information might have high payoffs. This idea is further elaborated by Shrimpton in Chapter 13.

Communities might also play a critical role in improving preschool child health and nutrition through decentralized loci for information dispersion and implementation of policies that require difficult-to-obtain household or individual information. The success of monitoring small loans through imposing responsibility on small groups of borrowers may be instructive in this regard. Placing responsibility on the borrowers appears substantially to lower the risks of moral hazard, shirking, and default, which are very expensive when monitored by government agencies. Perhaps this model could be expanded by using small groups of households with preschool children who already belong to a local microcommunity, defined by proximity and other relevant characteristics, to reinforce, for example, the growth-monitoring and safe water practices associated with improved preschool child health. Such microcommunities might lessen shirking and dropouts and provide critical information, some of which is unlikely to be available at a more centralized level, to governments for policy implementation.

Governmental Policy, Household Behavior, Information, and Preschool Child Health and Nutrition

Governments must make policies on the basis of available, often limited, information, even if the policies only amount to decisions to gather more information. Information concerning the many dimensions of household behavior as it relates to preschool child health and nutrition is especially scarce. The interactions among governmental policies, household behavior, and information, their separate and joint effects on preschool child health and nutrition, and the possibility of changing preferences as part of the effort to improve child health and nutrition are addressed here.

Household Income and Health and Nutrition. Until recently, most analysts and policy makers believed that increasing the income of the very poor was the most effective way to improve their health and nutrition status. The World Bank (1981, p. 59), for example, forcefully articulates this view: "There is now a wide measure of agreement on several broad propositions. . . . Malnutrition is largely a reflection of poverty: people do not have income for food. Given the slow income growth that is likely for the poorest people in the foreseeable future, large numbers will remain malnourished for decades to come. . . . The most efficient long-term policies are those that raise the income of the poor." Governmental policies to alleviate malnutrition through income enhancement would probably involve redistribution of income to the poor through transfers and subsidies of items, such as basic staples, consumed largely by the poor and schemes to increase their income, such as investment in their human resources, employment schemes for low-skilled workers, transfer of assets (such as land), and development of new technologies (such as for the semiarid tropics) to increase productivity.

Strong challenges to this conventional wisdom have been raised. The "revisionist" view is that improved nutrition in response to increased income (at least for calories) is very low even for poor people. Many characteristics are valued in food other than nutrients, and these are considered in making marginal food purchases. Therefore, with increased income, the tendency is to increase food expenditures considerably (i.e., by about 8 percent for a 10 percent increase in income), primarily on more expensive, rather than more nutrient-dense, food. People often assume that these marginal food choices are well-informed because of the physical characteristics of the foods, such as taste, texture, variety, status, odor, appearance, and processing, which are not necessarily positively correlated with basic nutrients. This possibility was suggested by Shah (1983), Behrman and Wolfe (1984), and Lipton (1983), among others.

The conventional wisdom that increased income results in greater caloric intake persisted until some studies questioned whether prior studies, which appeared to buttress the conventional wisdom, might have upward biases in their estimated responsiveness to income and demonstrated considerable biases for particular developing-country samples. For example, Behrman and Deolalikar (1987) argue that many studies ignore possibly important intrafood group substitution associated with income increases because of aggregation of foods. For rural south India, they estimate a calorie response to a 10 percent income increase to be closer to 1 than 8 percent. Bouis and Haddad (1992) argue that the standard procedures may overestimate the income responsiveness of nutrient intakes because of two types of measurement error: (1) the difference between nutrients available to the household and those that are consumed by household members increases with income because of food provided to others (e.g., workers, guests, mendicants), plate waste, and so on, factors often ignored; and (2) food purchases and total expenditures are used to represent income in many studies.[7] Their estimates for the rural Philippines suggest, once such measurement errors are taken into account, less than a 1 percent calorie increase for a 10 percent income increase, that is, only about one-tenth of the estimate obtained from standard methods that ignore these measurement errors. Bouis (1994) notes that the weight differences across income classes observed in poor societies are not sufficient to be consistent with very large nutrient-income responses.

[7] Food expenditures are a major part (usually about 70 percent) of total expenditures for poor households. If they are misreported, total expenditures are likely to be misreported in the same direction, creating an overestimated association between the two.

This issue is under debate, but the conventional wisdom, that calorie-income responses are substantial, has been challenged. The perception that such responses are fairly small has become increasingly widespread. Even if this revisionist view fails to stand the test of time, as of this writing the general perception that increased income will induce increased nutrient intake among poor populations has clearly changed substantially. Academic studies have provided new information that has altered considerably such perceptions and, with them, the information basis for policy formulation. Governmental policies that seek to increase nutrient intake of poor people through increased income, no matter how well justified on other grounds, appear much less sound than they did a short time ago. More careful studies are needed on this subject.

Information about Price Responses and Governmental Policies Related to Preschool Child Health and Nutrition. Governmental policies can affect household behavior that pertains to preschool child health and nutrition through market prices in a myriad of ways. They range from direct subsidies of health-related goods and services (e.g., basic staples, inoculations, drugs) to altering the prices (e.g., through exchange rates, tariffs, export restrictions) that the poor can command for items they produce. In designing such policies, therefore, it is important to know whether the household price responsiveness is likely to be large or small in matters related to child health and nutrition.

Studies of household behavior tend to suggest that our knowledge regarding the size of price responses is incomplete. Akin, Griffin, Guilkey, and Popkin (1985) studied the determinants of the decision of whether and what type of medical practitioner (e.g., public, private, traditional) should be used in the Philippines. Their data include extensive monetary and transportation-related prices (both time costs and monetary costs) for the alternatives. They found almost no significance for any of their price variables. Taken at face value, such results suggest that governments cannot induce substantial changes in these forms of health-related behavior through altering the prices directly related to curative health services.

Other evidence, however, points toward important and substantial price responses in demands for nutrients and other health-related goods and services. For nutrients, for example, Behrman and Deolalikar (1990), Pitt (1983), Sahn and Alderman (1988), Pitt and Rosenzweig (1985), and Alderman (1987a) report significant responses for samples in India, Bangladesh, Sri Lanka, and Indonesia. Their studies suggest that concerned governments should be aware of the impact their policies have on food prices, which are perhaps more important than income. But the significant price responses in each of these studies, with exceptions primarily for the basic staples, are more often positive than negative. That is, increases in the prices of nonstaple foods apparently tend to improve intakes of basic nutrients by inducing substitution of lower-cost, nutrient-dense foods. This result is somewhat surprising and, if validated in further work, suggests the need for more subtlety in food price policies than often has been displayed. This issue seems serious enough to warrant further research for policy formulation.

With respect to demands for different types of curative health care, studies have reported large and significant negative effects of price increases in terms of time and money: Birdsall and Chuhan (1986) for Mali; Mwabu (1989) for Kenya; Gertler, Locay, and Sanderson (1987) for Peru; and Gertler and van der Gaag (1988) for Peru and the Ivory Coast. These results are in sharp contrast to those reported by Akin et al. (1985). Gertler, Locay, and Sanderson and Gertler and van der Gaag argue that the difference is because earlier studies were misspecified by imposing a priori the same price response at a given health level for poorer as for richer individuals, rather than a larger one for poorer people, as would be predicted by economic household theory if demand for health increases with income. This may be part of the explanation for the differences in the estimates across studies, though some of the studies reporting large price responses do not allow for such a pattern (e.g., Birdsall and Chuhan, 1986). It would be useful to obtain further information about price responses and whether the different results reflect simply differences in research procedures, contexts, or preferences across household groups. Also, existing studies may be biased because the samples are usually limited to those who report that they were sick in a given time interval, which would seem to lead to selectivity bias because such a group is hardly random. Finally, it would be useful to better integrate the exploration of the determinants of health care choices (prices and other factors) with the impact on health per se. Often, investigators consider in isolation only the health care choices, which do not necessarily relate closely to health outcomes. For example, Wolfe and Behrman (1984) find that schooling for Nicaraguan women significantly affects their health care choices but does not affect a latent variable representation of their health status.

Studies report higher price elasticities for health care demands for poorer than for richer households. Alderman (1986) surveyed a number of food and nutrient demand studies and reports a similar tendency for both. Some studies seem to suggest that a greater price response for the poorer than for the richer implies that increasing prices or user charges, as advocated in a number of instances by the World Bank, will have relatively negative effects on the poorer. Yet the implications of standard economic modeling may be just the opposite: those who can substitute most readily for a commodity whose price has risen tend to have the highest price responses and to lose the least as a result of the price increase, provided the loss of income is compensated. To avoid misinterpretation of this statement, it should be emphasized that it refers to the pure price effect, which is what the studies that are surveyed here purport to estimate. In addition to the pure price effect, an increase in food or other health-related input prices may reduce income, which also may cause a reduction in the consumption or use, but that is not at issue here.

Food price policies are not the only social policies related to preschool child health and nutrition that may be informed by household demand studies. Jimenez (1990) provides surveys of pricing policy for health and education in developing countries. He concludes that the efficiency gains from user charges for selected types of health and education (i.e., those whose benefits accrue to the individuals concerned, such as hospital care and university education) could be substantial. In these cases, the elimination or lessening of subsidies probably improves efficiency because of a lack of positive externalities and public good characteristics, though some might question whether merit goods are involved. He adds that the impact of increased user charges need not be inequitable, since present distribution of subsidies tends to be highly skewed toward higher income groups, who obtain greater access to more costly social services even if they are uniformly free for all. Under these circumstances, the expansionary effect of fee increases for selected services (and, if possible, for selected individuals) may actually improve equity in the distribution of public resources.[8] Increased equity may improve the average health and nutrition of preschool children because the children of the poor generally are at particular health and nutrition risk.

Changing Preferences through Information. Policy-induced improvements in information might have high returns, but preferences such as those related to dietary prescriptions might limit their effectiveness. What if the effectiveness of an information policy can be increased (at least by some measures) by introducing propaganda designed to change the dietary preferences? This possibility points to a class of basic welfare problems and questions that should be considered in making policy decisions. In the interest of improving health and nutrition, such an attempt might be justified.

The policy object, presumably, is not simply to make people healthier and better nourished but to increase their welfare as a whole. Would health gains more than offset any welfare losses resulting from the encouragement (persuasion) of people to violate traditional, perhaps religious,

---

[8] Whether or not equity actually is improved depends on the uses of the resources that are freed from discontinuing the subsidies.

dietary prescriptions? Underlying this question are even more fundamental questions. If preferences are indeed changed through governmental provision of information, how can it be known whether the people whose preferences have been changed are better or worse off? Alderman (personal communication) has suggested that if households elect to participate in an activity, knowing that their preferences may change as a result, then it can be deduced that they were made better off by the change according to their dynamic preferences. This deduction seems valid, but it does not cover the cases (as Alderman recognizes) in which the preference changes are not elected but are induced by outside interventions, households have imperfect information about the nature of the induced preference changes, or that raised by the following question: what if they are worse off according to their previous tastes and better off according to their ex-post preferences? For preschool children the situation is even more complicated because many actions affecting them reflect not their own preferences but those of others, such as of their parents. How does one weigh their parents' perceptions of what is best for them against those, say, of public health officials?

These questions are difficult indeed, and it is not clear that social scientists can properly make the necessary value judgments. It seems inappropriate to impose blindly one's own values on others or to assume that the cost of violating or changing traditional beliefs or practices is necessarily small relative to the potential gains in preschool child health. It is useful, however, to be aware of the distinction between information that expands people's awareness of options, which seems unambiguously to improve their welfare (although a value judgment—more choice is better—has been made here, it seems unlikely that the cost of choosing among several options could be so great as to reduce someone's welfare: one can always simply ignore the expanded set of choices and not be worse off), and propaganda/social marketing efforts to change people's preferences "for their own good," which raises the conundrum of questions posed here. These and related issues are further discussed in the two chapters that follow.

Conclusions

Information has important effects on child health and nutrition on at least three levels: households, communities, and governments. Information is not likely to be produced sufficiently by private entities unless there are public subsidies because of the difficulties for private entities in capturing the rewards from producing and disseminating information.

More schooling, particularly of women, seems to improve the information relevant to child health and nutrition that is used at the household level; but the long lags and high costs raise the question of whether there are not more effective and more immediate means of improving household information than schooling young girls; further, in most studies schooling in part apparently is representing factors such as ability, motivation, and habits learned in childhood rather than the effects of schooling per se. At the community level there are important information flows in two directions, from households to governments and other organizations regarding needs related to child health and in the opposite direction regarding new procedures and options; the latter flows might be improved through adopting the small-group monitoring model that has been successful for credit allocations. At the level of governmental policies, careful academic studies have improved the basis of policy decisions—for example, by shifting the emphasis from income to price responses for basic health and nutrition through new studies. If information changes tastes, difficult issues are raised about welfare effects and the desirability of related policies.

4

Nutrition Education in Developing
Countries: An Examination of
Recent Successful Projects

Maria Teresa Cerqueira and Christine M. Olson

Starting in the 1950s, the importance of nutrition education as a component of health programs grew such that by the late 1970s nutrition education was included in approximately 90 percent of health and nutrition programs (Karlin, 1976; Austin et al., 1978).

Nutrition education is both a practical and an academic field and is concerned with improving people's lives and with generating a scientific knowledge base from which to do so. In the developing world, nutrition education as a practical field dates from about 1950, yet few nutrition education projects have been evaluated or appear in the scientific literature (Zeitlin and Formación, 1981). Thus the scientifically developed knowledge base of nutrition education rests largely on programs conducted in the United States and other developed countries.

Overview of Major Reviews of the Literature

Since the 1960s five major reviews of the primarily North American (English-language) scientific literature in nutrition education have been done; these are by Swope (1962); McKenzie and Mumford (1965); Whitehead (1973); Levy, Iverson, and Walberg (1980); and Johnson and Johnson (1985). Those of Whitehead (1973) and Johnson and Johnson (1985), the most inclusive, will be discussed here.

Whitehead reviewed the English literature in nutrition education through 1970. She examined 269 items in great detail and reached the following conclusions:

> There is evidence that nutrition education which purports to improve dietary habits can be expected to do so within carefully defined limitations. (p. 132)

> Problem-solving is an effective way to influence what people do about their dietary intakes and their food supply. (p. 133)

> Discussion-decision is more effective than is admonition by lecture as a method of influencing what people do about dietary habits and nutrition problems. (p. 134)

> Effective nutrition education, based on recognized needs, is cooperatively planned, conducted, and evaluated by individuals concerned in homes and communities and schools; such education is supervised by adequately prepared nutrition educators. (p. 134)

Whitehead concludes that nutrition education can be effective in changing behavior when changing behavior, rather disseminating information, is the clear intention of the program. And she contends that the literature supports the conclusion that active involvement of the learner in defining the nutrition problem and in designing and implementing the program is a key factor in the success of the program.

Evaluating three programs, the Food . . . Your Choice school nutrition education program, the Supplemental Food Program for Women, Infants, and Children (WIC), and the Expanded Food and Nutrition Education Program (EFNEP), Johnson and Johnson (1985) concluded that nutrition education results in a marked increase in knowledge about nutrition, some increases in positiveness of attitudes toward eating nutritiously, and constructive changes in participants' patterns of food consumption.

The evaluators feel that their results are widely generalizable and have been consistent throughout seventy-four years of nutrition education research. Johnson and Johnson (1985) also point out that a consistent shortcoming of research in nutrition education has been the failure to use theoretical models to explain how nutrition education programs positively affect knowledge, attitudes, and behavior regarding nutrition. They call for a systematic program of high-quality research to validate theoretical models that can be operationalized in actual nutrition education programs. They also call for future research to address the relative efficiency of a variety of instructional methods appropriate to nutrition education.

On the basis of the primarily North American English-language nutrition education research literature, it seems that it is time to move beyond the relatively simple question, Can nutrition education result in change? The answer is clearly yes, particularly when educational strategies actively involve the learner. This literature indicates the strong need for theoretically based intervention research that compares various educational strategies in producing desired nutrition-related behavioral outcomes. As Olson and Kelly (1989) note, however, the difficulties of designing and implementing such research should not be underestimated.

What major conclusions do reviews of research literature from the developing world present about nutrition education? Since 1980 four major articles and monographs on the state of nutrition education in the developing world have been written (Zeitlin and Formación, 1981; Gussow and Contento, 1984; Israel and Tighe, 1984; Hornik, 1985). The second is an analysis of the *field of nutrition education*, rather than a review of the literature. The third is primarily an extensive annotated bibliography of the nutrition education literature. Only the works of Zeitlin and Formación and of Hornik are syntheses of the research literature. These have recently been supplemented by an analysis of eight case studies in nutrition communications (Achterberg, 1991).

Zeitlin and Formación's review was part of a larger project that included a mail survey, field studies, and a literature review to gather and integrate information to present a representative, but not exhaustive, review of major nutrition interventions. The goal was to identify salient factors that planners should consider in designing nutrition interventions. Zeitlin and Formación drew the following conclusions: Although none of the existing evaluations of effectiveness of nutrition education is unflawed, all evidence tends to point in the same direction: well-managed nutrition education programs can, at a relatively low cost, bring about behavior changes that contribute to improved nutritional well-being. Moreover, for policy purposes, it is possible to generalize and conclude that the following major design characteristics favor cost-effectiveness: (1) absence of commercial promotion that contradicts nutrition education themes; (2) community-level programs; (3) combination of face-to-face and mass media channels; and (4) education of all vertical levels involved in nutrition policy and implementation.

Hornik (1985) carried out a literature review to provide decision makers with information on what works to improve nutritional conditions in different settings. As he stated,

The central questions here are straight-forward: Under what circumstances is there a role for nutrition education? In what content/behavior areas, with what educational methods, and for which populations is there evidence that education is an affordable, logistically feasible and effective intervention? Is it possible that nutrition education can stand on its own or is it valuable exclusively as a component of a comprehensive nutrition intervention? (p. 19)

Hornik points to the need for extending the coverage of nutrition education beyond the reach of health services and for improving the quality of nutrition information. He reasons that mass media approaches to nutrition education might more effectively address these needs than face-to-face strategies because of the lack of trained nutrition education personnel. Hornik identifies certain nutrition problems—low rates and short duration of breastfeeding among women in urban areas, low energy intakes of young children during weaning, and the treatment and prevention of diarrhea—that may be particularly amenable to educational interventions.

The Approach of This Review

Hornik raised important questions that have not been fully answered by research in nutrition education in the developing world. These questions are the focus of this review. To facilitate a systematic analysis of the literature, we have developed an analytical framework for examining nutrition education projects.

The framework is used to analyze five successful nutrition projects from the developing world in an effort to understand the reasons for their success, to identify their common characteristics, and to describe the variability across the projects on what characteristics are considered to be related to success. The findings of this analysis are offered as hypotheses that require further testing. To draw definitive conclusions about the importance of these characteristics for success, it would be necessary to do additional work, including an examination of unsuccessful projects to determine whether the characteristics were lacking. The problem with carrying out such a contrast, however, is that only extraordinary projects get published. They are typically funded by organizations from outside the country with more money and more technical expertise than is usually available. The characteristics associated with success in these projects may not be the same as those associated with success in smaller-scale, locally based programs.

The analytical framework highlights planning and implementation issues that are typically considered outside the scope of nutrition education. This was done in recognition of the importance to success that Whitehead (1973) and Zeitlin and Formación (1981) place on program management issues such as personnel training and supervision.

The projects were selected from a review of the literature, information provided by professionals in the field, and unpublished reports from various organizations. The criteria for final inclusion were that the project had an implementation period of at least four years and results of the impact on health and nutritional status were available. The projects selected for analysis were the Narangwal and Tamil Nadu projects from India (Kielmann et al., 1983; Berg, 1987a; Brems, 1987; Chidambaram, 1989); the Indonesia Nutrition Communication and Behavior Change program (NCBC); the Applied Nutrition Education Program (ANEP) from the Dominican Republic (Zeitlin et al., 1984; Griffiths, 1984; USAID, 1988); and the Iringa Nutrition Program from Tanzania (Ljungqvist, 1988; WHO-UNICEF, 1989; Latham et al., 1988; Yambi et al., 1989). These programs are described in greater detail in the Appendix. All of the programs claim some degree of improvement in child nutrition or health status and are generally considered successful.

The Analytical Framework

Table 4.1 lists the characteristics that were used to examine the nutrition education programs and projects selected. These characteristics reflect the major issues raised in the reviews of nutrition education discussed earlier in this chapter as well as the authors' combined experience in developing and implementing nutrition education programs in a variety of settings and contexts.

This approach faced several limitations. A full description of the planning, implementation, and evaluation activities is available for few nutrition education programs. Detailed descriptive information about the program setting or context and the communication or education strategy are commonly lacking. Mass media campaigns sometimes lack an evaluation of impact on biological parameters such as nutritional status (Hornik, 1988, 1989; Manoff, 1985, 1987; Hollis, 1986), and nutrition education usually is not the sole intervention but only one component of a larger intervention scheme.

Brief Description of Comparative Criteria

The basic philosophical assumptions of the model and theory undergirding the program, whether implicit or explicit, are crucial to understanding the nutrition education program as it is actually implemented (Olson and Kelly, 1989). This chapter will assess the models and theories guiding the development of nutrition education programs in developing

Table 4.1. Characteristics examined in the nutrition education programs

Key program and content characteristics	Basic components
Model and theory	Program philosophy Political support Sector priorities
Duration	Years (plan/operation)
Context	Social and economic conditions and setting
Needs assessment	Focus Method of identification
Intervention	Health goal Purpose Type and components
Administration and infrastructure	Organization Leadership Resources and coverage
Training and supervision	Purpose and concepts Method and curricula Location and length Reinforcement and frequency Monitoring and feedback
Communication and education strategy	Theory base Methods and dimensions Content and messages Channels Media and materials

countries. We will analyze the influence that the medical model, commonly used to guide interventions implemented in the health sector, has had on nutrition education.

An important aspect of planning in many nutrition education efforts, the needs assessment, is particularly weak. Nutrition education is often difficult to evaluate because of the lack of adequate baseline information collected as part of the needs assessment. The purpose and nature of the educational intervention are also likely to influence the chances for success (Whitehead, 1973).

The quality of the training and supervision of the people carrying out the nutrition education program, as well as the administration and infrastructure needed to implement it, are key to achieving cost-effective results. These components are particularly important to include in the analysis because, as Hornik (1985) maintains, the lack of trained personnel makes face-to-face approaches unfeasible in much of the developing world. Whitehead (1973) noted the need to have education supervised by adequately prepared nutrition educators.

The communication and educational strategies, including their theory base, are reviewed in particular detail because they are unique to educational nutrition interventions. The content of nutrition education messages, as well as their delivery channels, are considered important to success and will be reviewed. The evaluation methods and outcomes are not discussed here.

Analysis of the Projects

In Table 4.2 a summary of the major differences and similarities among the projects is presented. In this section a more detailed analysis of the projects will be presented using the categories in the analytical framework as an organizing tool.

Program Model and Theory

Most nutrition education worldwide is implemented within primary health care. Thus both the delivery and the content of nutrition education have been influenced by the general principles of the medical model in which the treatment (nutritional counseling) is a prescription for curing a disease; the patient follows the instructions, and this advice is the solution to the problem. In addition, nutritional science, rather than the clients' concerns, usually dictates the content of nutrition education (Gussow and Contento, 1984). Patients do not actively participate in planning the "cure," nor is their socioeconomic context considered, because diseases rather than people are the focal concern. Thus nutrition education in the form of prescriptive information is delivered to mothers of malnourished children (Hoorweg and McDowell, 1979; Hoorweg and Niemeijer, 1980a, 1980b).

In recent years the patient's role in complying (or not complying) with the treatment has been considered in interventions based on the medical model. But the basic assumptions of this approach to nutrition education are that medical experts still determine the actions to be taken, and the population's main role is passive. Since the declaration of the official policy of Primary Health Care with Alma Ata (WHO-UNICEF, 1978) many efforts have been made to build a participatory model of health services, promoting a more dynamic and active role of the population in the assessment of its problems and the development and implementation of solutions. Somewhat surprisingly, the nutrition education literature has few examples of projects in primary health care settings that are guided by these more participatory approaches.

Table 4.2. Analysis of the selected case studies

Characteristics	Narangwal	Tamil Nadu	Indonesia	Dominican Republic	Iringa
MODEL	Medical services	Community development	Social marketing	Social marketing	Social mobilization
DURATION	6 years	6 years	6 years	4 years	5 years
CONTEXT	Rural High grain production	Rural Urban Low income	Rural Urban Low income	Rural Low income	Rural High farm production
NEEDS ASSESSMENT	Epidemiologic	Nutritional	Qualitative	Qualitative	Triple-A
Problem of Interest	Malnutrition and infections	Malnutrition Mortality	Feeding practices	Feeding practices	Malnutrition Mortality
Health goal	Reduce mortality	Reduce malnutrition	Improve growth	Improve growth	Reduce mortality
INTERVENTION					
Type	Multiple	Multiple	"Single"	"Single"	Multiple
Components	Combination nutr./health	Selective feeding Growth monit. Nutr. educ.	Nutr. educ. Growth monit.	Nutr. educ. Growth monit.	Problem solving Growth monit.
Purpose	Provide services	Support mothers' capacity	Support mothers' capacity	Support mothers' capacity	Build local collective capacity
ADMINISTRATION	Top-down	Top-down	Top-down	Top-down	Bottom-up
INFRASTRUCTURE	Built health center	Built nutrition center	Used existing facilities	Used existing facilities	Built health and child care facilities
Coverage:	3,000	800,000	52,000	8,700	46,000
Children	150	9,000	2,000	120	350
Workers/children	1 to 100	1 to 100	1 to 100	1 to 60	1 to 150

TRAINING	On-the-job Delivery of services Data collec. 6 weeks Theory and practice	On-site Administra. Suppl. feed. Growth monit. 6 weeks Community development	On-site Administra. Growth monit. Communication 15 days Behavior change	On-site Administra. Growth monit. Communication 12 days Promotional	On-site Empowerment Build AAA capacity Ongoing community development
Continued Education: Type Frequency	Meetings 2x month	Meetings 2x month	Short sessions —	Meetings 1x month	Meetings 2x month
SUPERVISION Frequency (supervisor per worker)	Supportive 1x week 1 to 12 FHW	Supportive 2x month 1 to 10 CNW	Supportive 1x month 1 to 20 Kaders	Supportive 1x month 1 to 10 Prom.	Supportive 2x month 1 to 12 VHW
COMMUNICATION/EDUCATION **STRATEGY** Theoretical base	"Persuasion" Structuralist functionalist	"Persuasion" Structural functionalist	Social marketing Structural functionalist	Social marketing Structural functionalist	"Persuasion" Historical Materialism Dialectic
Channels	Face-to-face Individual counseling	Interpersonal Individual and group	Face-to-face Individual and group	Face-to-face Individual and group	Interpersonal Individual, group, mass assemblies
Media Materials	None None	Films Posters Flipcharts	Radio Action posters Weight graph	Audiocassettes Flash cards Weight graph	Films Newsletters Manuals Weight graph

The Narangwal project (Kielmann et al., 1983) is a good illustration of a well-planned and well-designed program that emphasizes medical expertise in solving public health and community problems (a medical model–based program). This project focused on providing medical services and extending the physician to the community. Participants were passive recipients of a service.

In Tamil Nadu (Brems, 1987; Greene, 1989), the main thrust of the program was multiple community interventions structured to improve the nutritional status of infants and reduce malnutrition. This program followed a community development model. Community participation was conceptualized as the need to get full cooperation and acceptance of the community for project implementation. The program did not envisage any major role for the community in needs assessment, planning, supervision, or evaluation of the program (TINP, 1989).

In Indonesia (Zeitlin et al., 1984) and the Dominican Republic (USAID, 1988), the fundamental purpose was to improve weaning practices. The projects used a social marketing approach and thus audience participation was a major element.

A major difference among the four case studies presented thus far is the amount of participant involvement in defining the nutrition problem and the design and implementation of the program. In Narangwal and Tamil Nadu, active participant involvement was limited. In Indonesia and the Dominican Republic, participants were more involved.

Because all four projects were successful, the reader could appropriately question the importance of basing a program on a model or theory that stresses true audience or community participation. In response to this question, it is important to note that in the Narangwal project (Kielmann et al., 1983), "an important part of the selection process was to assess the potential level of cooperation in each village and to negotiate with the villagers until they were willing to accept whatever combination of service interventions was assigned to their village according to the research design. All village leaders agreed without reservation to help persuade all families to participate in all of the survey and measurement activities that were necessary for this to be an effective research enterprise" (p. 14). Thus, in some ways, the project was almost guaranteed success because only villages with interested, motivated people had the opportunity to participate. In Tamil Nadu, only 16 percent of nonworking group member mothers participated in nutrition education sessions and demonstrations. This low rate could be related to the nonparticipatory nature of the model guiding program development.

The Iringa Nutrition Program in Tanzania (Ljungqvist, 1987; Jonsson et al., 1988; Yambi et al., 1989) presents an example of a model and theory base whose main purpose is "to develop the capacity at all levels of society to assess and analyze nutrition problems and to design appropriate actions" (Ljungqvist, 1987, p. 9). The intrinsic difference is that it emphasizes collective action and problem solving on all social levels. The focus of the model is social mobilization rather than individual behavior change or service delivery. This approach has characteristics that are similar to the empowerment process model developed by Freire (1971, 1973, 1974). Health or nutrition education based on empowerment focuses on group efforts to identify problems, critically assess social and historical roots of the problems, and promote structural change. Thus empowerment-based education involves more than improving the self-esteem, self-efficacy, or health behaviors of individuals (Wallerstein and Bernstein, 1988).

The fundamental thrust of all of the programs was to deliver a nutrition message or a service. The majority worked broadly within the health sector. Three case studies used models that focused on individuals. Two case studies appeared to use community development models: Tamil Nadu stressed self-help activities and cultural modifications; Iringa stressed social mobilization and structural, economic change. Tamil Nadu and Narangwal used relatively limited forms of client participation. The projects in Indonesia and the Dominican Republic included extensive client participation. The expectation in these four programs was to change individual behavior and cultural factors that determine malnutrition. The Iringa project was different in that it built community participation to identify social and economic problems that determine malnutrition. The expectation was that both individual and collective actions would solve nutritional problems.

The present review demonstrates that, in these extraordinary projects, the traditional medical model is being replaced by a more participatory model based on the premise that health is determined more strongly by life-style and economic and social conditions than by biomedical expertise and services. More participatory strategies in nutrition education are emerging even though many nutrition education programs are still delivered through primary health care. Whitehead's (1973) review indicates that this shift is likely to result in more successful nutrition education programs. Whether the shift detected in these projects is also occurring in smaller-scale local programs is a question that merits further study.

A second observation is that two quite different philosophies about the purposes and approach to nutrition education are beginning to emerge. One stresses building individual capacity to analyze various problems, make appropriate decisions, and take action. The other stresses identifying specific practices as causes of malnutrition and designing behavior modification programs to change these practices. The latter includes motivating individual behavior changes within the given socioeconomic constraints. The former emphasizes building the collective capacity for community development including the promotion of social and economic growth. The relative merits of each philosophy in guiding the development of nutrition education programs in a variety of sociocultural contexts is an issue that needs in-depth study.

Duration of the Projects

The nutrition education programs reviewed have been in operation for a longer period than most projects. Tamil Nadu reported that a two-year extension of the traditional four years of funding allowed the program to develop adequately and permitted the assessment of major outcomes, which would be impossible in a shorter time period (Greene, 1989). In Indonesia, the first two years were needed for planning, development of infrastructure, training of two thousand volunteer nutrition workers (kaders), and setting up the village growth-monitoring program. Two more years were needed to develop the communication strategy: identifying the specific behavior and practices, testing concepts, and elaborating the messages. This brief review leads us to an obvious but often forgotten point: significant behavior changes and impact on health and nutrition conditions cannot be expected in four-year programs. Adequate time for planning and implementation is important, especially for programs based on participatory learning, community development, and social mobilization models.

The Context

The social and economic context of the areas and households differed among the projects reviewed. Both the Narangwal project and the Iringa nutrition program were implemented in areas of apparent relative affluence. The Narangwal study was in the agricultural Punjab, an area with an abundant food surplus yet much malnutrition. Iringa was chosen because the infrastructure could support the implementation of such a program and also because it had better socioeconomic conditions than other districts but a high infant mortality rate (Yambi et al., 1989). The Tamil Nadu project was implemented in districts with serious nutrition problems. The infant mortality rate was high—125 per 1,000 live births, and the mortality rate of one- to four-year-old children was about 30 per 1,000 children. The baseline survey and case study results of the ninety communities in the ANEP project in the Dominican Republic report that incomes are extremely low. The evaluation report suggests that the incidence of malnutrition is low in this area, but the socioeconomic conditions are said to have greatly deteriorated in the last five years (Mora, 1989). The Indonesia NCBC project was carried out in five culturally diverse areas of the national nutrition and primary health program in the Kematan subdistrict. It is impossible to determine the extent to which the socioeconomic conditions associated with these projects influenced their success. The results of other studies may shed some light on this issue.

A pilot project developed in fourteen Philippine villages indicates that nutrition education has limited effects in improving nutritional status without an increase in household incomes (Garcia and Pinstrup-Andersen, 1987). The intervention scheme consisted of price discounts on rice and cooking oil and nutrition education. Results from the seventeen-month test period indicate that nutrition education had a small positive effect on increasing food consumption in households when it was accompanied by the subsidy. When nutrition education was provided without the food subsidy, however, no effect was detected. Multivariate analysis suggests that the nutrition education component of the scheme had no significant impact on household food expenditures and acquisition, but food consumption and the nutritional status of preschoolers were strongly affected, indicating that the nutrition messages increased the focus on children.

The interaction between the availability of resources within the household and nutrition education requires further study. Empirical evidence indicates that the availability of resources or an increase in income is not sufficient to assure adequate levels of nutrition, especially for women and children (Chapter 11 and McGuire and Austin, 1987). But education is not a substitute for food. When household income is low and quantities of food available are very limited, no amount of high-quality nutrition education will enhance food consumption and therefore possibly improve nutritional status. "There are limits to nutrition education because not every nutrition problem is an education problem" (Manoff, 1987, p. 68).

Experience and research have consistently shown that cultural beliefs often prevent full utilization of food resources. A challenge for nutrition education is to identify culturally acceptable ways of expanding the use of available food resources. In their review, Zeitlin and Formación (1981) point out the need to identify cultural beliefs and their associated behavioral sequences in designing themes and messages for nutrition education directed at alleviating malnutrition.

Needs Assessment

Many nutrition education projects have lacked an adequate preintervention study to focus the intervention on specific and meaningful objectives (Burkhalter, 1986; Hoorweg and Niemeijer, 1980a, 1980b). A practical information system, including adequate needs assessment, is needed to give the educational activities an appropriate focus.

In Indonesia, national and regional staff developed the needs assessment. They used a baseline survey to assess the communities' nutritional situation, and they took dietary information and anthropometric measures. Members of the target audience actively participated in identifying individual household behavior related to infant feeding practices and breastfeeding. In the Dominican Republic, the central staff and trained field supervisors developed both a baseline survey and case studies of 158 households. Target audience members also participated in identifying specific problems with weaning foods and infant feeding practices.

In the social marketing approach used in Indonesia and the Dominican Republic, active participation by the target audience was fundamental for the development and testing of the concepts, messages, and materials; it would have been impossible to identify specific household behaviors that might be modified through an educational intervention without audience participation.

In Iringa, a "Triple-A" conceptual framework (analysis, assessment, and action) was used to identify causes of malnutrition. Results of growth monitoring are discussed at the village council meetings, and decisions about how to solve problems are made at this level. Many intervention components were designed before the villages had the opportunity to conduct their own needs assessment (Pelletier, 1991b).

In Iringa, the impressive social mobilization of all elements of society and at all political and administrative levels would not have been possible without popular involvement in the analysis, assessment, and action process. Even when the interventions were in place, this process apparently acted as an extension of the needs assessment and as feed-forward for fine-tune planning. In contrast, neither Narangwal nor Tamil Nadu indicates that community participation was contemplated in the needs assessment or planning. The low coverage of pregnant and lactating women (43 percent) as well as of children with health care services could possibly have been improved with greater participation and community involvement in the needs assessment.

Many nutrition education programs lack an appropriate education-oriented needs assessment with a focus on behavior. The focus instead has been on the collection of quantitative information on morbidity and mortality. These data have traditionally been collected for the purpose of detecting long-term impact on health or for targeting a program to a specific geographical area. An education-oriented needs assessment may require more time and training of local workers to collect information on health behaviors amenable to educational interventions. A needs assessment with a combination of morbidity, mortality, and behavioral indicators could possibly promote both community participation in the identification and analysis of their own needs (and thus enhance the chances of educational success) and provide accurate data for monitoring and evaluation of the program's long-term impact.

Intervention: Health Goal, Purpose, and Components

The problem of interest in all of the programs was the reduction of infant malnutrition and mortality. The Narangwal project used health and nutrition services, including supplementary feeding and education, to reduce malnutrition and diarrhea. The health goal was to reduce infant mortality; the objectives were to see which combination of services (nutrition, health, family planning, child care, or integrated nutrition and health) achieved the greatest effect.

Tamil Nadu and Iringa have similar problems of interest: to reduce malnutrition and infant mortality. In Tamil Nadu, the nutrition services delivered included growth monitoring, education, and supplementary feeding. Local mothers were trained as community nutrition workers, and women's working groups were organized to support the project. The topic of interest was infant feeding and growth, and the purpose of the intervention was to teach the mothers how to improve their child's weaning foods and maintain adequate weight for age.

In Iringa, the purpose of the intervention was to strengthen the capacity of villages, from mothers to politicians, to analyze and assess the problem of severe malnutrition and its causes and then to take appropriate action. The intervention included growth monitoring, primary health care measures, improvement of water and sanitation, education, and infant care and feeding while mothers work away from their children. Local health and child care providers were trained and the village council monitored the activities.

The projects in Indonesia and the Dominican Republic focused on maternal and infant nutrition, specifically infant feeding practices. Intervention components were growth monitoring and education delivered by local volunteers in home visits and small group sessions. The focus was on individual behavior change, with emphasis on building maternal self-reliance and self-esteem.

The similarity in health goals and purpose across the projects makes it impossible to examine the relationship between these and success. The goals of reducing malnutrition and mortality were obviously viewed by program planners as requiring behavioral change and not ones that could be accomplished solely with information dissemination. Thus the results are consistent with Whitehead's (1973) premise that if program planners set behavior change as their goal for nutrition education, they are more likely to be successful in changing behavior than if they set information dissemination as their goal and hope it results in behavior change.

Administration and Infrastructure

The projects reviewed report different types of infrastructure and generally claim to have a supportive organization and reasonable funding conditions. The literature indicates that political commitment from national and local government is especially important for sustainability and expansion. All of the projects reviewed had extensive international funding.

The amount of expertise and technical assistance needed to support the program is another important issue. All projects had extensive technical assistance. The social marketing approach requires specialized training for workers involved in the planning and development of the communication strategy. This is an important aspect when considering the scaling up or replication of the experiences.

Geographic access to program services has been noted to be crucial to broad program coverage and is related to the infrastructure needed for program implementation (Hornik, 1985). The distance to and from the health center plays a major role in the frequency of the mothers' visits. In all of the projects trained local nutrition workers provided home visits and group activities in an accessible facility.

A fundamental aspect of the recent successful nutrition education programs is a solid and supportive health service environment and infrastructure. An effort is being made to address such constraints as distance and transportation, women's availability of time, and the problem of illiteracy. Recognizing that people go to the health centers for curative services, the projects reviewed have made extensive progress training local workers to develop community-based nutrition education activities. Resources to support community activities are also important because the regular hours of the health centers may be inadequate (Levinson, 1989).

In summary, political and governmental support, significant technical assistance, extensive outside funding, and many efforts to strengthen local, community-level capacity are common characteristics of the successful projects reviewed here. All of the programs either built or secured adequate physical facilities. The ratio of health workers to children, 1 per 60 to 1 per 150, is much higher than in many past unsuccessful programs. The experience of these programs illustrates that viability depends greatly on the program's capacity to generate a national and local political constituency, especially to address the issue of financial support.

Training and Supervision of Workers

In all of the programs reviewed, the program implementer was critical. This issue will be discussed in depth because personnel are considered to be the major limiting factor in face-to-face nutrition education (Hornik, 1985). The training of local workers and their supportive supervision are considered important components of the successful programs.

In Narangwal, family health workers (FHW) were selected who had "a high school education and training as a lady health visitor" (Kielmann et al., 1983, p. 52). Training was done on the job under the guidance of the physician. "A particularly effective pattern was established of alternating two weeks in the Center followed by two weeks in the field" (Kielmann et al., 1983, p. 52). Twice a month the FHWs of all the villages met at the Narangwal center for a full day of formal training sessions. "This pattern of continuing education was extremely efficient in augmenting knowledge and skills in direct relation to specific problems emerging from daily work" (Kielmann et al., 1983, p. 53).

In Tamil Nadu, local mothers with at least an eighth grade education were trained in two-month sessions in the community, or near enough to commute daily, with more than one-third of the time in the field. Emphasis was on program management and administration and interpersonal communications for interaction with the community. The community nutrition workers (CNW) were trained in survey techniques, weighing the children, delivery of nutrition education, and record keeping. The CNWs received periodic in-service training on the job and were assisted by village workers and the women's working group.

In Indonesia, local volunteers were trained to weigh the children and develop the growth-monitoring activities for the regular National Family Nutrition Improvement Program (UPGK) primary health program. Training varied from three to five days of intensive sessions in the village (two to three days of lectures and one to two days of practical experience usually scheduled with the first day of weighing). Technical supervision was done by health personnel at monthly meetings to discuss problems, plan activities, and review health and nutrition messages (Griffith, 1985a).

In the Dominican Republic, the regional supervisors were trained to supervise promoters in fieldwork (weighing and recording techniques and educational messages), train the local promoters on specific topics (growth monitoring, nutrition education, and information system), process data, distribute materials, hold community meetings, and follow up on malnourished children. The promoters were volunteer women from the community trained to carry out growth monitoring, give individual mothers nutrition messages, work with community groups to motivate and perceive needs of the community, and give group talks on various topics. A participatory methodology was used in training sessions with attention to feedback, learning by doing, role playing, and demonstration by others.

In Iringa, considerable resources have been invested in construction of multipurpose training centers, production of educational materials, and forming a regional team to train the district and village-level personnel. Training of local health workers for the health posts, traditional birth attendants, child care workers, and leaders at different levels has been done in preservice seminars and workshops.

Frequent and supportive supervision was crucial to success in all the projects reviewed. In Tamil Nadu, the supervisors visited the workers at least twice a month, and the ratio of supervisors to workers was 1 to 10. Supervisors, who received two months of training, made the final selection of the children for the supplementary feeding. They checked the children's weight, both the low registers and those reported as having regained. "Close supervision was oriented to motivation and problem solving, rather than fault finding" (Brems, 1987, p. 3).

In Narangwal, the public health nurses visited each FHW once a week and spent at least half a day in each village. The visits consisted of both informal training sessions and problem-solving consultations. Supervision was said to be "supportive and educational rather than punitive" (Kielmann et al., 1983, p. 46).

In the Dominican Republic, prompt feedback, including corrective measures by either the central staff or the regional supervisors, is part of a motivational supervisory process. The supervisors visit each of the six to ten communities under their charge every month, and they "clean and hand tabulate data for the nutritional surveillance and internal evaluation system" (USAID, 1988, p. 13). The supervisors hold community meetings to discuss the community growth chart every six months.

These programs relied heavily on community-based and trained human resources. Training emphasized field experience over the presentation of factual information. Adequate initial training and continuing education, including periodic reinforcements, refresher courses, and seminars or workshops, were provided. All of the programs claimed to have developed a system of supportive supervision, rather than emphasizing fiscal control of resources and so-called fault-finding supervision. This system of training and development and the use of local personnel appear to be key elements of success.

The Communication and Education Strategy

Little information is available on the specific theory of education, communication, or human behavior that guided the development of the nutrition education effort in the projects. The projects in Indonesia and the Dominican Republic were based on the concept of social marketing, using the results of a behavior-oriented qualitative needs assessment. Their purpose was to change behavior through learner-oriented, practical activities.

The theory that appears relevant to all of the projects is the diffusion of innovations.[1] All have a cognitive phase in which the target group is exposed to an innovative message or idea, and a persuasion phase, in which the local workers and target group interact to form a positive or favorable attitude or opinion about the new idea. Then a tentative decision is made about whether to adopt the practice. When the decision is positive, a trial implementation is the next step. Finally, depending on whether the new practice is perceived as compatible, useful, or having some relative advantage to the learner, it is either adopted or rejected (Rogers, 1983; Severin and Tankard, 1988).

With the advent of the mass media, some researchers developed what might be called the "magic bullet" or "hypodermic needle" theory of nutrition education. Proponents of this theory think that exposure of large numbers of individuals to new ideas through mass media can have massive effects. Although this theory has been largely discarded in development communication, many health and nutrition education projects invest significant amounts of capital in large, sophisticated mass media projects but achieve very limited if any real results in improving the health or nutritional status of the target audience (Hornik, 1985, 1987, 1988, 1989; Stevenson, 1988).

A major criticism of the "magic bullet, hypodermic needle" theory is that the messages are sender-oriented, that is, they reflect the sender's concept of what is relevant and important (Dervin, 1984). The role of the audience in determining program success points to the need for more receiver-oriented information (Dervin, 1984). A major contribution of the social marketing approach to nutrition education, embraced by the projects reviewed here, is that its messages are receiver-oriented (Manoff, 1985). The Indonesia and Dominican Republic projects have done this by following the methods of social marketing. Tamil Nadu and Narangwal appear to have attempted to accomplish this same goal by hiring local workers who are similar to the target audience and presumably would have the same concerns.

---

[1] Diffusion of innovation refers to the steps observed in the introduction of a new concept, product, or practice in a population. It was first observed with the adoption of hybrid corn

The Iringa project appears to be based on the socialist (Marxist) philosophy of historical materialism (McQuail, 1989). The Triple-A framework corresponds to the dialectic method.[2] Analyses of the underlying causes of malnutrition and assessments of the economic and sociopolitical conditions as determinants of food insecurity, low status of women, poverty, and infant mortality are made at all political levels. Stress on assessing the social and economic contradictions and the conflict approach to problem solving are also based on this theory. As mentioned earlier, this method has some similarities to empowerment educational methods.

Health planners and nutrition educators need to be able to predict which educational strategy will be effective for a particular purpose with a particular audience. It is somewhat disappointing that none of the projects attempted to test the usefulness of an explicitly stated theory in its nutrition education, nor did any of them compare educational strategies. As Olson and Kelly (1989) have stated, "From our point of view, the only way we, as a community of nutrition educators, will be able to get to the point of accurate prediction is through theory-building intervention research in nutrition education. Using and adapting theoretical frameworks from the social and behavioral sciences is one logical starting point for developing theory-building intervention research in nutrition education. Another approach is to start building a theory or model of nutrition education from atheoretical, qualitative research on nutrition-related behaviors. In our opinion, both approaches are needed. They are complementary and will hopefully converge in a theoretical model for effective nutrition education" (p. 284).

Content and Messages. Several reviews of the state of nutrition education agree that prepackaged information, talks, demonstrations, and visual aids are unsuccessful (Gussow and Contento, 1984; Israel and Tighe, 1984; Hornik, 1985). This top-down approach with preestablished content and sender-oriented messages, delivered in rigid classroom settings, has been severely criticized for many reasons, including its ineffectiveness (Drummond, 1977; Barth-Eide, 1980; Church, 1982; Praun, 1982; Uauy and Miranda, 1983).

Traditional nutrition education, obedient to the dictates of nutritional science, has also been criticized (Gussow and Contento, 1984). Its content is often said to be too theoretical. The use of food groups to teach nutrition concepts is considered irrelevant and out of context. Its suggestions

---

by Iowa farmers. The role of both mass media to build awareness and of interpersonal communication to adopt and maintain the new practice has been described (Rogers, 1983).

    [2] The dialectic method focuses on the unequal distribution of economic power as the cause of poverty and disease. It is one of conflict and confrontation, of contrasting situations of those who have versus those who have not.

are impractical and above and beyond the economic means of the audience, and the messages are mostly do's and don't's: "give infants high-protein foods" and "wash your hands before preparing foods," for example. Other messages on nutrients are mainly sender-oriented and do not reflect the needs of the receivers.

In recent years, appropriate needs assessment research to identify the cognitive and affective needs of the learners have improved both the content of the messages and the appropriateness of language and graphic symbols used. This research has also helped to segment the groups within the audience in order to tailor the messages to address specific situations.

The social marketing approach emphasizes the development and testing of messages that respond to the needs of the participants. In the Indonesia project, extensive concept testing was used to develop the messages. "Village families were involved in decisions that determined the practices the project selected to improve the nutrition of children and pregnant and nursing women." Families tried the proposed new practices and adapted them to their conditions, and the results of these trials were used to establish behavioral objectives. The messages and materials were then designed and tested (Zeitlin et al., 1984, p. v).

The project in the Dominican Republic generally followed a similar process. Qualitative research techniques were used to identify common causes of poor child growth in order to establish educational objectives and develop the messages and counseling materials. Focus group techniques were used to develop the messages for the laminas (teaching cards) and for program promotion. The educational messages addressed the major problems in feeding practices for breastfed versus bottle-fed infants, those who gain weight or not, and by age groups (0–4 months, 5–8 months, 9–23 months, and so on). The content dealt with improving weaning foods, addition of milk to cereals, introduction of complementary foods with a spoon rather than the baby bottle, and promotion of breastfeeding (USAID, 1988).

In the Narangwal project, the messages encouraged late weaning (beyond 18 months) and consistent supplementation starting at 4–6 months of age. "Every three months the FHW visits the households with children 0–3 years, and on the basis of the diet history information, she gives the mother instructions to correct the practices found to be faulty, and reinforces the need for breastfeeding and good feeding habits" (Kielmann et al., 1983, p. 49). Nutrition education classes for groups of mothers and traditional village midwives were occasionally held. These meetings were organized mainly for mothers of malnourished children.

In Tamil Nadu, communication was designed to encourage families to adopt a few specific practices to improve the nutrition and health status of their children. The importance of colostrum and breastfeeding, timely introduction of solid foods to supplement breast milk, home management of diarrhea, immunization, and improved hygiene were stressed.

In Iringa, the approach was to solve problems identified as having a negative effect on child growth. Community members were involved in the assessment of nutrition and health status of the village. Information was recorded in a register, discussed, and used to persuade the communities to take collective action to solve the problems. Individual families whose children were not growing well were counseled personally by the health worker and an appropriate administrative official. The nutrition messages were specific to each situation.

In summary, recent nutrition education programs have recognized the many influences on human behavior and the importance of the cultural context and have taken steps to understand this complexity and use it in the design of nutrition education content and messages. All of the programs reviewed indicate that content and messages were determined by the needs of the learners. Mothers were actively involved in developing and testing messages and finding solutions to everyday needs. Nutrition education has become more participatory in recognition of the crucial role of the active involvement in learning and behavior change. Home demonstrations involved workers and mothers in actually preparing the recommended foods. The results of these programs are entirely consistent with Whitehead's (1973) conclusions about the effectiveness of problem solving and active involvement approaches to nutrition education.

The Channels. The projects reviewed, as well as several others not included, demonstrate the superiority of a multichannel approach over either direct face-to-face contact or mass media alone. The social marketing projects have made a valuable contribution in creating educational programs with multichannel approaches. In the process, the difficulties of achieving national mass media coverage were also made visible. From both an economic and an access-to-prime-time perspective, getting into the mass media in developing countries is difficult. The use of local radio stations, "small media," and indigenous (folk) media has great potential that merits further exploration (Colle, 1977; Cerqueira et al., 1979).

An in-depth description of the multichannel approaches taken in the ANEP will illustrate the potential of this approach. In the Dominican project, the educational strategy included individual counseling in the home of each mother. During the visit the worker both discussed the growth chart and used a set of twelve flash cards with drawings and messages tailored to the age and condition of the child. For instance, for children 0–4 months that were not breastfed, emphasis was put on giving milk with cereals using a spoon because spoon-feeding is more hygienic.

The mother was asked what type of food the child was eating daily. The worker would then advise the mother to combine that food with milk and explain that combinations of foods are better for the child's growth. The child was then weighed, the results plotted and interpreted, and the mother's infant feeding practices reviewed. Ways to improve the weaning foods were discussed, and modifications were made if the mother reported difficulty following the recommendations. This was reinforced with twice-yearly group sessions to discuss the community growth chart and the children's progress. Stories were presented on flip charts and audiocassettes to build on mothers' awareness and concern for their child's health and growth (USAID, 1988). Evaluation results indicate that continuous interactions between the local workers and the mothers went beyond the home visits and group sessions.

As with ANEP, the other programs reviewed used several channels of communication. This approach allowed for greater exposure to the messages in several dimensions: seeing, listening, talking, and doing. The messages were heard on the radio or audiocassette and from the local workers. The concepts were discussed in group sessions. The growth charts provided a visible and concrete reference to the messages. The mothers themselves prepared the weaning foods, kept the growth chart, marked the action poster, and delivered a demonstration for other mothers. Although it is generally not possible to isolate the effects of the separate components on knowledge and practices, in Indonesia the radio messages together with face-to-face counseling augmented knowledge scores. Zeitlin and Formación (1981) cited a combination of face-to-face and mass media approaches as favoring cost effectiveness. A recent examination of eight case studies in nutrition communications strongly supports multimedia approaches (Achterberg, 1991).

The Materials. In the programs reviewed, face-to-face interpersonal communication by trained local workers with supportive materials (the action posters in Indonesia, the growth charts used by mothers, and the flash cards used by local workers in the Dominican Republic) was frequently used.

The systematic and supportive use of culturally appropriate graphic materials was an important part of the programs reviewed. During the development and pretesting of the messages, the production personnel visited with the mothers. The physical appearance of the people and their communities (surroundings, type of houses, furnishings, manner of dress, dishes, utensils, and the like) were considered in the drawings of posters, flip charts, leaflets, and other materials. This may have contributed to the audiences' identification with the educational message, as was reported for the social marketing projects, especially in Indonesia.

The Iringa project produced several films and quarterly newsletters to communicate program activities and exchange information among villages. Media and materials are said to have been instrumental in training and in social mobilization (Yambi et al., 1989; Jonsson, 1989). In Tamil Nadu, films, which were said to be very popular in the village cinema, were produced, but their contribution to the improvement of health and nutrition was probably not worth the high cost (Greene, 1989). The children's working groups relayed project messages via poems, songs, and skits. Traditional folk media put on skits and performances with nutrition messages. Films, filmstrips, slides, posters, flip books, flash cards, and pamphlets were developed. The evaluation results indicate that 48 percent of the respondent mothers had not seen any of these materials (Chidambaram, 1989). An early evaluation of the communications portion of the Tamil Nadu Integrated Nutrition Project points to a problem common to many health and nutrition interventions: more emphasis is placed on producing many different materials than on successful communication of health and nutrition messages (Berg, 1985).

In summary, these programs used various printed and audiovisual materials to maintain uniformity and accuracy in the information diffused by the local workers. The materials also reinforced the messages and the adoption of new practices, not merely illustrating the messages but as part of the "multiple dimensions" approach to involve the audience in the learning experience. The materials created in this way were more likely to achieve their goal than those that used a more passive approach.

Summary of Major Findings (Hypotheses)

The influence of the traditional medical model on the conceptualization and delivery of nutrition education is waning because of the lack of success of efforts based on this model. The movement is toward more participatory intervention models, including those that urge collective action. The Iringa project illustrates such a model within a socialist political context.

None of the projects explicitly described a theory of human behavior, communication, or education to guide the development of the intervention. The social marketing projects are the closest of any to theoretically based interventions. This lack of an explicit theory makes it difficult to explain why a program did or did not work so that in subsequent interventions appropriate modifications can be made. Also, the experiences of one project cannot build on another so that a model of effective education can eventually be developed. The need for theory-based nutrition education intervention projects in the developing world is critical.

Education-oriented (behavior-oriented) needs assessment that actively involves program participants is key to successful education intervention. The social marketing approach of extensive audience participation in identifying the behavioral constraints and elaborating message content is one such approach that is gaining widespread acceptance in topical areas as diverse as vitamin-A deficiency prevention and weaning practices (International Vitamin A Consultative Group, 1992; Griffiths, 1991). Others could certainly be developed and their effectiveness explored.

Multiple-component interventions are more likely to be effective than single-component interventions. It is a well-known adage of education that people are more likely to learn when they hear, see, and touch the object of their learning.

Nearly all the projects examined included growth monitoring. Growth monitoring basically generates information that an educator or an educated program participant can use for self-monitoring and reinforcing behaviors. Nutrition educators need information-generating tools such as growth monitoring that help people personally and concretely assess their own nutritional status.

This analysis indicates that educational interventions, possibly more than other types of interventions, require strong political support and an infrastructure for delivery. Compared with other interventions, particularly feeding programs, educational interventions are unlikely to build political support for their promoters. Empowerment education approaches may actually lead to popular unrest and dissatisfaction with current government policies related to food, health, and welfare.

Implementation of these projects requires the training and supervision of field-based educators. The decentralized, regional, flexible institutional organization and infrastructure is of central importance. All the programs appear to have had a comprehensive yet practical preservice training component. All made extraordinary efforts to train an extensive network of local personnel instead of relying on service delivery by urban-based and urban-trained health personnel. All projects used short sessions and emphasized community experience. Also significant is the supervision system. All of the projects reviewed claimed to have supportive supervision, with an emphasis in the continuing education of the workers rather than fault-finding or punitive, fiscal supervision.

5

Growth Monitoring as an Educational
Tool, an Integrating Strategy, and
a Source of Information:
A Review of Experience

Marie T. Ruel

The literature abounds with contrary opinions and "evidence" concerning the usefulness, the effectiveness, and the necessity of including growth monitoring and promotion (GMP) in primary health care (PHC) programs. Critics argue that the role of GMP should be seriously reconsidered and that more research is needed on its feasibility and cost-effectiveness (Gerein, 1988; Gopalan and Chatterjee, 1985; Nabarro and Chinnock, 1988), while supporters believe that current evidence is sufficient to support continued practice and implementation of GMP in a growing number of programs worldwide (Rohde, 1988; Rohde and Northrup, 1988; Griffiths, 1988a; Hendrata, 1987). Part of this controversy seems to result from a lack of consensus on what GMP really is, what it can potentially achieve, and how it should be evaluated. The first part of this chapter will attempt to clarify these aspects by reviewing the definition of GMP and its most common purposes. A clear understanding of the objectives of GMP will permit the identification of appropriate indicators to assess its performance and to evaluate its success in achieving its goals. This first step will provide the framework that will be used in the following section to review the empirical evidence. The purpose of the review is to compare, for each of GMP's distinct applications, the theoretical objectives and expectations with its actual achievements as experienced in various programs around the world. In this way, it is hoped that overall conclusions regarding the utility of GMP for unspecified purposes may be replaced by a clearer understanding of which aspects of GMP might be successful in a given context and what factors contribute to that success.

Analytical Framework

GMP has been defined as "the regular measurement, recording and interpretation of a child's growth in order to counsel, act, and follow-up results" (Yee and Zerfas, 1986, p. 1). The term "promotion" is added to "growth monitoring" to emphasize the action component of the activity. The above description makes it clear that GMP, which consists of measuring children, is not an intervention in itself but rather a process or strategy used to generate action. This distinction needs to be made if realistic outcomes are to be expected from the use of GMP.

A summary of the most common purposes of GMP and of the postulated mechanisms by which it is expected to lead to action is presented in Table 5.1. For simplicity, the purposes of GMP are divided into three broad categories: (1) an educational and promotional tool; (2) an integrating strategy; and (3) a source of information. Table 5.1 shows that whatever its specific purposes, GMP is consistently intended to lead to action. Therefore, it is inappropriate to evaluate GMP's performance solely on the basis of indicators of impact such as changes in the prevalence of malnutrition. GMP is a tool that aims to improve processes, motivate individuals or groups to take action, and/or provide information that will guide decision making. It should therefore be evaluated on the basis of its effectiveness in performing these tasks. The impact, in turn, should be seen as the consequence of the improved targeting, implementation, and delivery of specific interventions resulting from the effective use of GMP. In other words, the additional (and potentially synergistic) effect on a child's nutritional status obtained by including GMP in a PHC package will depend on how effectively GMP has motivated action and behavioral change (educational, motivational tool), guided the choice of appropriate interventions (source of data for screening), and facilitated the targeting, implementation, and delivery of appropriate interventions to at-risk children (source of data and integrating strategy). The framework of analysis adopted in this chapter focuses strictly on processes and ignores the usual indicators of impact. Each of the three proposed objectives of GMP (Table 5.1) is reviewed separately with an emphasis on (1) what GMP is expected to do when used for this purpose and what conditions or processes are necessary to achieve it and (2) what is the empirical evidence concerning (a) how well these conditions appear to be met in practice and (b) how well GMP has achieved its goals.

A clear distinction is made throughout this review between clinic- and community-based GMP programs because these two types of programs differ greatly in their strengths and limitations with respect to design, implementation and evaluation.

Review of Experience

GMP as an Educational and Promotional Tool

Expectations and Conditions Necessary to Meet Them. Through the use of growth charts, GMP is said to make malnutrition visible to both health workers and mothers (Griffiths, 1985a) and to facilitate the formulation of individualized advice to meet the specific needs of each child. Thus GMP is said to "make nutrition education action-oriented, specific, and relevant; and thus more effective" (Hendrata, 1987, p. 10). By strengthening the communication component of nutrition education (NED), GMP is expected to improve the process of NED and its impact on behavior change. As a motivational tool, GMP can be used to promote adequate growth in children and make it the goal to be achieved by mothers, health workers, communities, and governments: GMP can "create a mass awareness of the importance of the growth problem and a mass demand for its solution" (Grant , 1987).

The operational steps that should take place for the successful use of GMP as an integral component of the NED strategy are to be sure that (1) the workers have adequate knowledge and skills to conduct the GMP activities properly; (2) the health workers have the time and communication skills necessary to transmit the information to the mothers; (3) mothers understand the messages taught to them and can translate the information into action; and (4) health workers and mothers discuss together feasible solutions and actions to be taken, considering mothers' time and available resources. For GMP to create mass awareness about growth in children, active community participation by members and their leaders is highly recommended (AED, 1988).

Review of Empirical Evidence. Little is known of the additional impact on behavioral change and on children's nutritional status obtained by the inclusion of GMP in a NED intervention. A study conducted in Ghana and Lesotho in the late 1970s failed to show any association between the intensity of use of growth charts and maternal knowledge and practices, and a child's nutritional status (Pielemeier et al., 1978). More recently,

Table 5.1. Summary of the various purposes of GMP and of the postulated mechanisms by which it is expected to lead to action

Purposes of GMP	Mechanism	Action
EDUCATIONAL AND PROMOTIONAL TOOL		
For individuals, communities, governments, policy makers	Increased knowledge, interest, awareness, motivation, and commitment	Better management of health and nutrition problems. Ability to: Assess the nature of the problem, Analyze the potential solutions, and Act on it[a]
INTEGRATING STRATEGY		
For improved coverage and delivery of health services	Increased motivation and interest	Increased participation rates and regularity of attendance
	Better integration, organization, and delivery of health services	Improved coverage and delivery of health services
INFORMATION SOURCE		
For screening	Identification of at-risk children	Targeting of appropriate interventions
For program monitoring and evaluation	Process and/or impact evaluation	Decisions and actions taken by program managers following the analysis of data (i.e., allocation of resources, targeting and choice of interventions)
For health and development planning (surveillance)	Assessment of trends, needs by geographic area, regions, functional, and socioeconomic groups	Decisions and actions taken by planners and policy makers following analysis of data (same as for monitoring and evaluation)

[a]This Assessment-Analysis-Action process has been described as the Triple-A cycle (Government of Tanzania et al., 1988).

results from a clinic-based GMP and NED program in Lesotho showed that nutrition education significantly improved maternal knowledge but that growth charts were not necessary for obtaining such an effect (Ruel et al., 1992; Ruel and Habicht, 1992). Similar results were obtained in India, where growth monitoring was not more successful than nutrition education alone in improving children's growth (George et al., 1992). The results of these two studies suggest that GMP may not be necessary for nutrition education programs conducted under ideal conditions. It remains to be seen, however, whether GMP improves the quality and impact of nutrition education in programs conducted under usual field conditions.

The next section will briefly review the more anecdotal evidence of the use of GMP as an educational and promotional tool in both clinic- and community-based studies. The emphasis will be on assessing the likelihood that GMP can be a powerful educational tool at present, considering the way it is generally used, and the extent to which the conditions necessary for its success appear to be met.

Clinic-Based Studies

1. Health Workers' Skills in Conducting GMP. The personnel usually responsible for GMP in clinics undoubtedly can learn to use the technology involved efficiently if they are given appropriate training (Ruel et al., 1991). A common mistake, however, is the tendency to undertrain the clinic staff, assuming that their relatively high level of education should enable them to pick up these tasks with only minimal training. In the Philippines, 52 percent of the health workers conducting GMP activities had received one day or less of special training; in Haiti and Zaire, only 47 percent and 68 percent of health workers, respectively, had received any previous training (PRICOR, 1989a). Observations from clinics reveal unacceptable rates of errors at all levels of the GMP process (Marquez, 1988; PRICOR, 1989a, 1989b; Gopalan and Chatterjee, 1985; Cape, 1988; Serdula et al., 1987; UNICEF, 1983a, 1984b) Results from PRICOR's systems analysis in four countries demonstrated that measurement errors accumulate dramatically from inaccurate weighing procedures and errors in recording, plotting, and age determination (PRICOR, 1989a). These inaccuracies, often attributed to overcrowding of the clinics and time constraints, might also reflect the inappropriate training and supervision of the health personnel and their related lack of interest and motivation (Reid, 1984).

2. Time, Communication Skills, and Motivation of Workers to Inform Mothers. Assuming that health workers can weigh, measure, and plot accurately, the next important step is to communicate this information effectively to the mother, using the growth chart and the specific growth pattern of the child to discuss problems and feasible solutions. This is the stage at which the educational potential of the growth chart and of the whole GMP process can be realized. In clinics, however, this step is typically the one that receives the least attention and time (Reid, 1984; Marquez, 1988; Gerein and Ross, 1991). A common observation from clinics is that immediately after plotting the child's weight on the growth chart, the health worker closes it and hands it to the mother without any comment about the child's progress (Reid, 1984; Ruel, observation). PRICOR's study in four countries showed that only 10 to 20 percent of all mothers whose children were weighed received any individual counseling. In clinics in Papua New Guinea and Zaire, 71 percent and 64 percent, respectively, of the consultations took less than two minutes, during which time the child was weighed, examined, vaccinated, and treated (Reid, 1984; Gerein and Ross, 1991). In Togo, the verbal exchange between mothers and staff ranged from eleven to ninety seconds with a median of forty-six seconds (PRICOR, 1989b). Although the time spent with mothers does not necessarily reflect the quality of the social interaction and the intensity of the educational effort, the extremely short contact time documented in these studies speaks for itself.

Growth charts and GMP results also appear to be rarely used for group education in clinics. The quality and content of group education has been shown to vary markedly between clinics, depending mainly on the personality and qualities of individual staff members, including conviction, dedication, training, and teaching ability (Pielemeier, 1982; Gerein and Ross, 1991; Hoorweg and Niemeijer, 1980a, 1980b; Reid, 1984). Obviously, if the results of GMP are not used to teach mothers, either individually or in groups, and to discuss with them some specific behavior-oriented solutions to improve their children's growth, the educational potential of GMP is lost. This seems to be the case in most clinic settings.

3. Mothers' Understanding. Given this situation, the question of whether mothers can understand the charts and the educational messages presented to them seems irrelevant. The question should relate more to process issues—given the way the teaching is conducted (or not conducted) in clinics, can it possibly have an impact on knowledge and behavior? From the available evidence described above, a significant impact appears unlikely.

4. Participation of Mothers. Active participation of mothers in clinic and GMP activities is usually not encouraged (Gerein and Ross, 1991; Reid, 1984; PRICOR, 1989b; CRS-USCC-The Gambia, 1989). Mothers have been described as "passive recipients of services" (Gerein and Ross, 1991, p.673), and the NED is perceived as something mothers must endure to receive their food ration (CRS-USCC-The Gambia, 1989).

Community-Based Studies

By contrast, in community-based studies GMP is primarily used as an educational and motivational tool both at the individual and community levels (Tamil Nadu, NCBC, ANEP, and Iringa).[1] The conditions necessary

---

[1] See Table 5.2 for the list of community-based programs reviewed and references consulted.

Table 5.2. Community-based programs reviewed and references used

Name of project	Country	References used
Iringa	Tanzania	Government of Tanzania et al., 1988 UNICEF, 1989a Pelletier, 1991b
ANEP (Applied Nutrition Education Program)	Dominican Republic	USAID, 1988 Shrimpton, 1989
Tamil Nadu	India	Bhan and Ghosh, 1986 Berg, 1987a Brems, 1987 Ghosh, 1988 Shekar, 1991 Mathew, n.d. Shekar and Latham, 1992
ICDS (Integrated Child Development Scheme)	India	Mukarji, 1985 Gopaldas, 1988 Ghosh, 1988 Subbarao, 1989 Anonymous 1, 1989
UPGK (National Family Nutrition Program)	Indonesia	UNICEF, 1984a National Family Planning Coordinating board (BKKBN) et al., 1986 Anonymous 2, 1989
NCBC (Nutrition Communication and Behavior Change Component)	Indonesia	Manoff International, 1984

for the successful use of GMP as a vehicle for NED seem more likely to be met in these programs than in clinic settings.

1. Health Workers' Skills in Conducting GMP. Health workers in various community-based programs have demonstrated impressive levels of understanding and skills in conducting GMP activities, in spite of minimal formal education (ANEP, Tamil Nadu, National Family Nutrition Program [UPGK], Integrated Child Development Scheme [ICDS]). The community-based programs reviewed here, however, are unique with respect to the amount of time dedicated and the quality of the training and supervision of their health workers. Initial training lasts two, three, and six months in Tamil Nadu, ICDS, and Iringa, respectively, and is followed by in-service training. Most programs also include techniques to develop communication skills and motivation of the workers (NCBC, Tamil Nadu, ANEP; Ghosh, 1988).

2. Time, Communication Skills, and Motivation of Workers to Inform Mothers. In the studies reviewed, community workers were said to be highly motivated, dedicated, and enthusiastic (Ghosh, 1988: ICDS, Child in Need Institute [CINI], Tamil Nadu, ANEP, NCBC) and well-known and appreciated by their communities (Iringa, ANEP, Tamil Nadu). Time for communicating and interacting with mothers is a less serious limitation than in clinic settings because home visits are often part of the workers' regular activities. It remains to be seen, however, whether the workers are using this time efficiently.

3. *Mothers' Understanding.* There is sufficient empirical evidence to show that mothers can understand educational messages and growth charts if the teaching is done appropriately (Ghosh, 1988; Chaudhuri, 1988; Arole, 1988; Hendrata, 1985; Ruel et al., 1990, 1992). Many of the community programs reviewed use well-designed communication strategies, and their effectiveness in improving knowledge, motivation, and interest of individuals and communities is well documented (ANEP, UPGK, Tamil Nadu, Iringa).

4. *Participation of Mothers and Communities.* Most community-based GMP programs encourage the involvement of mothers and communities in the process of GMP (Ghosh, 1988; Chaudhuri, 1988; Priyosusilo, 1988; Arole, 1988; Rohde et al., 1975; Berg, 1987a; Rohde and Northrup, 1988) and in deciding on actions to be taken for children at risk of malnutrition (Shrimpton, this volume; Chaudhuri, 1988; Ghosh, 1988; Cowan, 1988; Priyosusilo, 1988; Arole, 1988; Griffiths, 1985b; Ashworth and Feachem, 1986). The goal is to develop a mass awareness about the importance of growth and to enable mothers and communities to make better use and management of the resources at their disposal. The level of community participation in three of the projects reviewed (Tamil Nadu, Iringa, Indonesia) is discussed at length in Shrimpton (this volume) and will not be addressed here. As a motivational tool GMP has been used successfully in at least four of the projects reviewed (Iringa, ANEP, NCBC, Tamil Nadu). The Iringa project achieved remarkable success in raising interest and awareness about nutrition at all levels, from individuals and households to communities and higher government officials (Pelletier, 1991b). In this program, however, the GMP activities were accompanied by a much larger mass media and training effort directed at all levels of government and society than is usually seen in community-based programs.

GMP as an Integrating Strategy

Expectations and Conditions Necessary to Meet Them. "Growth Monitoring offers a way of uniting the low cost actions outlined by the child survival initiative into a synergistic whole which could improve child survival" (Grant, 1987, p. 65). As an integrating strategy GMP has the potential to improve child survival and growth by reducing morbidity as a result of a more efficient delivery of health services and through increased food intake as a result of the more effective delivery of NED and of its greater impact on maternal feeding practices. Improvements can be expected from increased coverage and quality of the services delivered and potentially from a synergism among the various interventions. The process indicators of GMP's effectiveness as an integrating strategy include changes in immunization coverage, delivery of oral rehydration solution packages, use of family planning, number of sick children referred and treated by the medical staff, attendance and regularity of attendance at clinics or health posts (where applicable), and others.

Two conditions are necessary for GMP to be an effective promoter of other health and nutrition services: (1) the rate and regularity of attendance at the health delivery point must be improved by the inclusion of GMP and (2) other health and nutrition services must be available and properly delivered to the intended beneficiaries (Ashworth and Feachem, 1986).

Review of Empirical Evidence

Clinic-Based Studies. None of the clinic studies reviewed mentioned increased attendance rates or coverage of PHC services attributable to GMP. No information was found on the availability of other health and nutrition services or on any of the process indicators mentioned above.

Community-Based Studies. With reference to the UPGK program, Hendrata (1987, p. 13) reports that "weighing has been able to create a forum through which other PHC activities are being conducted. The availability of those services has in turn made the weighing program more attractive for mothers." The potential for GMP to create a forum through which other PHC activities can be delivered in the communities is very promising.

Most of the programs reviewed do not provide any comparative data about the coverage of PHC activities in project and nonproject areas, but some reports mention positive changes associated with the implementation of their program in immunization coverage (Iringa, Tamil Nadu, Haiti: Genece and Rohde, 1988; and KB-Gizi: National Family Planning Coordinating Board et al., 1986), the distribution of vitamin A and iron supplements (ICDS), the number of home visits (Iringa, ICDS), the number of medical checkups for malnourished children (ICDS), the distribution of ORS packages (Haiti: Genece and Rohde, 1988), and the use of contraceptives (KB-Gizi: National Family Planning Coordinating Board et al.,

1986). It is impossible, however, to determine the specific role of GMP relative to other components of the package in achieving these positive changes in the coverage of health services. More information is needed to determine how crucial GMP is in this process.

GMP as a Source of Data

The data generated by GMP activities can be used for various purposes. At the individual level, they can be used to assess the adequacy of a child's growth and guide the targeting of appropriate actions. This use of GMP for screening and targeting is universal. At the program or national level, the data can be aggregated and used for monitoring, evaluation, and surveillance purposes.[2]

The important difference between the use of GMP as an educational tool and as an integrating strategy and its use as a source of data is in the quality of data required. For GMP to be a useful screening tool, children must be measured with sufficient accuracy to minimize misclassification and maximize the cost-effectiveness of targeting. Similarly, if the data are to be aggregated and used for evaluation and surveillance, higher accuracy in the measurements will ensure higher precision of the estimates of prevalence and of changes in prevalence over time. By contrast, if GMP is used simply to create interest and awareness about growth or as an integrating strategy, the data do not need to be of such high quality for GMP to achieve its motivational objectives.

For Screening at the Individual Level

Expectations and Conditions Necessary to Meet Them. GMP is most commonly used as a screening tool for targeting interventions. The rationale for using the repeated anthropometric measurements collected during GMP activities for screening at-risk children is that they allow the early detection of growth faltering in children, which in turn improves the chances of success and the cost-effectiveness of interventions.

The following elements are necessary for effective screening:

- The coverage of the population screened must be as complete as possible. *High* and *regular* attendance rates at the screening sessions is necessary. Equally important is that there are no self-selected portions of the popula-

---

[2] The term "monitoring" refers to the internal (within project) use of the data for management and as a source of information about processes. The term "evaluation" refers to impact evaluation, and the term "surveillance" refers strictly to national nutritional surveillance. These distinctions, often blurred in practice, are made here to facilitate discussion.

tion not attending, especially among the most needy. If those who do not attend are the poorest, least educated, and most malnourished, the children most at risk are likely not to be screened, in spite of a potentially high overall coverage of the population.

- Misclassification must be minimal. That is, the number of false positives (normal children misclassified as being underweight) and false negatives (underweight children misclassified as normal) must be minimized.
- The cost of screening must be low compared to the cost of providing the intervention indiscriminately to all children.
- Screening must lead to appropriate targeting of age- and situation-specific interventions to children identified as at risk.

These four principles apply to any screening tool. The following section will assess how well GMP fulfills these conditions and hence how adequate it may be for screening.

Review of Studies

Clinic Studies

1. Population coverage. Clinics typically cover only a small proportion of the total child population of a country (Test et al., 1987). Self-selection in attendance is a well-recognized problem in clinic studies and affects both the rate and regularity of attendance of mothers (Gerein and Ross, 1991; Ashworth and Feachem, 1986). The extent to which it results in discrimination against the most needy is difficult to assess from available evidence and is likely to vary from one context to another.

2. Minimize misclassification. The process of determining a child's weight-for-age is fraught with potential for error, and, as a consequence, a large proportion of children are misclassified. In Papua New Guinea, 25 percent of the children weighed during a GMP session were misdiagnosed as a result of random measurement errors at various steps of the process (Cape, 1988). Systematic errors also occur and may result in even greater misclassification problems. In Botswana, noncalibrated scales caused an overestimation of all weight values by 0.4 kg, which in turn resulted in an underestimation of the malnutrition prevalence by about one-half (UNICEF, 1983a). At the individual level, misclassification implies that a large proportion of the at-risk children are not screened and do not receive appropriate attention, whereas many of those who receive it do not need it and are unlikely to benefit from it.

3. Cost of screening. No assessment of the cost of screening with growth monitoring, compared to the use of other methods, appears to have been done. Because of the controversy around the usefulness of growth monitoring as a screening tool, alternative, potentially cheaper methods have been proposed such as the child's age (Gerein and Ross, 1991; Henry et al., 1989), socioeconomic status indicators (Mukarji, 1985; Gopalan and Chatterjee, 1985), and arm circumference (Zerfas, 1975; Nabarro, 1983; Huffman et al., 1985).

4. *Follow-up action.* Very little information was found on the targeting and delivery of specific interventions to children classified as at-risk by GMP. Most clinic-based programs are designed to offer some group nutrition education, individual counseling, medical referrals, and food supplements when available (Capone, 1977). In general, the targeting of these interventions is poor and does not take into account the specific needs of each child. The few studies that examined targeting of nutrition education and of individual counseling showed that the time spent with mothers was generally not influenced by the child's nutritional and health status (Gerein and Ross, 1991; Ashworth and Feachem, 1986; PRICOR, 1989a, 1989b). In Zaire, no individual counseling was given to approximately one-third of mothers of at-risk children (PRICOR, 1989a; Marquez, 1988; Gerein and Ross, 1991), and of those who received counseling, 22 percent were given the wrong information. Mothers of poorly growing children were also more likely to be misinformed than mothers of children whose growth was adequate. These results suggest that targeting of interventions following screening with GMP is generally poor in clinics.

Community-Based Studies

1. *Population coverage.* Community-based programs generally have higher attendance rates than clinic-based programs, particularly because of the reduction in travel time. Still, many programs operate through a "weighing post" or community center, and self-selection remains a problem (Zinn and Drake, 1988).

2. *Misclassification.* Although community workers from various programs have demonstrated a high level of competence in conducting GMP activities, their accuracy in measuring and classifying children has rarely been assessed. One study done in the Iringa project showed an average misclassification rate of 26.7 percent resulting from errors in age determination and errors from rounding weights to the nearest digit fraction (Zinn and Drake, 1988). Considering that all other sources of errors related to measurement were ignored in this analysis and that the program was thought to have an excellent field protocol compared to similar programs, this is a gross underestimate of the usual error rate. These results indicate that GMP might be an inefficient screening tool.

3. *Cost of screening.* Most programs do not separate the cost of GMP from the cost of the entire package of interventions. It is also impossible

from most programs' cost analysis to estimate the training and supervision costs of the GMP activities.

4. *Follow-up action.* All community programs reviewed provided a clear description of the protocol used in identifying malnourished or at-risk children. Most programs included home visits for individual counseling and nutrition education to allow regular follow-up of the children and to ensure favorable interaction between health workers and mothers, but information about the health workers' effectiveness in detecting at-risk children and in providing them with the appropriate interventions was generally scarce. As pointed out by Gopalan (1987), when projects show a positive impact, people assume that these efforts (home visits, referrals, nutrition education, and others) are being made properly, but sufficient information on this most crucial aspect is rarely available. The Tamil Nadu program was the only one among those reviewed that routinely collected the type of process data needed to obtain information about the percentage of malnourished children covered by the targeted interventions. The data showed, for instance, that 95 percent of the screened children did receive the food supplements intended for them, a performance that is believed to be particularly high compared to other programs.

In general the actions planned for the at-risk children seem less standardized in community-based than in clinic-based studies. Although some programs offer a supplementary feeding program for all malnourished children, the education component seems generally more flexible and intended to be child- and situation-specific. In this regard the Iringa program has the most impressive system for tailoring a specific action plan to each malnourished child. The village health worker and some members of the village health committee visit the families of malnourished children at home to Assess the nature of the problem, Analyze potential solutions, and recommend appropriate Actions (Triple-A cycle). This approach is innovative in that it involves parents in the characterization of the problem and in the design of feasible solutions to attack it. The success and problems with the solutions adopted are discussed in subsequent follow-up visits, and modifications are made when necessary (Pelletier, 1991b).

Use of Aggregate Data for Monitoring, Evaluation, and Surveillance

Expectations and Conditions Necessary to Meet Them. Using GMP as a source of data leads to the expectation that the monthly weighings will provide information that can be recorded and aggregated for any level (community, district, region, national) to guide decisions about the program itself, about the allocation of national resources, and about health and policy planning. The data should be accurate, collected and aggregated regularly, efficiently directed to the central levels, and processed and analyzed in an appropriate and timely manner. The conditions specific to the purposes of monitoring, evaluation, and surveillance, respectively, will be discussed in the following three subsections.

For Monitoring

Clinic Studies. The management and administration of the Catholic Relief Services' food distribution program in Africa is based entirely on clinic-based GMP data (CRS-Africa Regional Office, 1979). The weighing information is aggregated monthly in the clinics and sent to the headquarters, where it is processed and used mainly for accounting and decisions concerning the allocation of the food rations. For such administrative purposes, a simple head count could replace the GMP data. If the data were to be used to examine regional and clinic differences in malnutrition prevalence and to guide decisions about reallocation of resources, two major problems would be encountered. First, accuracy in the data collection, recording, and processing would need to be greatly improved. Second and even more important, the enrollment criteria would need to be standardized. For instance, if some clinics apply a given screening mechanism more strictly than others (i.e., enroll only children <80 percent weight-for-age), the malnutrition prevalence estimates obtained for these clinics reflect their success in reaching the needy children and not the true prevalence of malnutrition in this population. Thus these data should not be used to compare malnutrition prevalences between clinics and geographical regions. In practice, these comparisons are often made and used for decisions about resource allocation.

Community Studies. An in-depth analysis of the monitoring and information system of three of the projects reviewed is available in separate papers: ANEP (Shrimpton, 1989), Iringa (Pelletier, 1991b), and Tamil Nadu (Shekar, 1991) and will not be discussed here. All three information systems rely heavily on the weight data from GMP activities.

The UPGK's monitoring system also uses GMP data but focuses on weight gain rather than attained weight. The stated objectives of this system are to "monitor UPGK activities and use the data for inputs in the planning, supervision, and evaluation of the program" (Anonymous 2, 1989, p. 3). A review of this system highlighted various problems of data collection and processing as well as inefficient use of the information generated. According to this report, the system fails to provide feedback of the information to the communities, and the data are used almost exclusively for national reporting (Anonymous 2, 1989). The problems encountered in UPGK are not uncommon and raise the important question about the feasibility of using the same health workers for the delivery of services and for operating ongoing monitoring systems (Teller et al., 1985).

For Evaluation

Most clinic- and community-based programs have attempted to use GMP data to evaluate impact. These efforts are generally fraught with internal and external validity problems, such as measurement errors, inappropriate comparison groups, and biases due to confounding that result from weaknesses in various design aspects. These problems are not specific to GMP programs and are simply noted here, and the reader is referred to the general literature on quantitative evaluation for a thorough discussion of these issues (Habicht et al., 1984).

Evaluation of GMP programs is generally difficult because of the absence of a control group (a group not participating in GMP) or the lack of comparability between the control (nonparticipants) and the study group (participants). When comparison groups are inappropriate, it is impossible to attribute the differences observed between groups to the intervention itself without controlling for plausible alternative explanations. A partial solution is to control statistically for potential confounding factors in the analysis. This is rarely done in GMP evaluations, mostly because of the absence of necessary information.

For Surveillance

The use of GMP data has been suggested as an efficient way to obtain information for national nutritional surveillance. These data are expected to allow the assessment of the prevalence of nutritional problems, the identification of at-risk groups, and the monitoring of trends.

Review of Studies. Only data from clinic studies appear to have been analyzed for their accuracy, validity, representativeness, and, hence, usefulness for nutritional surveillance. In a workshop held in Botswana in 1984, representatives from seven African countries discussed their experience and problems with their clinic-based nutritional surveillance system (UNICEF, 1984b). Inaccuracies in data collection, recording, and reporting; delays and irregularities in sending the data to the central office; and self-selection of clinic attenders were the most common difficulties reported. Efforts to strengthen health workers' training and supervision were proposed as means to improve the accuracy of data collection and processing. Still, the problems related to the lack of representativeness of the clinic population as a consequence of self-selection and the differential application of targeting criteria remain unsolved.

Attempts have been made to assess the validity of clinic data by comparing prevalence estimates obtained from clinic-based surveillance systems with estimates from national surveys (UNICEF, 1983a, 1983b, 1984b; Trowbridge et al., 1980; and Serdula et al., 1987). The two sources of data generally provided substantially different estimates of prevalence. Although most studies concluded that clinic data were not providing accurate estimates of overall prevalences and of regional differences, more skeptical researchers questioned the accuracy of the national surveys themselves.

Conclusions

GMP can potentially be extremely useful in PHC programs, particularly for education, motivation, and to promote other health services. Since the mid-1980s there has been remarkable improvement in design and implementation of GMP, which has led to a greater emphasis on community-based programs. Active involvement of mothers, families, and communities at all stages of the design, implementation, and evaluation of the program, as well as intensive training and regular supervision of health workers, appear to be key to success. In community-based programs, GMP also appears to be an efficient promoter of health services. Improvements in immunization coverage, in the distribution of ORS packets, vitamin A, and iron supplements, and in the frequency of home visits and medical checkups have been documented following the implementation of GMP programs.

The usefulness of GMP data for screening at the individual level or for monitoring, evaluation, and surveillance at the aggregate level appears less promising. From the review of both clinic- and community-based studies, it appears that in usual field conditions, the data collected during growth-monitoring activities have a high rate of measurement errors which diminish its utility for screening children, targeting appropriate interventions, and providing useful estimates of prevalence or impact. More research in this area is needed to determine whether, and at what cost, problems of measurement errors can be overcome and to assess the feasibility of combining the educational and motivational objectives of GMP with its use as a source of data. The relative incompatibility between service delivery and data-collection objectives has been documented before: cumbersome reporting systems are said to distract health workers from using the data to counsel and motivate mothers (Teller et al., 1985).

If the complementarity between the use of GMP for education and its use as a source of data cannot be achieved harmoniously, then a choice needs to be made between these two purposes. This decision should be made according to the main purpose for which GMP is used in a specific program and should be based on a clear understanding of the strengths and weaknesses of GMP in achieving either of these goals.

Research Priorities

The continued strong interest in GMP and the differences of opinion concerning its objectives suggest key issues for future research.

Operations Research and Feasibility Studies

In countries where GMP has already been implemented, operations research should be used to improve the effectiveness of existing programs by examining processes, identifying problems, and designing and testing the feasibility and sustainability of alternative solutions to the identified problems (Teller, 1986a; Blumenfeld, 1985; PRICOR, 1989a, 1989b).

Comparison of GMP with Alternative Approaches and Cost-Effectiveness Studies

A comparison of programs with and without GMP, within a specific context, is crucial to determine whether GMP should be included in a particular PHC package or in a specific program or country, specifically, whether it increases the effectiveness, delivery, population coverage, and impact of a particular package of interventions. The same approach could be used to compare the cost-effectiveness of alternative tools and strategies with the use of GMP for each of its particular objectives.

A related question of interest would be to assess the specific role of the various components of GMP in the process of educating and motivating, that is, the role of weighing, of the chart, of the interaction between health workers and mothers, and so on. It would be interesting to know if NED alone is sufficient to produce the same results, given the same level of resources and effort and, more important, whether cheaper and simpler educational tools could replace GMP. This question is important not only to continue to strengthen NED methods but also to apply the most important principles of GMP as a communication strategy to other problems.

Research on Time Costs and Savings

Much more information is needed on the time cost of GMP for mothers and health workers. In the context of PHC activities, information is needed on the time costs associated with the involvement of health workers in GMP. This includes the time used for conducting all the steps of GMP with accuracy and competence as well as the training and supervision time necessary to achieve an acceptable level of quality. Mothers' time also needs to be addressed, considering both the time costs of attending GMP sessions and the time saved by reducing and preventing children's illnesses (Leslie, 1989a).

Research on Contextual Factors

Zinn and Drake (1988) used a novel and relevant approach to assess the importance of various contextual factors in the success of GMP programs in five countries. Overall, their results suggested that implementation was generally more successful in areas where the need for the intervention was less. The authors concluded: "The more a community needs growth monitoring, the more difficult it will be to successfully implement. The more difficult it is to successfully implement, the greater the resource expenditure required for successful implementation. And to complete the loop, the greater the need, the greater the potential effectiveness" (Zinn and Drake, 1988, p. 98).

Postnote

After this chapter was written, UNICEF conducted an evaluation of the UNICEF-supported growth-monitoring activities in seven case study countries—China, Ecuador, Indonesia, Malawi, Thailand, Zaire, and Zambia. The mandate of the evaluation was to document whether the information generated by growth monitoring for assessment and analysis did, in practice, lead to action. In the context of UNICEF's nutrition strategy, growth monitoring was seen as a strategy to assist families and communities in getting the necessary information to help them with their decision-making process. Details about the design and results of the evaluation and the future directions of UNICEF relative to advocacy of growth monitoring are discussed in length in Pearson (1993). Conclusions and recommendations made at two meetings on growth monitoring held in Kenya in 1992 are also presented in this report.

UNICEF's evaluation confirms the general success achieved in most GMP programs in teaching mothers and health workers the appropriate use of the technology involved (e.g., scales, growth charts). The evaluation concludes, however, that in all seven study countries "few actions—either at household or at community levels—aimed at improving the nutritional status of children, based on discussion stimulated by growth monitoring, were reported by caretakers of children and monitors" (Pearson, 1993, p. ii). Other limitations of GMP related to the use of the data for decision making at regional and central levels are discussed in the report, namely the problems of low coverage, lack of representativeness of the data, and the competition for health workers' time and resources. Overall, UNICEF's evaluation corroborates most of the conclusions derived in the present chapter from the review of earlier studies.

An important conclusion from UNICEF's evaluation is that the information generated by growth monitoring is not sufficient to stimulate the cycle of Assessment, Analysis and Action (Triple-A cycle) necessary for decision making either at family, community, or central levels. Alternative strategies, which may or may not include growth-monitoring processes, have been adopted by UNICEF in response to this evaluation in the newly designed nutrition information strategy (UNICEF, 1993c).

6

Child Caregiving and Infant and Preschool Nutrition

Patrice L. Engle

Most interventions to improve the health and nutritional status of children rely at some point on the caregivers' compliance with or support of the intervention. The more limited the economic resources, the more important will be the establishment of functioning child-caregiver interactions and caregiver behavior. Much of the nutritional and public health research, however, does not employ a model that provides a theoretical framework for conceptualizing the caregiver's role and interaction with the child. This chapter presents a transactional model for child development that is widely employed in developmental psychology and illustrates how it can be applied to nutritional interventions.

"Child care" as used here refers to a range of caregiving behaviors that directly affect a child from infancy through roughly six years, such as feeding, bathing, comforting, responding to distress, protecting from harm and infection, seeking medical treatment, nursing, stimulating cognitive development, and providing an emotionally positive environment (Engle, 1992). These behaviors are normally performed by the mother but may be done by any family member, other caregiver, or institution. This chapter examines whether the way these behaviors are undertaken—with what energy, thought, or investment—influences children's nutritional status. All caregiving acts are assumed to involve social processes that form the basis for future interactions. As Lipsitt, Crook, and Booth (1985) observe with respect to the behavior of feeding, "(a) the human baby, like other

The comments of Sue Crockenberg, Ernesto Pollitt, Kathy Gorman, Per Pinstrup-Andersen, Kay Dewey, Harold Alderman, David Pelletier, Ken Brown, and Marian Zeitlan on the ideas in this paper are appreciated.

infant mammals, depends completely upon a social relationship for its nutritional requirements and thus the maintenance of life and physical well-being, and (b) the style and quality of caretaker-infant interactions are determinative of other (nonfeeding) interactions and subsequent feeding behavior, including preferences and aversions" (p. 485).

Some public health researchers have acknowledged the importance of these behaviors but are unclear how to assess them or use them in interventions. For example, Mosley (1984) concludes: "It is within the family, where the modern (generally Western) health systems interact with the traditional social systems, that most health interventions succeed or fail. And so it is on this crucial interaction that policy-relevant research is needed. Yet it is precisely in this area, where biomedical and social science must join together to define and solve the problems, that research has been most neglected" (p. 19).

Research on these microbehaviors can be time- and money-intensive. Using the theoretical perspective described here may lead an investigator to include a broader range of variables, to target interventions more precisely, and to include the developmental stage of the child in planning descriptive and intervention studies. Although careful observational research is time-intensive, practice trials, ethnographic studies, and focus groups can provide initial information on child-caregiver interactions.

The Transactional Model

For many years, the view that undernutrition is caused by a lack of food, combined with infection, dominated thinking about nutrition interventions. Undernutrition was thought to be caused primarily by household resource constraints. Since the 1970s numerous investigators, often from a social science perspective, have argued for the need to develop a more complex interactional model to explain undernutrition of children (e.g., Pollitt, 1973, 1988; Hepner and Maiden, 1971; Bell, 1971; Galler et al., 1984; Bentley et al., 1993; Engle, 1994). As Ricciuti observes (1981, p. 119), "Unfavorable early childcare practices and dysfunctional patterns of caregiver-infant interaction may contribute to an increased risk of malnutrition, growth retardation, and suboptimal behavioral development. There is growing evidence that the altered nutritional status of the infant or young child, as reflected in physical appearance, general demeanor, and behavior, may also significantly affect the manner in which the mother or other primary caregivers respond to and care for the child" (see also Chávez et al., 1975; Graves, 1978). Ricciuti (1981) concludes that intervention strategies limited to supplementary feeding have much less effect on children's development than those that combine cognitive stimulation and feeding.

The eventual nutritional status of the child depends not only on food availability and household resources but also on the constitutional strength or vulnerability of the child (Werner, 1988), the environmental conditions (caregiver, family, social support, and cultural beliefs), and age-appropriate shifts and changes in the child's developing systems of self-regulation and control (Lipsitt et al., 1985). Child growth and development result from a transaction, a continual and progressive interplay between the child and the environment, which tend to alter each other.

The transactional model emerged in part from Sameroff and Chandler's studies of at-risk infants in developed countries (Sameroff, 1979, 1981). Before 1975, high-risk infants were viewed as having biomedical problems that would directly affect their outcomes. In their 1975 study, Sameroff and Chandler found that early biological risk was less important than socioeconomic and familial factors. They postulated the existence of social self-righting tendencies, which operate postnatally through social systems to produce a psychologically normal child, despite early risk. These processes were parallel to self-righting biological mechanisms (Waddington, 1966).

A study of language development of low-birth-weight children in the United States illustrates the transactional model (Rocissano and Yatchmink, 1983). The authors hypothesize that these children have a "limited capacity" to respond—either to their own internal messages or to messages from the environment. The child at risk must direct more attention to autonomic functions that are being stabilized. A mother can take some of the burden off the child by being extremely responsive and may be able to enhance the child's learning capacity. If she is not attentive to her child's cues, however, learning opportunities will be lost, and the child will develop more slowly than a normal child. Mothers of premature infants, who are oversolicitous but not responsive, can set in motion a passive style among their infants. Mothers who are depressed or grieving at the vulnerable condition of their children may similarly be unable to facilitate the child's cognitive growth (Rocissano and Yatchmink, 1983).

The authors recommended that mothers be helped to observe the infant and respond to his or her cues; rather than becoming overly intrusive, they can be taught to follow the child's lead. These findings could have direct application to interventions with undernourished children; the mother or caregiver who is responsive to requests for food may be more able to bring a child back to health or better nutritional status than one who provides food when the child is not receptive. The at-risk child has an increased need for the caregiver to be in sync with his or her needs (Pollitt and Wirtz, 1981).

Developmental Periods of the Child

Transactions change with the developing capabilities of the child. These changes are of two kinds: changes in the child's psychobiological processes and changes in the child's environment. During the first five years of a child's life, the conditions that compromise growth and development vary tremendously. The relative importance of the mother's time in caregiving and the nutritional benefit of environmental resources will also vary with the child's age. The "developmental niche" or social context of the child (Super and Harkness, 1986) will also change with age.

During the first six months, the child's behavior gradually shifts from reflexive, obligatory control to a voluntary or deliberate response system (McGraw, 1943). With the acquisition and refinement of voluntary behavior, behavioral development is increasingly embedded within social relationships (Lipsitt et al., 1985; Wachs and Gruen, 1982). Supplementary feeding, a process that depends on social support and may form the basis for many social interactions, usually begins during this first year.

During the second and third years of a child's life, the benefits of increased family resources become more evident, but so do the costs of an inadequate environment. Rates of malnutrition and infection peak in the second year (13–24 months) (Gordon et al., 1967; UNICEF, 1993a), and the proportion of children dying matches or exceeds the total dying in the following three years (Puffer and Serrano, 1973). Changes occur in the child's behavior and the social context of rearing that enable the child to become mobile but not to have the cognitive structure to understand important health-related distinctions (where to deposit feces, for example); or the child becomes capable of self-feeding without understanding what foods are appropriate and inappropriate. In many cultures, exclusive maternal care is replaced by care by other family members, and family competition begins (Werner, 1988). "Many weaning customs of nonindustrialized peoples potentiate malnutrition" (Cassidy, 1980, p. 109). Customs common during this period, such as restricting "strong" or protein-rich foods, allowing competition for food with older children or the preferred sex, or separating the child from the mother for a period of time, tend to result in malnutrition.

Beyond the age of thirty-six months, the child is motorically and cognitively more capable of self-care, self-feeding, and avoiding harm. In many societies, children at age three or four are not really "cared for"; they are initiated into the culture of children and may even become fledgling caregivers to younger siblings (Werner, 1984). They may have developed the skills to obtain food for themselves and the wisdom to protect themselves a little from pathogens in the environment. Socioeconomic factors become increasingly significant (Johnston et al., 1980).

Child Effects

Characteristics of the child such as gender, parentage, attractiveness, disabilities, or other idiosyncratic effects predispose her or him to undernutrition by influencing the caregivers' response (e.g., Gokulanathan and Kannarkat, 1969; Okeahialam, 1975). For example, girls are more likely to be malnourished than boys and are less likely to be taken for medical treatment in South Asia (D'Souza and Chen, 1980; Chen et al., 1981).

Studies of intrahousehold food and resource distribution have shown how age and gender can influence the proportion of the family food that each child receives (Rogers, 1990). Although some studies have shown that children ingest significantly less food than adults within a household, this difference tends to disappear when between-meal eating is included (Harbert and Scandizzo, 1982; Engle and Nieves, 1993). In South Asia, however, girls receive a smaller share of the household's diet (Abdullah and Wheeler, 1985; Brown et al., 1982).

A vicious cycle linking children's low birth weight or sickliness with failure to thrive (FTT) has been found in the United States (Lozoff, 1989). Mothers of FTT children tend to come from more abused backgrounds, and children who become FTT tend to be low-birth-weight infants, children with feeding difficulty, or children perceived as sickly (Lozoff, 1989; Kotelchuck and Newberger, 1983).

Once a child is mildly or severely malnourished, behaviors typical of undernourished children may undermine the developing child-caregiver transaction, such as a high-pitched irritating cry (Zeskind, 1983), disorganized sleep/wake patterns (Peirano et al., 1989), poor suckling ability (Pollitt, 1973), less responsiveness or energy (Pollitt, 1973; Ricciuti, 1981; Zeskind and Ramey, 1978), and more frequent illness (Wachs et al., 1988; Greene et al., 1983). Malnourished children have been found to be less securely attached to their mothers than adequately nourished children (Valenzuela, 1988, 1990). They may also use environmental supports, such as the presence of their mother, in different ways from well-nourished children; presence of the mother may facilitate the well-nourished child's exploration but not the poorly nourished child's (Wachs et al., 1988). Some mothers have been found to respond to an undernourished child with increased physical contact and more time spent breastfeeding (Galler et al., 1984), yet increased holding entails risks because it has been associated with passivity and with lowered cognitive development (Munroe and Munroe, 1984; Sigman et al., 1989).

Caregiver Effects: Maternal Behaviors

Just as the child plays a major role in establishing the responsive relationship, the caregiver also has a major role to play and, at least initially, has the larger role (Wachs et al., 1988; Cohen and Parmelee, 1983). Educational level and nutritional status of the mother have been found to be associated with caregiving behaviors in developing countries (Mosley, 1984; Zeitlin et al., 1990). Other variables awaiting investigation are physical stress, mental health or absence of depression, health status (presence of anemia or other nutritional deficiencies), and maternal management style.

Education. Despite overwhelming evidence relating increased maternal education with improved child survival rates, improved child health, and better nutritional status, little is known about the actual mechanism through which these effects occur (see Chapter 3). Most work has focused on the relationship between education and fertility. Kasarda, Billy, and West (1986) and Caldwell, Reddy, and Caldwell (1983) hypothesize that education changes women's self-image and increases their desire to forge ahead; therefore they have fewer children. LeVine (1987) suggests that education changes the mother's investment strategy from letting the child develop on its own to the more controlling, time-intensive child rearing that is often coupled with a desire for fewer children. How five or six years of schooling can lead to these dramatic effects needs to be investigated.

Depression. Estimates worldwide of incidence of depression suggest that it is widespread (Sartorius, 1974) and that women report greater emotional distress than men (Paltiel, 1987; Murphy, 1976), although treatment rates are higher for men than women in developing countries (Weissman and Kierman, 1977; ICRW, 1989). Taub (1989), using the Center for Epidemiological Studies depression scale, found that 35 percent of poor slum dwellers in Montevideo, Uruguay, reported depressive symptoms.

Rutter (1990) reviewed twenty years of research in the United States linking maternal depression with lack of adequate care and supervision of children, more medical problems and accidents among children, and more time spent in mutual child-caregiver negative states. Many studies show an impaired pattern of synchronicity in interactions, which seems to be related to the depression itself rather than to associated family risk factors (e.g., Breznitz and Friedman, 1988).

Given the substantial effects of maternal depression in the United States and its prevalence in developing countries, it could be a factor in under-nutrition among preschool children, although no studies linking the psychological health of the mother to the nutritional status of the child were found. Engle (1989) reported an association between higher somatic symptoms of stress and preschool children's lower height-for-age in three hundred women in a periurban area of Guatemala. Zeitlin et al. (1990) reported that their most predictive variable for higher child nutritional status and growth rate in Bangladesh was the mother's "happy" mood state, rated according to operationally defined criteria and observed over several visits. The causal direction is unclear; poor nutritional status of children could be either a cause or a consequence of depression or a consequence of family risk factors, which in turn are related to undernutrition.

Caregiver's health. Few studies have examined effects of maternal nutritional status or health on child care behaviors. Scrimshaw and Scrimshaw (1989) found an association between a mother's hemoglobin levels and infant mortality rate. McCullough et al. (1990) found associations between low levels of Egyptian mothers' vitamin B_6 in their milk and less responsive patterns of caregiver-child interaction at three to six months of age, controlling for confounding variables. Maternal depletion, overwork, and exhaustion are likely to be associated with less active and energetic caregiving. In periurban Guatemala, 50 percent of mothers of young children reported feeling tired "all of the time" (Engle, 1989). A mother's involvement in volunteer community development activities correlated with poorer health and nutritional status of her children in Lima, Peru (Anderson, 1989).

Caregiver's abilities. Dettwyler (1986) found that individual differences in maternal attitude, consisting of beliefs that children should be called to meals, that food should be tailored to their interests, and that medical care should be sought for illnesses, correlated with child growth, whereas socioeconomic variables did not. Zeitlin, Mansour, and Boghani (1990) have developed a methodology to discover the child care "microbehaviors" used by successful or "positively deviant" mothers to teach these strategies to other mothers. For example, in Bangladesh, actively feeding finger foods was associated with better nutritional status in children (Zeitlin et al., 1990). This strategy was then taught to other mothers who did not actively feed their children finger foods.

Although there are clearly differences in caregivers' abilities to provide adequate care, no appropriate metric for "caregiver's competence" has been developed. The construct itself needs further definition. It is probably multidimensional and covers a wide range of acceptable behaviors. The construct should include both knowledge of an appropriate child care activity and the willingness, ability, or motivation to perform it. Those who use the construct should recognize that caregiving which results in a healthy, well-nourished child is the result of interaction between caregiver, support system, and child, not the quality of a particular individual.

Caregiver Effects: Alternative Caregivers

Alternative caregivers provide much care. It is now widely recognized that even without income-generating activities, mothers' work loads may be too great to allow additional time for more caregiving (e.g., McGuire and Popkin, 1990). Also, the incidence of mothers of young children working for income is increasing. For example, in one town in Guatemala, Engle (1989) reported that the proportion of mothers working had increased from 25 percent to 33 percent over ten years, but the fastest-growing group of working mothers were those with infants, for whom the rate changed from 12 percent to 30 percent. Maternal work for earnings in developing countries is not new, but some of its new forms (leaving the home for extended periods to work in places where the child is excluded) are different.

Leslie's (1988, 1989b) review of twenty-five studies from sixteen developing countries found no conclusive evidence linking maternal employment with poorer nutritional status of children. Those studies that did find effects of maternal work on children did not control for other potentially confounding variables, such as poverty, limiting the possibility of making causal statements. Much research has also been hampered by viewing work as a dichotomous variable and failing to consider age of the child, the social context (work and child caregiving conditions), and maternal and child characteristics.

Studies that have examined effects of maternal work as a function of the age of the child, controlling for potentially confounding variables, have reported a negative association between maternal work for earnings and children's nutritional status during infancy (Engle and Pedersen, 1989; O'Gara, 1989), particularly when work begins before the child's second month of life, a finding not observed when mothers were home for the first three months of the child's life (Vial et al., 1989). In the second and third years of life, however, workers' children tend to be nourished as well as or better than children of nonworkers, controlling for socioeconomic variables (Engle, 1991; Engle and Pedersen, 1989; La Montagne et al., 1993, in Nicaragua; Engle, forthcoming).

Although surprisingly few studies have examined the effect of alternate caregivers on children's nutritional status (Joekes, 1989), there is evidence from a few studies that have controlled for potentially confounding variables of associations between type of alternate caregiver and children's nutritional status. Caregiving of children by teens and by young children has been found to be associated with less food intake (Lung'aho and Pelto, 1983; Wachs et al., 1988) when food was not limiting and poorer nutritional status (Engle, 1991, in Guatemala; Engle et al., 1993, in Nicaragua).

Negative associations between mothers' working at home and the nutritional status of children has been reported by several investigators (O'Gara, 1989, in urban Honduras; PMPA and Manoff, 1986, in Indonesia; Joekes, 1989; Engle, 1991, in Guatemala). Ethnographic data from these studies suggest that under the pressure of work, mothers working at home are less responsive to their children because of the pressure of work and may be less able to provide a positive interactive environment for their children than nonworkers.

The role of fathers in providing child care has been neglected in research in southern countries. Data from the north suggest that fathers living in the home spend less than one-third of the time mothers spend in child care, and their time appears to be oriented toward play rather than physical care (see Engle and Breaux, 1994, for a review). Fathers' absence is frequent in many areas. For example, a recent study in Barbados found that in a sample of 303 teen mothers, only 23 percent of eight-year-old children were still living with their biological fathers (Russell-Brown, Engle, and Townsend, 1994).

Social Support

Sameroff and Seifer (1983) suggest that parental knowledge, attitudes, or understanding can buffer the effects of economic and social stress on a family. Social support has often been considered an important contextual variable that reduces the negative impact of life stress (Crockenberg, 1988; Repetti et al., 1989). Exploration of these buffering effects might provide ideas on which one could develop an intervention.

An Application of the Transactional Model: Feeding Behavior

Despite an extensive body of literature on infant and child feeding, the actual behaviors surrounding feeding have received relatively little attention (Lipsitt et al., 1985). Yet feeding is essentially a social process. It involves the interactions of caregiver and child over an extended developmental period. It can be viewed from the transactional perspective as influenced by the child's characteristics, such as appetite, and the caregiver's characteristics, such as knowledge, health, or energy, within the context of resource and food limitations. Feeding can be viewed both as a cause and a mediator of better nutrition and as a mechanism to enhance caregiver interactions leading to cognitive development and socioemotional well-being.

A number of investigators who have found that increases in income or supplementary feeding programs alone are relatively unsuccessful in increasing children's nutritional status have begun to examine the actual feeding situation for young children (e.g., Grantham-McGregor et al., 1989). Others have come to observe behaviors around feeding only after field experiences indicated that they were important determinants of food ingestion (e.g., PMPA and Manoff, 1986; Brown et al., 1986).

The studies reviewed here are from Nigeria (Brown et al., 1986), Peru (Bentley et al., 1991; Bentley, 1992), Mexico (Garcia et al., 1990a, 1990b; Zeitlin et al., 1989), Nicaragua and Guatemala (Engle et al., 1993; Engle et al., forthcoming), Bangladesh (Zeitlin et al., 1990), and Mali (Dettwyler, 1986, 1987). Each attempted to determine the role of the child's demand or the mother's feeding behavior in nutrient ingestion, nutritional status, or both. This is a new area of research, and the studies tend to be correlational, descriptive, and generally have not yet developed data-collection methodologies that would meet stringent criteria for reliability or validity of assessment techniques. The only studies that used multiple regressions, controlling for confounding variables, were Bentley et al. (1991), Zeitlin et al. (1989, 1990), and Engle et al. (1993). Only Engle et al. (1990) reported interobserver reliability and consistency in behaviors over time. Data analysis presents difficult problems because of the nonnormality of many variables. These studies are consistent with each other, however, and have revealed important behaviors and beliefs that have implications for interventions.

Age Transitions

Lipsitt et al.'s (1985) research shows that babies are "keenly sensitive in the first few hours of life to subtle changes in gustatory stimulation" (p. 491); although their behavior is primarily reflexive, they show a marked preference for sweetness. During the first six months infants shift from primarily reflexive control of responses to voluntary control. Dislikes appear even on first food presentation and become stable by the second year of life. Patterns of offering and acceptance of food during the initiation of complementary feeding probably lay the basis for feeding in the future; however, the process has been little studied in the psychological literature.

The studies summarized here sampled children from 3 to 36 months, except the Garcia et al. (1990a, 1990b) studies (33–60 months) and Engle et al.'s (1990) Guatemalan study (12–60 months). None of the studies examined age differences specifically, but some controlled for it in regressions.

Child Effects: Appetite and Refusal

Most of these investigations reported that children were not eating all of the food offered to them (Garcia et al., 1990a, 1990b; Engle et al., 1990; Brown et al., 1988; Zeitlin et al., 1990). This food leaving may be a function of poor-quality, low-nutrient-density food, poor-tasting food, child illness and loss of appetite, inappropriate timing of food, failure to assist the child, or the caregiver offering too much food initially. These results suggest that in many cases of undernutrition, food availability per se does not appear to be the limiting factor in food ingestion. Not surprisingly, studies have found associations between finishing food and nutritional status. Zeitlin et al. (1989, 1990) found that in 123 Bangladeshi children (4 to 33 months old), the more often they finished their food, the higher their nutritional status. Engle et al. (1990, 1993) also reported that food refusal was associated with lower height-for-age and weight-for-age among 80 Nicaraguan children aged 12 to 18 months.

Illness-associated anorexia may explain some of these findings. Bentley et al. (1991) examined children's refusal during episodes of diarrhea, during convalescence, and after recovery. Children's acceptance of food increased significantly during good health compared to diarrhea. This study is methodologically strengthened by using each child as its own control. Anorexia is a major factor in limiting child intake (Bentley et al., 1993).

Caregiver's Behaviors: Active Feeding Behavior

Several studies have reported significant associations between the caregiver's active role in child feeding and the child's food ingestion or nutritional status. Zeitlin, Houser, and Johnson (1989) observed feeding behavior of 74 children aged 8 to 22 months in Mexico for thirteen hours on three different days. All the mother's actions about feeding and all the children's actions, whether accepting or rejecting of food, were coded, using five-second time sampling. They found significant associations between feeding activity of mother and child's height-for-age z-score (HAZ) and change in HAZ over a five-month period, controlling for confounds.

Dettwyler (1986) followed 136 children aged 4 through 36 months in a periurban community in Mali. She categorized mothers according to a maternal attitude scale, representing four attitudes: calling children to meals, trying to make foods children like, purchasing small treats, and using medical care and found that this combination of attitudes was a better predictor of child weight-for-age than socioeconomic status. Hepinstall et al. (1987) observed mealtime behavior of 4-year-olds in poor families in London. Poor growth was associated with lack of parental supervision of meals, irregular mealtimes, and parental indifference or anxiety. Klesges et al. (1983, 1986) in the United States showed that parental encouragement to eat correlated with the amount of time the child spent eating and the child's weight.

In Bangladesh, using a time sampling as in the Mexican study, with 175 children ranging in ages from 4 through 34 months, Zeitlin et al. (1990) concluded that "the personal energy and resources that mothers invested in feeding their babies were significant determinants of size and growth" (p. 25). Feeding variables associated with weight gain over a six-month period were the mother's investment in breastfeeding (e.g., doing nothing else while breastfeeding, lying down while breastfeeding), bottle-feeding, and active feeding of complementary foods.

Gender may affect food ingestion through differential caregiver feeding behaviors. For example, among Mexican-American mothers in the United States, Olvera-Ezzel, Power, and Cousins (1990) reported significantly more encouragement to eat for males than for females. Similar differences were found in Santa Maria de Jesus, Guatemala (Bentley et al., 1992) and Nicaragua (Engle et al., forthcoming).

Nutritional status may be more highly associated with child demand than adult active feeding. Garcia et al. (1990a, 1990b) concluded that children in their sample had considerable control over the amount of food ingested and its selection. Those who requested feeding more often than the median (nine times per day) ingested significantly more kcal and kcal/kg than those who requested food less often. Among 1- to 5-year-old children in Guatemala, Engle et al. (1990) also reported evidence of child regulation of diet; a significant predictor of food ingested at a meal was the number of requests before the meal and the number of requests for more food during the meal. Parental encouragement was unrelated to food ingestion. In Nicaragua, poor nutritional status of 12- to 18-month-old children was associated with child refusal but was unrelated to maternal encouragement to eat (Engle et al., 1990, 1993). The importance of child demand in food ingestion was also seen in Egypt and Kenya (Wachs et al., 1992).

The discrepancies between studies may be related to the effects of illness on appetite. If maternal encouragement is greater when children refuse food, and food refusal is associated with lower nutritional status, maternal active feeding will not be related to nutritional status. Bentley et al.'s (1991) Peruvian findings are consistent with this picture. When children were ill with diarrhea, they refused food, and mothers were active in caregiving. When children were healthy, however, maternal encouragement to eat was minimal; only 36 percent of mothers encouraged children. The Zeitlin studies included only healthy children; children ill with diarrhea were excluded. In future studies, maternal feeding behavior should be examined separately for ill and healthy children because the significance of maternal feeding behavior may be quite different.

Maternal feeding behavior tends to be passive in many cultures (e.g., Bentley et al., 1992, in Guatemala; Engle et al., forthcoming, in Nicaragua; Grantham-McGregor, Schofield, and Haggard, 1989, in Jamaica). In southwestern Nigeria, however, Brown et al. (1988) found that 85 percent of mothers feed their children by hand or by forcing from 6 months through 11 months, with the percent declining with age. Children who refuse food can be force-fed a liquid pap. In a sample of ten children from 6 to 24 months, much more force-feeding was observed when children had diarrhea than when they were healthy.

Beliefs about Feeding

One issue that has received little attention is parental attitudes and beliefs about children's self-feeding. In Engle et al.'s (1990) Nicaraguan study, 41 percent of the mothers felt that children should be able to eat alone at 12 months, although standard child development texts recommend that a child cannot eat with a spoon alone at that age. Dettwyler (1986, 1987) observed similar attitudes toward children's self-regulation in Mali: it is believed that children should be in charge of the amount they eat because only they know they are hungry. Families believed that children will eat when hungry; if they do not want to eat they should not be forced to eat. Children are not helped to eat but use their fingers from the family pot when they are ready. Similar attitudes were reported in Malaysia (Wolff, 1965) and Papua New Guinea (Malcolm, 1974). In Indonesia, the Weaning Project (PMPA and Manoff International, 1986) also found mothers reluctant to feed a child who was apparently not hungry.

A mother's belief that she can encourage a child who refuses food to eat was associated with better child nutritional status in Nicaragua (Engle et al., forthcoming). This attitude toward feeding may be associated with mother's education; mothers with more education have been found to adopt more active caregiving (LeVine, 1987). In Bangladesh, the less educated mothers tended to leave much of the impetus for development up to the natural patterns of the child, whereas the more educated mothers took a much more active role in controlling, feeding, and stimulating the child (Zeitlin et al., 1990). Even beliefs associating food and health may not be widely held. Mull (1991) in Pakistan reported no strong association between the two, little monitoring of what children eat, and little encouragement. These beliefs were also not associated in the Rukwa area of Tanzania (Wandel et al., 1992).

These studies provide evidence that food availability in the household is a relatively poor measure of actual food intake over the course of the day. To improve prediction, variables to consider as well are (1) feeding timing and frequency, (2) food quality and caloric density, (3) child appetite and child refusal, (4) active feeding behaviors by caregiver, and (5) beliefs about children's feeding. Examining attitudes of caregivers about self-feeding by children could be an important clue for intervention. A laissez-faire belief about feeding, particularly during illness or periods of anorexia, could be a significant risk factor.

Interventions

A transactional model has been presented as a framework for linking the standard inputs of food availability and infection with nutritional status through caregiving behaviors. At first glance, the model may seem too complex; however, adopting this perspective can have several immediate applications. First, before an intervention, a descriptive study could include characteristics of the child, the caregiver's behavior and beliefs, and the social environment as well as the more standard measures of resource availability. Second, the developmental period of the child in terms of control over the feeding process would be essential to consider. Third, interventions that ignore the within-family process would be less likely to be recommended. Fourth would be a greater likelihood to couch nutritional interventions in an integrated program of child development, including cognitive, social, and affective development, because these changes would in turn improve the quality of caregiving the child might receive. Finally, this model would tend to lead to the development of lower-technology interventions that would be implemented at the household level and would include community participation and would have effects on the caregivers.

The studies on feeding behavior provide several examples of how interventions could be altered by including the transactional framework. Bentley et al. (1991) observed that educational messages to mothers about diarrheal control often encourage them to feed a child during an episode of diarrhea, assuming that the mothers are trying to "starve" the children.

Her research showed that, on the contrary, mothers were trying to feed their children, but the children were refusing the food. A more appropriate message would have focused on how to feed a reluctant child. In Nicaragua (Engle et al., 1990), mothers did not begin to encourage active feeding until the end of the meal, although the child's refusal partly into the meal was significantly associated with lower nutritional status. An intervention strategy might include helping the mother to read refusal cues throughout a meal and begin to enhance her child care.

Specific recommendations based on this research model would either enhance or complement existing interventions or suggest different interventions. All of these interventions need not be delivered in face-to-face training; some may operate through a mass media or social marketing project. Interventions stemming from the application of this model can be grouped into three main categories:

(A) Increase child's responsiveness
    (1) nutritional rehabilitation programs
    (2) child stimulation programs
(B) Increase caregiver's resources
    (1) enhance the main caregiver's ability to be a good caregiver through improved health, social support, reduced work load, increased empowerment, employment training, or formal education
(C) Enhance within-household interactions
    (1) focus on modifying specific behaviors, such as using more finger foods, weaning food preparation, handwashing, feces disposal
    (2) modify beliefs and behaviors regarding caregiver-child interactions, such as responsiveness to child cues, control over eating events, or beliefs about feeding
    (3) develop the abilities of alternative caregivers to provide care

Interventions less likely to be effective in improving children's nutritional status are technological solutions, such as the production of a perfect weaning food, or programs that do not enhance a child-caregiver role, such as institutional day care. In a World Bank working paper, Chernichovsky and Zangwill (1988) emphasize that whether or not a nutrition program will work depends on behaviors within the household, although the interventions they describe (food stamps, supplementary feeding, income transfer), which aim to increase food availability, do not consider intrahousehold processes.

Child-Centered Interventions

Interventions to alter children's behavior have often been successful but expensive. In Canada, Ramsay and Zelazo (1988) were able to rehabilitate five hospitalized failure-to-thrive infants who refused food by nasogastric feeding combined with social and tactile stimulation, first by a therapist and later by the caregiver. The behavior modification intervention resulted in establishing positive caregiver-child interactions. In Colombia, a combined nutritional and social stimulation program with low-income preschool children for six hours a day, five days a week, for at least a year resulted in nutritional and cognitive gains three years later, compared with a control group (McKay et al., 1978). In a longitudinal study of early nutritional supplementation in Guatemala, supplemented children were taller and brighter as adolescents (Pollitt et al., 1993).

These intervention efforts may be particularly effective for high-risk children, as one might suspect from the transactional model. When the child is less able to stimulate caregiving, caregivers trained to stimulate the child will facilitate interaction. For example, in the United States, Zeskind and Ramey (1978) placed low socioeconomic status infants in an intensive eight-hour-per-day child care program and located controls who stayed home with their mothers. Half of each group were fetally malnourished (low ponderal index). There were no differences in maternal involvement or twenty-four month test performance between fetally malnourished and normal children in the day care treatment group, but the fetally malnourished children who were cared for at home had significantly lower test scores than normal controls and the experimental children.

Although ideal programs appear to have beneficial effects on children's development, institutional day care (not community-based programs) in developing countries rarely provides this benefit, yet it is very costly. Systematic evaluations of the effects of these programs on children are lacking. An evaluation of thirty-five Guatemalan day care programs found problems of cultural inappropriateness, lack of funding, inexperience with methods of handling children in groups, and an absence of parental involvement in the programs (Engle and Garcia, 1989). Day care use was uncommon; the most common form of alternate care was from family members.

Interventions to Enhance the Caregiver Role

Targeting the caregiver (mother or alternate) rather than the child would lead to different interventions. If initial descriptive work suggests that many of the mothers are depressed or physically ill, an intervention could involve support groups for women, skill training, health improvement, or self-esteem building. Training may vary by caregiver type.

Although recommendations for strategies to support the caregiver or reduce work loads have been made based on correlational evidence (e.g., formal education, labor force participation), the number of careful intervention studies based on this hypothesis are limited in developing countries. In the United States, Slaughter (1983) found that enrolling poor black women in support groups was at least as effective for changing children's cognitive level as specific skill training in a home visiting program. Whether social support groups or other alterations in women's health (physical or mental) would have similar effects on children's cognitive or nutritional development in a developing country is open for investigation.

Interventions to Enhance Child-Caregiver Interactions

Interventions that have attempted to improve children's cognitive development by improving the mother's caregiving skills have been shown to result in improved levels of cognitive development and even long-term nutritional effects. In Jamaica, Grantham-McGregor et al. (1987) instituted a home visiting program with previously malnourished children and children previously hospitalized for other reasons. The results indicated that cognitive differences between the previously malnourished and the control children disappeared after three years for children in the home visiting program but remained for those without the program. Play and exploratory behavior of the home visited and control children was similar, whereas the nonvisited children reflected the abnormal behavior patterns often associated with severe malnutrition (Grantham-McGregor et al., 1989). Differences in child behavior were much more marked than differences in mothers' behavior. The authors explain these results in terms of a transactional model.

Improving caregivers' interacting abilities may have nutritional benefits. In a carefully executed investigation, Super, Herrera, and Mora (1990) found effects of a combined nutritional and home visiting program on children's nutritional status three years after the termination of the intervention program. The authors attribute the surprising long-term "sleeper effect" of the home visiting program to changes in parental attention to processes of development and family function, such as a possible increase in interest on the part of the father in the child's development.

Alternate caregivers can be trained to provide improved care. The Child to Child Programme (Aarons et al., 1979), which has extended to sixty countries, involves schoolchildren in learning about nutrition and health care and empowers them to work with peers and their younger siblings. There is some evidence that it has resulted in changes in siblings' behavior (Otaala et al., 1988; Knight and Grantham-McGregor, 1985).

Community-based early stimulation programs for children from impoverished environments, using paraprofessionals, can result in significant changes in children's cognitive development, particularly if they are begun when the child is under three and the mother or primary caregiver is involved (see Pollitt, 1984, for an extensive review).

The Iringa project in Tanzania (funded by the Joint Nutrition Support Group) included community-level day care to provide frequent and regular feeding of children. Rather than supply supplementary foods, mothers were taught how to use existing foods to meet the children's nutrient needs. Because the project operated through community participation, it was possible to develop culturally acceptable child caregiver arrangements. Finally, the project identified a need for women to control the income generated from their labors in order to meet household food and nutritional needs. This project is an excellent example of the incorporation of a within-household perspective into a larger effort.

Zeitlin et al. (1989, p. 2) observe that "weaning food programs that have focussed on behavioral change, using social marketing methods, such as the Nutrition Education and Behavioral Change Component of the Indonesian Nutritional Improvement Program [Zeitlin et al., 1984] and the Applied Nutrition Program in the Dominican Republic [USAID, 1988] have tended to have a more measurable impact on anthropometric status than supplementary feeding programs where the focus was on food distribution."

Promising Directions and a Research Agenda

A theoretical understanding of within-household processes is necessary if we wish to continue to improve child health and nutritional status. This understanding can lead to examining the difference between what people do and what they say they do. Ethnographic interviews have revealed belief structures that make the intensive caregiving recommended for improving nutritional status unlikely to occur. How these beliefs are reflected in behavior and vary by culture needs to be investigated. The theory may also suggest additional variables to investigate, such as the caregiver's beliefs about feeding, the child's appetite, or maternal and child responsiveness.

Research is also needed to determine how much information is necessary to evaluate a household's behavior. Can an assessment be made in a day, an hour, or fifteen minutes? Are behaviors reliable over time? With which behaviors will a survey response prove adequate and for which is it imperative to observe? What behaviors can a caregiver reliably report?

What cultural factors determine accuracy? As an example, Engle and Lumpkin (1992) evaluated the recall accuracy of Guatemalan and Californian young adults and found that 66 percent of their activities could be recalled accurately. Assessments of this type can help pinpoint the amount and timing of data necessary to collect.

More research is needed in strategies for developing parental capacity to apply existing local or professional information. Most research has focused on developing knowledge about the appropriate interventions; relatively little has been done on determining the best strategies for creating behavior change in the household. Application of the techniques of behavior change, which relies on an analysis of behavioral contingencies before intervention, could provide a theoretical basis for intervention strategies for specific behaviors such as handwashing. Other strategies that deserve further investigation are belief change projects and child care. More information is needed about the risks inherent in various types of child care (care by a preteen sibling, a mother while working at home, or an institution), on the roles and competencies of other caregivers, including the father, and on intervention strategies targeted to caregivers other than the mother. Finally, a careful look at the father's responsibility for child care is overdue.

Information is needed on ways to improve the woman's life conditions, her openness to new messages, her willingness to try different strategies, her self-confidence in her child-rearing abilities, and the reasons for her investment in time and energy in her children. A final area needing investigation is support systems for the mother, including husband's attitude, and conditions that buffer the family.

These are complex problems and will require patience, an awareness of cultural differences, and a willingness to look at more "soft" data before solutions emerge, but without this phase the child development revolution of survival with dignity will be lost.

Summary

This chapter has reviewed evidence of the influences of child caregiving activities on infant and preschool children's nutrition and suggested ways that interventions can be improved through more attention to caring behaviors. Four major conclusions were reached:

1. Most nutritional and health interventions rely on the caregiver's compliance and caregiving behaviors. The poorer the economic conditions, the more important caregiving behaviors can be for child nutrition.

2. Child care activities cannot be thought of as a single variable or input to the child. Rather, child caregiving activities are part of a system of relationships among child, caregiver, and social and physical context. These relationships are part of an ongoing transaction. Both the child's characteristics and the caregiver's characteristics interact to develop a caregiving system that may or may not be adaptive. Not only does the caregiver affect the child, but the child's characteristics also alter the caregiving.

3. With economic development and urbanization, the content and context of child care activities are changing rapidly. Interventions need to consider alternative caregivers' skills and constraints.

4. Applying a transactional model to the development of nutrition interventions would (a) increase the range of variables considered to include both child variables and caregiver capabilities; (b) include age and developmental stage of the child as a central element in planning; (c) tend to focus on integrated child development; (d) prioritize community participative, local resource-based interventions that increase the capabilities of families to care for themselves; and (e) avoid inappropriate interventions that rely heavily on technology and external input.

5. Research to identify culture-specific and culturally broader dimensions of within-household behaviors and cultural beliefs related to nutrition is needed. More concern needs to be given to the quality of the research design, and there is a need for intervention trials in addition to correlational/descriptive studies. Finally, more quality control for the assessment of behavioral and psychological processes cross-culturally is needed.

7

Improving the Nutrition of
Women in the Third World

Joanne Leslie

Women's nutrition and health status is central to the quality of their lives and is a key determinant of the survival and healthy development of their children. Women are the main providers of nutrition and informal health care to other members of the household, as well as the main target of the majority of government-sponsored health and nutrition interventions. Therefore, strengthening women by improving their own nutrition and health status may be one of the best avenues for promoting the health and welfare of all in the Third World. Unfortunately, insufficient understanding of the extent, causes, and consequences of malnutrition among women has resulted in an inadequate allocation of resources, both private and public, to efforts to improve the nutrition of women.

The Special Nutritional Situation of Women

Gender is a key determinant both of the biological characteristics of an individual and of his or her social, cultural, and economic roles. The clearest gender-determined difference in responsibilities between men and women relates to women's reproductive function. The nutritional status of a woman (current and past) is an important determinant of the ease with which she will conceive and carry an infant to term, the likelihood that she and the infant will survive and emerge from the birth in good health, and her capacity to breastfeed successfully.

In addition to these specific reproduction-related consequences of women's nutritional status, however, poor nutrition contributes to poor

117

health among women before and after their reproductive years, constrains their economic productivity, and limits their capacity to achieve personal and social goals of importance to themselves and others. Although these nonreproduction-related consequences of malnutrition are significant for both men and women, their extent and severity, as well as the most appropriate approaches to eliminating or reducing them, differ significantly by gender. The long workdays put in by women in most developing countries, the key roles that women play in the production and preparation of food, the provision of health care in the home, and the care of children make it likely that current levels of malnutrition among women in the Third World have widespread and serious consequences for the welfare of the entire household (Himes et al., 1992; Leslie, 1989b; Holmboe-Ottesen et al., 1989).

Women as Targets of Nutrition Interventions

It can be argued that with the advent of primary health care, women have been overtargeted rather than undertargeted by nutrition interventions in the Third World. If one considers the target of an intervention to be the person expected to find out about and use a new service, or to assimilate and act upon new knowledge, then women have been the target of the majority of nutrition and health interventions (Leslie, 1989a). The difference between being the intended target and being the intended beneficiary of an intervention is significant.

Most nutrition interventions in the Third World have provided services and information designed primarily to reduce malnutrition among children. Even programs that include women among the intended beneficiaries usually limit their provision of services to pregnant and lactating women. Such programs leave the unfortunate impression that efforts to improve the nutritional status of women are undertaken solely to improve the nutritional status of children. Such an approach is likely to limit the effectiveness of nutrition interventions in several ways. First, many actions needed to improve nutrition-related reproductive outcomes can be more effectively implemented before women become pregnant and in some cases must be undertaken even before girls reach reproductive age (Abrams and Berman, 1993). Second, the indirect links between a mother's health and nutritional status and the health and nutrition of her children (i.e., her capacity to nurture her children emotionally and to carry out her domestic and income-generating work responsibilities successfully) may be equally or even more important than the direct, biological links during pregnancy and lactation (Leslie et al., 1988). Finally, while women are correctly

perceived as placing great importance on the survival and healthy development of their children, they also universally report considerable stress in
their efforts to meet their multiple reproductive, productive, and social
responsibilities (ICRW, 1989; Holmboe-Ottesen et al., 1989; Stinson,
1986; Birdsall and McGreevy, 1983). Therefore, both practically and psychologically, women are likely to respond better to programs that are
clearly designed with a genuine concern for their own welfare, in addition
to that of their children.

This chapter will summarize the information available concerning the
extent and major types of malnutrition affecting women in the Third
World; review current thinking about the causes of malnutrition among
women; look at problems that have arisen in connection with efforts
to influence the nutritional status of women, including household and
community practices as well as formal nutrition interventions; and offer
some conclusions and recommendations concerning policy and research.[1]

Malnutrition among Women in Developing Countries

This section provides an overview of the major nutritional problems
affecting women in developing countries, highlighting important geographic or age-related differences as well as significant functional consequences.[2] The major nutritional deficiencies of concern in the developing
world are protein-energy malnutrition (PEM), iron-deficiency anemia,
iodine-deficiency disorders (IDD), and vitamin A deficiency (ACC/SCN,
1992; Latham, 1987). All four major nutritional problems show gender
differentials in prevalence and severity at least for some important population subgroups. Three of these represent a more serious problem for females than for males: the prevalence of PEM is significantly higher among
females in South Asia (where almost half the world's undernourished
people live); and both iron-deficiency anemia and goiter are more prevalent among adult women than men, while vitamin A deficiency appears
to be more prevalent among boys than girls.[3]

[1] Information concerning women's nutritional status in developing countries based on
careful scientific research is limited, particularly concerning causes or consequences of malnutrition not linked to pregnancy or lactation. Therefore, the discussion in this chapter
draws not only on empirical findings but also on common sense, personal field experience,
and ethnographic reports of how women talk about their lives. Every effort has been made
to distinguish between generalizations and recommendations that are well supported by
empirical research and those that are less empirically based.

[2] Readers interested in other recent reviews of nutritional problems of Third World women
are referred to ACC/SCN (1992); McGuire and Popkin (1989); Adair (1987); and Soysa
(1987); as well as to the condition-specific references in the rest of this section.

[3] Because most available data on vitamin A deficiency concern children rather than adults,
and the risk appears to be higher among preschool-age boys than among preschool-age girls

PEM in childhood has not only severe short-term consequences, including increased risk of mortality and morbidity, poorer cognitive development and school achievement, and less energy for play and social development, but also serious long-term consequences, primarily associated with nutritional stunting. The consequences of nutritional stunting are particularly severe for females because short stature is a major risk factor for obstetrical complications and maternal mortality (Royston and Armstrong, 1989; Lettenmeier et al., 1988).

McGuire and Popkin (1989) compiled data from thirty-two studies that reported dietary intake data, anthropometric data, or both for women in developing countries. With few exceptions (e.g., Korea, Micronesia, and Singapore), these studies found women to be consuming only about two-thirds of the WHO-recommended daily allowance for energy (reported protein intakes were about as frequently above as below the WHO-recommended daily allowance). Women's average weight-for-height was, in most cases, well below the fiftieth percentile for small-frame women in the United States (McGuire and Popkin, 1989). More recently, the ACC/SCN compiled a data base on women's nutritional status based on 340 studies carried out since the late 1970s (ACC/SCN, 1992). Anthropometric indicators of nutritional status reveal a relatively low prevalence of PEM among reproductive-age women in China and South America but higher levels in the rest of the Third World. Regional variations in the main manifestations of PEM among women are notable and warrant further investigation. Overall, women in South Asia have the highest rates of PEM with over 15 percent stunted (height below 145 cm), over 40 percent with Body Mass Index (BMI) below 18.5, and over 60 percent with weight below 45 kg. Women in Southeast Asia and Middle America are equally stunted but less thin, whereas the opposite is the case with women in sub-Saharan Africa, where a small percentage of women are stunted, but over 20 percent have low BMI and seasonal weight losses are substantial.

A particular concern relates to the finding from studies that the energy intake of pregnant and lactating women only marginally exceeds that of nonpregnant, nonlactating women; the pregnant and lactating women in most populations studied are meeting an even smaller percentage of their estimated energy requirement (McGuire and Popkin, 1989; Pathak, 1987,

---

(Levin et al., 1990; Stanton et al., 1986), this chapter does not discuss the problem of vitamin A deficiency among women, except to note the severe social and economic costs associated with blindness resulting from vitamin A deficiency among both men and women. In addition, however, the growing evidence of a relationship between vitamin A deficiency and mortality among children suggests that studies of a possible similar linkage among adults should be undertaken.

cited in Bajaj, 1989). A study of nutrition and health status of Indian Tamil tea plantation workers in Sri Lanka found that pregnant women consumed less food than any other subgroup of females and that, while lactating women consumed slightly more than other groups of women, their intake was significantly below recommended levels, and they had high levels of anemia (Samarasinghe et al., 1990).

A substantial literature, and a certain amount of controversy, concerns the reproductive consequences of PEM among women. The long-term negative reproductive consequences of childhood PEM appear to be the most widely accepted. That stunted women are at higher risk of obstructed labor because of cephalopelvic disproportion is well established (Royston and Armstrong, 1989). The most severe consequence of obstructed labor is maternal mortality. But even among women who survive, there is increased morbidity, including vesico-vaginal fistulae, which cause extreme discomfort, high risk of infection, and frequently social ostracism (ICRW, 1989; Lettenmeier et al., 1988). In addition to these significant risks to women themselves, stunted mothers have higher rates of miscarriage, stillbirth, low-birth-weight infants, and infant mortality (Chatterjee and Lambert, 1989; Lettenmeier et al., 1988; Ravindran, 1986).

More debate concerns the short-term reproductive consequences of PEM. Research in the mid-1980s from The Gambia raised the possibility that women could produce adequate birth-weight infants at lower energy intake levels during pregnancy than the WHO-recommended allowances through compensatory metabolic adjustments (Durnin, 1987). These findings were not supported by more recent research from Kenya (Neumann et al., 1992). The Kenya research also reported surprisingly good birth weights in spite of low energy intake during pregnancy but found that there was no measurable metabolic adjustment. Instead, they found that, late in pregnancy, women doubled their inactive time (at the expense of critical economic activities) to compensate for inadequate energy intake. The Kenya research, as well as findings from related studies in Egypt and Mexico, also reports a significant positive association between maternal preconception nutritional status and infant birth weight and a positive relationship between maternal postpartum nutritional status and infant growth during the first six months (Neumann et al., 1992; Kirksey et al., 1992; Allen et al., 1992).

In addition to reproductive consequences, PEM can affect women's capacity for physical work. As with reproductive consequences, both the long-term effects of childhood malnutrition on adult productivity and the effects of current PEM must be considered. The long-term effects of childhood malnutrition, acting through reduced muscle mass and therefore reduced aerobic capacity, have a reasonably well-established negative effect on the productivity of men engaged in strenuous activities such as cutting cane or moving earth (Martorell and Arroyave, 1988; McGuire and Austin, 1987). It is reasonable to hypothesize similar effects for women, although some researchers cite evidence suggesting that women are more efficient at producing work for a given body mass than are men (Edmundson and Sukhatme, 1990; Svedberg, 1988).

Few studies have directly investigated the effects of current nutritional status on work among women. Jones, Jarjou, Whitehead, and Jequier (1987) reported that Gambian women with low body fat stores were more efficient at carrying loads than women with higher body fat content. Kennedy and Garcia (1993) found a positive effect of both being taller and having a higher BMI on the work capacity of women in sugarcane farming households in Kenya.

Behavioral and perhaps metabolic adaptations can be made in the face of low energy intakes (Thomas et al., 1989; Edmundson and Sukhatme, 1990). But there may still be substantial losses in productivity and quality of life and no physiological reserves laid down for future periods of stress or dietary deprivation. An important area for future research concerns the productivity and quality of life effects of improving energy intakes or reducing energy expenditure among women, particularly those engaged in strenuous household or market work (Bajaj, 1989; Holmboe-Ottesen et al., 1989).

Iron-Deficiency Anemia

Anemia, which in developing countries is primarily a result of iron deficiency, is undoubtedly the most widespread nutritional problem among women.[4] Extremely high prevalence rates are reported for low-income women in tropical areas (30 to 50 percent), but significant prevalence rates (10 to 15 percent) are reported even among higher-income women living in temperate zone developing or industrialized countries. As with PEM, the most severe situation is found in South Asia, with over 60 percent of pregnant women and almost as high a percentage of nonpregnant women in their reproductive years found to be anemic (ACC/SCN, 1992). Other regions of the Third World show a lower prevalence and a bigger difference between pregnant and nonpregnant women. Even in South America, however, the region with the lowest prevalence of anemia, over 20 percent of nonpregnant women and about 30 percent of pregnant women are anemic.

[4] Folate deficiency, particularly during pregnancy, as well as vitamin B_{12} deficiency and malaria, may also cause or contribute to anemia among women.

The normal physiologic iron losses among reproductive-age women (as a result of shedding of surface cells, unavoidable gastrointestinal blood loss, menstrual blood loss, lactation, and most significantly the increase in blood volume and fetal/placental iron requirements during pregnancy) make it inevitable that, without supplemental iron, women in this age group will become anemic. Where these unavoidable losses are compounded, as in many developing countries, by a limited intake of absorbable iron, extremely closely spaced pregnancies, blood loss from hookworm infection, or malaria, the prevalence of anemia among women is substantially higher.

Iron-deficiency anemia has severe consequences among women in both their reproductive and productive roles. Maternal mortality rates are significantly higher among anemic women, as are prematurity and infant mortality rates (Royston and Armstrong, 1989; Lettenmeier et al., 1988; Bothwell and Charlton, 1981). Maternal mortality associated with anemia may be caused directly by oxygen starvation of the tissues, particularly the heart muscle, the much lower tolerance for blood loss of anemic women, or the less effective functioning of the immune system in anemic pregnant women (Royston and Armstrong, 1989; Levin et al., 1990).

In addition, although direct evidence concerning the effect of anemia on women's physical work capacity is limited, research on men shows a clear association between iron-deficiency anemia and reduced work capacity (Martorell and Arroyave, 1988). Studies of female tea workers in Sri Lanka and Indonesia have found that anemic women who received supplementary iron were significantly more productive than a comparison group of unsupplemented women (Levin et al., 1990; Bothwell and Charlton, 1981; Edgerton et al., 1979). Because low-income rural women in the tropics experience the highest rates of iron-deficiency anemia (along with other forms of malnutrition and morbidity) and have among the most physically demanding work responsibilities (including weeding, threshing, pounding, fetching fuel, and hauling water), anemia among women probably accounts for a significant loss of productivity and therefore of family welfare.

Iodine-Deficiency Disorders

The most widespread and well-studied of the iodine-deficiency disorders are goiter in adolescents and adults and congenital abnormalities in infants born to iodine-deficient mothers. Increasing attention has been paid to the (partially reversible) impaired mental function that can result from iodine deficiency in both school-age children and adults (Hetzel, 1988; Bautista et al., 1982). In addition, a general apathy and lack of initiative among iodine-deficient adults is widely reported (Hetzel, 1988). Kochupillai and Pandar (cited in Levin, 1987) measured significant increases in village income in China attributable to initiation of salt iodination.

IDD are of particular concern among women for two reasons. First, the range of functional consequences is broader for women than for men because it includes severe negative reproductive outcomes for both mothers and infants. Rates of miscarriage, stillbirth, infant mortality, and congenital abnormalities such as deafness, cretinism, and less severe mental retardation are all higher among infants of iodine-deficient pregnant women (Hetzel, 1988). Maternal mortality from cephalopelvic disproportion is higher among cretinous women (ICRW, 1989). In addition to this broader range of functional consequences, the prevalence of goiter appears to be higher among females than males. Simon, Manning, and Jamison (1989) summarize data from nineteen studies that show a consistent pattern of higher prevalence of goiter among women; the sex differential first appears in adolescence and becomes much more pronounced among adults. Although more research is needed, the studies they review suggest a pattern of goiter prevalence peaking in both sexes during adolescence but then declining significantly in males after adolescence. The prevalence of goiter seems not only to remain high among adult women, but also the severity of goiter increases in females with age. Although the reasons for the higher prevalence and greater severity of goiter among women are not well understood, the finding of a similar pattern from different parts of the world (including industrialized as well as developing countries) suggests that at least part of the reason is biological, perhaps aggravated by socioeconomic or behavioral factors.

Biological and Social Determinants of Malnutrition among Women across the Life Cycle

The following discussion of biological and socioeconomic determinants of malnutrition among women first examines the causes of malnutrition among preschool and school-age girls; next, nutritional issues specifically relevant to the adolescent period; and finally, important determinants of malnutrition among adult women, including maternal depletion and various socioeconomic factors affecting women's nutritional status.

Childhood Discrimination and Malnutrition

Gender differences in the long-term consequences of childhood malnutrition could arise either from differences during childhood between boys and girls in the causes or extent of malnutrition or because the experience of having been malnourished as a child presents different risks to men and women during their adult years. The evidence suggests that both of the above are true, at least in some regions.

Ravindran (1986) summarizes much of the literature through the mid-1980s on evidence of parental sex preference in the Third World and of discriminatory feeding and health care practices. The review finds widespread evidence of an expressed preference for sons on the part of parents. Among the countries for which comparable data were available (based on the World Fertility Survey), several (all, except Korea, located in either South Asia or the Middle East) are classified as having a strong preference for sons; many others (including quite a number in West Africa) have a moderate preference for sons; a similar number (including many Latin America and Caribbean countries) have equal preference; and only two (Venezuela and Jamaica) have a slight preference for daughters.

As Ravindran is careful to point out, however, an expressed preference for one sex over the other does not automatically lead to discriminatory allocation of household resources or patterns of care. Indeed, a recent review of fifty different data sets with data on twenty sub-Saharan African countries finds that, with the notable exception of Nigeria, neither anthropometric nor mortality data suggest a pattern of discrimination against females (Svedberg, 1988).[5] It is primarily in those countries of South Asia showing a strong preference for sons (e.g., India, Nepal, Pakistan, and Bangladesh) that consistent evidence of widespread discrimination against girls can be found, resulting in marked sex differences in mortality, morbidity, and malnutrition.

Many studies, in addition to those summarized by Ravindran (1986), show widespread evidence in South Asia of less adequate feeding of girls relative to boys (particularly in circumstances of scarcity); a decreased propensity to seek health care for girls than for boys; and poorer nutritional status of girls compared with boys (Behrman and Deolalikar, 1990; Abdullah, 1989; Gertler and Alderman, 1989; Chatterjee, 1989; Behrman, 1988a, 1988b; Babu et al., 1988). Most of the studies from South Asia that have documented gender bias in nutrition have reported only dietary intake data, but a few have also included anthropometric data. A 1981 study of sex bias in family allocation of food and health care among preschool-age children in Bangladesh found 26 percent of girls to have

---

[5] Svedberg concludes that more evidence points toward discrimination against boys, and he hypothesizes that this is related to a recognized greater efficiency of females in food production, which is reflected in or at least consistent with bride price rather than dowry being widespread in sub-Saharan Africa (see also Alderman, 1990, who reports higher rates of malnutrition among boys in Ghana).

attained less than 85 percent of the standard height of age compared with only 18 percent of boys (Chen et al., 1981).[6]

Other negative consequences of childhood discrimination against girls, which can affect many aspects of women's lives including their adult nutritional status, are underinvestment in girls' education, early marriage and childbearing, and lowered self-confidence and self-esteem (Ravindran, 1986). For example, several investigators have noted that where adult female dietary intake is poorer than that of males, the discrimination is partially if not completely self-inflicted; that is, by adulthood many women in South Asia appear to have accepted a self-sacrificing role that dictates meeting their own needs last (Samarasinghe et al., 1990; Holmboe-Ottesen et al., 1989; Rao Gupta, 1985).

Nutritional Risks and Opportunities during Adolescence

Adolescence presents many risks as well as important opportunities for the nutrition of girls in developing countries. All adolescent girls face some nutritional risks simply by virtue of reaching a certain age or stage in their maturation, while other risks are faced only by sexually active adolescent females.

With menarche, the iron requirements of adolescent girls rise significantly, increasing the risk of iron-deficiency anemia. Although surveys have not documented as consistent a pattern of gender differentials in anemia rates among adolescents as among adults (see DeMaeyer and Adiels-Tegman, 1985), this may be because the gender difference in iron needs among younger adolescents is less than among older adolescents and adults, as well as because the majority of adolescent girls have not yet experienced the substantially increased iron demands of pregnancy. Nonetheless, biological changes that begin in adolescence set the stage for significantly higher rates of both iron and iodine deficiency in adult women.

Sexual maturity also brings about changes in the risks faced by girls and the cultural expectations placed on them, which may be directly or indirectly detrimental to their nutritional status. Simply the potential for becoming pregnant, the inconvenience of being in a public place during menstruation, and the belief in some cultures that menstruating females

---

[6] While the vast majority of studies find a clear pattern of discrimination against females in South Asia reflected in mutually reinforcing evidence of gender differences in mortality, nutritional status, access to health care and education, and cultural practices such as the dowry system or ritualized expressions of regret at the birth of a daughter, a few have called attention to the existence of heterogeneity even within South Asia (Behrman, 1992) or raised questions concerning the interpretation of the discriminatory behaviors (Kakwani, 1986; Pitt et al., 1990).

are unclean are sufficient to place significant limitations on the options open to girls, particularly those living in rural areas (Soysa, 1987; Ravindran, 1986). The dramatic declines in female school participation rates between primary and secondary school that occur in most developing countries may be attributable, in part, to a concern to avoid inappropriate sexual activity or a preference for early marriage (Leslie and Jamison, 1990). The widespread cultural constraints on the freedom of postmenarcheal girls to leave their home or compound may also limit their access to seasonal fruits, commercially prepared foods, or other nutritionally significant sources of dietary diversity (Ravindran, 1986).

Beyond the nutritional risks associated with normal maturation, particular nutritional risks are associated with premature fertility. Several studies, in both industrialized and developing countries, have assessed the nutritional risks and reproductive outcomes of adolescent mothers. Much of this literature has been summarized and reviewed by Olson (1987a, 1987b). Although there are confounding effects of primiparity, prematurity, and differing socioeconomic circumstances, it appears clear that, even adjusting for these factors, adolescent girls (particularly those who are still growing themselves, a process that continues for at least four years postmenarche) are at risk of poorer reproductive outcomes, in part for nutrition-related reasons.

The higher rate of low-birth-weight infants born to adolescent mothers is attributable to the combined effects of shorter average maternal height, competition for nutrients between the mother's growth needs and the growth needs of her fetus, and poorer placental function among adolescent mothers (Scholl et al., 1990; Olson, 1987a; Frisancho et al., 1985). Adolescent girls must gain more weight than older mothers in order to have normal-sized, healthy babies (Olson, 1987a; Geervani and Jayashree, 1988). In addition, controlling for nutrient intake and other confounding variables, concurrent pregnancy and growth in low-income adolescent girls have been found to have a significant negative effect on micronutrient status of adolescent mothers themselves (Scholl et al., 1990).

Although there are both fewer studies and less consensus concerning the risks, if any, of lactation during adolescence, several findings point to possibly significant differences in breastfeeding performance between adolescent and nonadolescent mothers. A study from India found lower weight gain during pregnancy and greater weight loss during lactation among adolescents compared with nonadolescent mothers (Geervani and Jayashree, 1988). Studies by Chan et al. (1987) suggest a higher loss of bone minerals among lactating adolescents, although their findings have been challenged (Olson, 1987b). And finally, a study of Jamaican infants hospitalized for malnutrition found that the longer a child had been breastfed, the older he or she was at hospital admission, but for a similar length of breastfeeding, the babies of adolescent mothers were admitted at a younger age (Bailey, 1981). Considering the high rate of births to adolescents, the substantial energy cost to mothers of lactation, and the importance of successful breastfeeding to infant survival and growth in developing countries, questions concerning lactation among adolescent mothers would seem to warrant considerably more attention than they have so far received.

Recent years have seen a lively debate over the extent to which stunting during the early preschool years can be partially reversed by catch-up growth during the adolescent period (Martorell et al., 1994; see Chapter 2 in this book). It is clear that when previously malnourished children are moved into substantially better environments, dramatic improvements in physical stature can occur (Proos et al., 1992 cited in Martorell et al., 1994; Graham and Adrianzen, 1972). It also appears that more modest catch-up can occur when environments remain essentially unchanged. One example comes from a cross-sectional comparison of height at different ages between rural and urban Kenyan children (Kulin et al., 1982). At age ten, the rural children were much shorter: 12 centimeters for boys and 20 centimeters for girls. Because the pubertal growth spurt and sexual maturation were delayed in the rural sample, their growth spurt continued longer, and by age seventeen for girls (eighteen for boys) there were no longer significant differences in height between the urban and rural samples. The authors hypothesize that, with increasing age, the children were able to obtain relatively more food for themselves and thus caught up in height growth (Kulin et al., 1982). The case for focusing on adolescence as a period of potential catch-up growth is further strengthened by the observation that the average secular increase in height in Europe and North America has been greatest for adolescents (2 to 3 cm per decade) compared with 1 to 2 cm per decade for children and about 1 cm per decade for adults (Eveleth and Tanner, 1976).

Maternal Depletion

The existence of a maternal depletion syndrome was hypothesized by Jelliffe and colleagues based on observations of premature aging among women in the New Guinea Highlands (Jelliffe, 1966; Jelliffe and Maddocks, 1964). Although little subsequent research was undertaken to investigate the specific conditions under which such a syndrome could develop or how widespread it was in the developing world, there has been a recent renewal of interest in the question of maternal depletion (Merchant and Martorell, 1988; Winikoff and Castle, 1987). Winikoff and

Castle conclude from their review of the literature that there is no convincing evidence for the maternal depletion syndrome as a clinical entity and that widespread malnutrition among women in developing countries is more attributable to hard physical work and poverty than to any nutritionally detrimental effects of reproduction per se. While agreeing with Winikoff and Castle that the evidence is far from conclusive, Merchant and Martorell conclude that there is strongly suggestive evidence that the energetic costs of pregnancy and, even more, of lactation, particularly when incurred in a pattern of frequent reproductive cycling (i.e., with little or no recuperative time when a woman is neither pregnant nor lactating) do take a cumulative toll on maternal nutritional status (Merchant and Martorell, 1988).

Several empirical studies shed additional light on the possible nutritional costs of reproduction on mothers. An analysis of nutritional supplement consumption among actively reproductive Guatemalan women reported a significant negative effect on maternal fat stores of concurrent lactation and pregnancy (which occurred among half the pregnant women) and a significant positive effect on maternal fat stores of nonpregnant nonlactating intervals of six months or more (Merchant et al., 1990). Adair et al. (1990) analyzed anthropometric data from a large sample of lactating Filipino women and found that prolonged lactation contributed significantly to short-term depletion of maternal energy reserves (as measured by both weight-for-height and triceps skinfold thickness). A positive association between parity and maternal weight in this sample was interpreted as indicating no long-term depletive effect of reproduction (Adair et al., 1990). Contrary to the finding in the Philippines of no long-term negative effects, however, studies from both Bangladesh (Huffman et al., 1985) and Ghana (Alderman, 1990) report a negative association between parity and women's nutritional status, although it is not clear if this is directly related to either pregnancy or lactation.

Undoubtedly, much of the apparent nutritional stress of reproduction is caused by the strenuous work load during pregnancy and lactation of women in most parts of the developing world. A review of literature on the combined impact of diet and physical activity on pregnancy and lactation concludes that women in the developing world, including those who are pregnant and lactating, are frequently engaged in moderate to high levels of physical activity that are not offset by increases in energy intake. The review concludes that this imbalance between energy intake and energy output is reflected in low weight gain during pregnancy, impaired intrauterine growth, and decreased ability to sustain milk production (NAS, 1989b). Holmboe-Ottesen, Mascarenhas, and Wandel (1989) point to a number of studies that show lower pregnancy weight gain during the peak agricultural season, emphasizing that this is owing to the combined effects of low energy intake and high energy expenditure. As noted earlier, however, research in Kenya found that in the face of inadequate energy intake, during times of high energy need such as the last trimester of pregnancy and the first six months of lactation, women were able to reduce activity levels as a partial compensatory strategy (Neumann et al., 1992).

The specific issue of bone demineralization as a result of lactation is more extensively investigated (Chan et al., 1982, 1987). Although conflicting findings have been reported in the literature, the weight of the evidence suggests that prolonged lactation can cause significant bone demineralization, leading to an increased risk of osteoporosis and bone fracture. Wardlaw and Pike (1986), for example, found no difference in shaft bone mass but a significant (20 percent) reduction in ultradistal-bone mass in women with a history of prolonged breastfeeding, compared with women who breastfed for shorter periods of time. These and similar findings have been reported from studies of women living in industrialized countries who had adequate calcium intakes. This finding suggests that women in certain parts of the developing world, such as Asia or the Middle East, who have small bones and limited dietary sources of calcium may be at high risk of bone demineralization associated with lactation.

The Socioeconomic Context of Malnutrition among Women

The proximate determinants of women's nutritional status—dietary intake, morbidity, reproduction, and activity levels—are influenced by a range of social, cultural, and economic factors, which indirectly determine women's nutritional status by operating through one or more of these proximate determinants. Among these, the three most frequently hypothesized to be significant are level of education, status of women in society, and income earned or controlled by individual women.

Education. The evidence linking higher levels of maternal education with improved child survival and nutritional status is extremely strong (Cleland and van Ginneken, 1988; Ware, 1984; Cochrane et al., 1982), although the extent to which the association represents causality and the specific mechanisms through which women's education may affect the health and nutrition of children are only beginning to be elucidated (Cleland and van Ginneken, 1988; Behrman and Wolfe, 1989). Although it seems reasonable, given the strong effect on child nutrition, to assume that higher levels of education would also be reflected in better nutritional status of women themselves, questions about the strength of the link between women's education and their own nutritional status are indirectly raised by the finding of a significantly stronger effect of maternal education for child than for infant mortality (Cleland and van Ginneken, 1988). To the extent that infant mortality is a better proxy for maternal nutritional status than is child nutrition, this suggests the possibility of a somewhat more limited effect of women's education on their own nutritional status than on that of their children. Behrman and Wolfe (1987b) examine the effect of women's education on their own health and nutrition status in Nicaragua. The main goal of their analysis is to estimate the residual effect of education on health and nutrition outcomes after controlling for the effects of unobserved childhood endowments, and they conclude that there is a significantly stronger residual effect of education on women's nutritional status than on their health status.

Status of women. The multifaceted and culture-specific nature of the status of women, as well as the need, in many cases, for political and legal remedies to improve their status have caused many in the health and nutrition fields to hesitate to investigate this factor as a determinant of women's health or nutrition. Important exceptions include Royston and Armstrong (1989) and Soysa (1987).

Two aspects of the status of women appear to be particularly relevant as indirect determinants of their nutritional status. The first is sex bias in intrahousehold food allocation, which is a particularly significant problem in South Asia. The second is the cultural importance of childbearing to women's status and to their fulfillment of family expectations. Whether it is to achieve standing vis-à-vis her mother-in-law, to demonstrate her husband's virility in the eyes of the community, to provide generational continuity for religious reasons, to produce one or more sons to carry on the family name, or for other culture-specific reasons, women are usually under considerable pressure to produce children. In some settings, women are expected to have as many closely spaced children as possible (Royston and Armstrong, 1989; Soysa, 1987; Caldwell and Caldwell, 1987). In the face of such deep-seated expectations concerning reproduction, even if households are aware (or can be made aware) of possible negative effects of excess fertility on women's health and nutritional status, such concerns may have limited influence on fertility patterns.

Income. Both women's income and their control over household income have been found to influence child nutrition positively (Holmboe-Ottesen et al., 1989; Leslie, 1989b; Blumberg, 1988), but once again empirical evidence concerning the effect of women's income or their control of income on their own nutritional status is limited. A particular difficulty in predicting the effect of women's work on their nutritional status is that work patterns are likely to affect energy expenditure as well as income or food production.

In a study of the intrahousehold allocation of nutrients in a community in rural south India, Behrman and Deolalikar (1990) analyzed the effect of income and food prices on individual dietary intake. Two findings concerning nutrient intakes of women in this study are particularly interesting. One is that when food prices rose, the nutrient intakes of girls and women were adjusted downward more than those of boys and men. Another finding was that although increased female wages were associated with an improvement in the nutrient intakes of most household members, little positive effect was found on the nutrient intakes of women themselves (Behrman and Deolalikar, 1990).

Research by Kennedy (1993) among women in sugarcane farming households in Kenya found that there was no significant association between increasing household income and either the women's total time ill or the women's BMI. Part of the explanation appeared to be that the increased income from sugarcane production was more likely to be controlled by men and to be spent on nonfood expenditures such as housing, education, and transportation.

An interesting difference between urban and rural women emerged from a study in the Philippines of work, income, and dietary intake. Among urban women, income was found to have a positive effect on dietary intake; an additional 200 pesos (US$10) per week was associated with an increased intake of about 250 kcal/day. Among rural women, however, although level of income earned was not significantly associated with dietary intake (in part because there was little variability in rural women's incomes), working women consumed on average 250 kcal/day less than nonworking women (Adair et al., 1990). Because the magnitude of the income effect on dietary intake is small in many studies and because women's work can increase their energy expenditure as well as income, careful local research will be required to clarify the relative importance of work status, income, and income control as determinants of women's nutritional status.

Actions Intended to Influence the Nutrition of Women

The proximate determinants of women's nutritional status are influenced not only by socioeconomic factors but also by practices and interventions specifically intended to affect health and nutrition. These nutrition-influencing actions can be conveniently (although not always neatly) subdivided along two dimensions (see Figure 7.1). One dimension

Figure 7.1. Matrix of actions directly influencing the nutritional status of women

	Origin	
	Household and community practices	Formal nutrition services and interventions
Target: Entire Household	Example: Avoidance of meat for religious reasons	Example: Iodization of salt
Women only	Example: Dietary limitations during pregnancy and lactation	Example: Provision of iron or ascorbic acid supplements to women

distinguishes the initiator or implementor of the action, dividing nutrition-influencing actions into community and household practices on the one hand and formal nutrition and health care interventions on the other. The second dimension distinguishes the target of the action, dividing behaviors and interventions intended to influence the nutrition of the entire household from those specifically directed at women.

The nutritional status of women may be equally or more strongly influenced by actions intended to influence the nutrition of the entire household, through, for example, increased crop yields, higher incomes, food price subsidies, better nutrition knowledge, food fortification, reduced intestinal parasites.[7] Discussion in this chapter, however, focuses on nutrition-influencing actions targeted specifically to women: first, community and household practices intended to influence the nutrition of women; and second, formal nutrition interventions targeted to women.

Household and Community Practices

All cultures have dietary practices that are traditionally recommended during pregnancy and lactation, although there is wide variation in the substance of these practices and the diligence with which they are followed

[7] A useful overview of household and community practices that affect household nutrition (including different food categorization systems, the effect of religious beliefs and ceremonies on food consumption, and culturally required food sharing) can be found in Soemardjan (1985). A detailed examination of the major formal nutrition interventions (including supplementary feeding, nutrition education, food fortification, formulated foods, and food price subsidies) is available in a seven-study series, *Nutrition Intervention in Developing Countries,* coordinated by Austin and Zeitlin (1981).

(Pillsbury et al., 1990; NAS, 1982). Given the increased nutrient needs of women during pregnancy and lactation, an issue of particular interest to health and nutrition professionals is the extent to which culturally recommended practices during pregnancy and lactation increase or decrease the likelihood that women will meet their dietary needs.

In a review of research from developing countries concerning the extent to which women modify their diets during pregnancy, Brems and Berg (1988) cite findings from eighteen different cultures in which food intake is consciously restricted to facilitate easier labor and delivery. They conclude that deliberate restriction of food intake during pregnancy is likely to have a small but significant effect on birth weight, thus perhaps partially accomplishing the objective of facilitating childbirth.[8] Unfortunately, because the research they review focuses on infant outcomes, the authors are unable to reach any conclusions concerning the effect of deliberate food restriction during pregnancy on women's postpartum nutritional status.

In addition to cultural recommendations regarding an overall increase or decrease in food intake during pregnancy, particular foods may be encouraged or discouraged by traditional beliefs concerning maternal cravings, deliberate attempts to "mark" (or avoid marking) the fetus in a particular way, or an effort to protect the health of the mother (Brems and Berg, 1988; Adair, 1987; NAS, 1982). Although such dietary practices vary greatly from one culture to another, two food preferences during pregnancy across a number of cultures—a craving for dairy products and a distaste for caffeinated beverages and alcohol—are likely to be beneficial for the health of both women and infants (Adair, 1987; NAS, 1982). An issue of concern, however, is the fairly widespread practice of discouraging consumption of animal-source foods during pregnancy. A number of studies have found that meat, or meat from particular animals, is specifically withheld, sometimes from women in general but most frequently from pregnant or lactating women (Adair, 1987; Soysa, 1987). Research from Kenya (Neumann et al., 1992), Egypt (Kirksey et al., 1992), and Mexico (Allen et al., 1992) suggests that animal-source foods are important for maternal and infant nutritional status, although it may be the micronutrient content of these foods more than their protein content that is significant for reproductive outcomes.

The literature on dietary practices during pregnancy is reasonably large, but information on dietary practices during lactation is more limited.

---

[8] Because difficulty during delivery is mainly related to infant head circumference (and food restriction has little effect on head circumference), however, important obstetrical benefits are unlikely. Costs for both maternal and infant nutritional status are more likely.

To the extent that specific foods have been reported as encouraged or discouraged during breastfeeding, it is usually only during a specific, fairly short, postpartum period (corresponding in many cultures to a time designated for ritual cleansing and recuperation) rather than throughout lactation. Thus nutritional impact is likely to be relatively limited (Adair, 1987). Nonetheless, the absence of any evidence of household or community practices that encourage increased food consumption throughout lactation (a time when women's energy requirements are even higher than during pregnancy) is cause for concern, particularly in light of the data reported earlier showing limited increases in the energy consumption of women during pregnancy.

Women's Use of Formal Nutrition Services

It is increasingly evident that, in addition to problems of availability, there is serious underuse of health and nutrition services in the Third World (Royston and Armstrong, 1989; Leslie and Rao Gupta, 1989; Stinson, 1986; Akin et al., 1985). The extent of underuse seems to be more serious for preventive than for curative care, and most nutrition interventions fall into the category of preventive care. In addition, although the data are limited and not always consistent, underuse of health services (relative to their needs) appears more widespread among women than among men (Gertler, 1990; Chatterjee and Lambert, 1989; Leslie and Rao Gupta, 1989; Stinson, 1986).

Akin et al. (1985) review and analyze a large number of studies of determinants of demand for primary health care in the Third World. They conclude that some key factors limiting demand for primary health care services are perceived low quality, the provision of preventive care when curative care is desired, and the continuing availability and preference for traditional health care providers. Leslie and Rao Gupta (1989) find that certain factors emerge as particularly critical in determining women's use of maternal care services. First, women appear to have a stronger preference than men for traditional health care providers, in part because many rural women feel less comfortable than do men interacting with formal institutions, and in part because a large percentage of traditional health care providers are female. In addition, distance and inappropriate transportation present a greater barrier to women's than to men's use of health and nutrition services, both for cultural reasons and because women are often encumbered by pregnancy and young children. Also, to the extent that women, particularly in rural areas, are less likely to have access to or control over cash, lack of money is more often a deterrent to their use of services.[9] A final important impediment to the use of health services is the opportunity cost of women's time. Giving up a day or half a day of work to seek care, particularly when women do not perceive themselves to be ill (as is usually the case during pregnancy, lactation, or chronic malnutrition) is likely to seem too high a price to pay.

The effectiveness of supplementary feeding programs for pregnant and lactating women depends on the extent of their participation and the extent to which they share the supplement with other family members or substitute the supplement for their normal dietary intake. Although good participation rates have been achieved in a few programs for pregnant and lactating women, a high level of convenience seems to be necessary (McGuire and Popkin, 1989; Leslie and Rao Gupta, 1989). An analysis of determinants of compliance with nutritional supplements during pregnancy based on data from Guatemala and Indonesia found that characteristics of the intervention, such as its duration and the distance the woman had to travel to receive the supplement, were more strongly associated with participation than characteristics of the women themselves (Rasmussen et al., 1990). One interesting observation on determinants of participation in supplementary feeding comes from Project Poshak in India, where participation rates were found to be higher among lactating than pregnant women, apparently in part because of a reluctance to proclaim pregnancy publicly and in part a desire to avoid a large infant (Gopaldas et al., 1975; cited in Hamilton et al., 1984). The widely reported tendency on the part of women to share their food ration with other family members or to substitute the ration for regular household diet has been addressed in some programs by carefully targeting the neediest women, providing a food less likely to be shared or substituted (e.g., powdered milk) or providing appropriate nutrition education concerning the need for increased food consumption by pregnant and lactating women (Kennedy and Knudsen, 1985; Chávez et al., 1981).

Although fortification of foods with iron can be successful in preventing iron-deficiency anemia at a population level, interventions to prevent or treat iron-deficiency anemia among women in most developing countries are usually based on the distribution of ferrous sulphate tablets to pregnant women.[10] The oral administration of iron sometimes causes gastrointestinal side effects, which can have a negative effect on women's

---

[9] Although many health and nutrition services in developing countries are nominally provided for free, money is usually required for transportation, prescribed drugs or laboratory tests, and unofficial "fees" (Leslie and Rao Gupta, 1989).

[10] Other successful but less frequently used approaches are intramuscular iron injections and provision of vitamin C supplements to enhance the absorption of dietary iron.

participation in iron supplementation programs. Placebos have also been reported to "cause" gastrointestinal problems among pregnant women, and some clinicians and researchers feel that part of the discomfort attributed to iron supplements is actually due to the pregnancy itself (Simmons, personal communication). A recent review of interventions to control iron deficiency concluded that problems of irregular supply and poor monitoring were much more significant causes of limited program effectiveness than were reported side effects of iron tablets (Gillespie et al., 1991).

Conclusions and Recommendations

A lack both of good epidemiological data on nutritional status among adults and of appropriate reference standards (particularly for women during times of rapid tissue change such as pregnancy or lactation) make it difficult to estimate precisely the extent of malnutrition among women in the developing world. Conservative calculations suggest, however, that among adult women (fifteen years or older) living in the Third World, 458 million suffer from iron-deficiency anemia, about 450 million are stunted as a result of childhood malnutrition, about 250 million are at risk of disorders resulting from severe iodine deficiency (almost 100 million have frank goiters), and almost 2 million are blind because of vitamin A deficiency (World Bank, 1993). A problem of this magnitude cannot be ignored; it also cannot be dealt with by a few narrowly targeted feeding programs for pregnant and lactating women on the one hand, or by relying on the long-term effects of broad-based economic development programs on the other.

The lives of women in developing countries differ from those of men for both biological and socioeconomic reasons. In some parts of the developing world, most notably for the one-fourth of developing-country women who live in South Asia, these differences place women at significantly higher risk than men of malnutrition and mortality. Even in countries where women's risk of malnutrition does not appear to be greater than men's, differences between women and men in the causes and consequences of malnutrition and in the constraints they face in trying to improve their nutritional status necessitate a gender disaggregated approach to analyzing nutrition problems and to developing appropriate policies and interventions.

Enhanced female education is likely to be one successful approach. Efforts to expand access to primary and secondary education and to reduce gender differentials in school participation are likely to improve women's nutritional status substantially through delayed childbearing, improved work opportunities, and better dietary practices and use of health and nutrition services.

If further research confirms that supplementary feeding targeted to adolescent girls can reduce the prevalence of permanent stunting, such interventions could be provided (at least in part) through schools. Although relatively expensive, the potential benefits of supplementary feeding to promote catch-up growth of girls during adolescence would be large because such benefits would include reduced morbidity and mortality of mothers and infants and increased productivity of women in their domestic and market work throughout their adult years.

Improvements in the nutritional status of adult women should also be pursued through technologies to reduce energy expenditure. Such efforts will be particularly important during times of high stress, such as the last trimester of pregnancy, the first six months of lactation, and the preharvest agricultural season or periods of seasonally high food prices. Wells, fuel-efficient stoves, grain hullers, bicycles, and plows are a few examples of technologies that could substantially reduce energy expenditure among women, while at the same time increasing their productivity, thus potentially improving their nutritional status in two ways.

The importance of women's nutritional status to their own health, productivity, and quality of life, to the survival and healthy development of their children, and to other family members who depend on women's domestic and market work warrant immediate serious efforts to reduce malnutrition among women, even while multidisciplinary biomedical and social science research continues to quantify more adequately the precise dimensions of the problem (Leslie, 1992). Fortunately, there appear to be feasible avenues for intervention, many of which involve modifying or strengthening ongoing development activities rather than mounting separate programs.

8

Do Child Survival Interventions Reduce Malnutrition? The Dark Side of Child Survival

Sandra L. Huffman and Adwoa Steel

In the last decade, international agencies have developed activities to prevent deaths from a few selected, highly prevalent illnesses among children (Warren, 1988). Prevention of deaths from diarrhea-induced dehydration and immunizable diseases became the central focus of most child survival activities. Other interventions that are part of the child survival package are improved infant and child feeding (breastfeeding and appropriate weaning), growth monitoring, family planning, female education, and food supplementation. Control of acute respiratory infections has recently been added to the child survival strategy.

Of the 12.9 million deaths occurring annually in children under five years of age, over 25 percent are related to underlying malnutrition (UNICEF, 1993b; Pelletier, 1991a; World Bank, 1993). Thus interventions that directly improve child growth may also further reduce mortality. Interventions focused on reducing morbidity also have a potential to improve nutritional status of young children. This chapter assesses whether child survival interventions have led to improvements in nutritional status of young children. The following interventions are discussed: (1) oral rehydration therapy; (2) measles immunization; (3) control of acute respiratory infections; and (4) improving infant and child feeding by promotion of breastfeeding and of improved weaning practices.

Not surprisingly, these topics are similar to those discussed in Feachem's (1986) review of cost-effective interventions potentially useful in preventing diarrhea or its impact on mortality: breastfeeding, weaning educa-

Figure 8.1. Child survival interventions and child growth

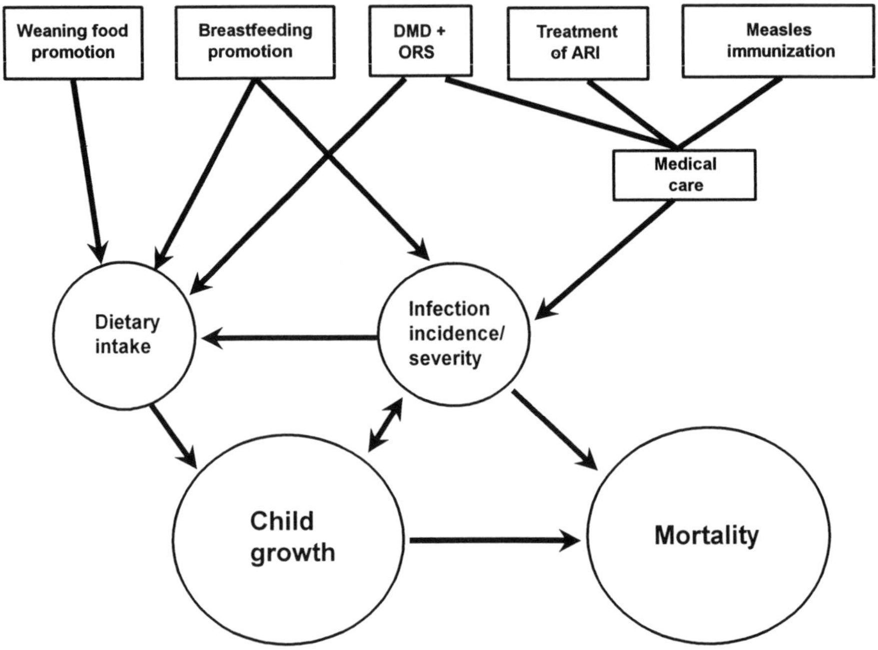

tion, and measles immunization, among others. Other child survival interventions are treated in other chapters and are not dealt with here.

Child survival interventions can affect growth through dietary intake and infections (Figure 8.1). Dietary intake can be enhanced by improved child feeding, including increases in exclusive breastfeeding and appropriate weaning. Infections are associated with increased metabolic rates, anorexia, and decreased nutrient absorption so reduction of infection could affect dietary intake and growth. Infection load can be reduced through several mechanisms: immunization prevents illness; treatment and improved nutritional status can decrease the severity and duration of illness; and reductions in some infections and improvements in nutritional status can enhance the immune status.

Malnourished children have higher rates of morbidity and mortality than well-nourished children. Malnutrition is related to decreased cellular immunity (Kielmann et al., 1983; McMurray et al., 1981) and an increased incidence (Sepúlveda et al., 1988; El Samani et al., 1988; Tomkins, 1981) and/or duration of illness (Black et al., 1983; WHO/CDD/EPI, 1988). Studies in Bangladesh, India, and Papua New Guinea have shown increased mortality rates with decreased weight-for-age, height-for-age, and weight-for-height levels (Pelletier, 1991a; Chen et al., 1980; Heywood, 1982; Kielmann and McCord, 1978; Trowbridge, 1985), and fatality from many illnesses is higher among malnourished children (Koster et al., 1981; Lehman et al., 1988).

High malnutrition rates are generally correlated with high infant and young child mortality rates. Where effective health services are widespread, however, such as in Kerala or Sri Lanka, malnutrition rates may remain high in the presence of declining mortality (Krishnan, 1985). This is the dark side of child survival, and it carries implications for the quality of life of surviving children.

Oral Rehydration Therapy

One of the most frequent causes of mortality and malnutrition is diarrhea. Three million deaths among children under five years are caused by diarrhea, which accounts for 25 percent of all deaths among children (UNICEF, 1993b). Cases of diarrhea in young children are estimated at 750 million to 1 billion each year (Gadomski and Black, 1988). The effect of diarrhea on child growth is well documented (Chen and Scrimshaw, 1983; Tomkins, 1981; Guerrant et al., 1983; Black et al., 1983; Rowland et al., 1988). Diarrhea causes decreased nutrient absorption, decreased dietary intake, and increased catabolism. Recent studies have shown, however, that when energy intake is adequate, diarrhea does not have a negative effect on growth (Lutter et al., 1989, 1992).

Oral rehydration therapy (ORT) programs are expected to include both the promotion of oral rehydration solution (ORS) to prevent dehydration and dietary management of diarrhea to enhance feeding during and following diarrhea. Few if any ORT programs have emphasized prevention of diarrhea to any great extent.

ORS Promotion

The use of ORS to prevent and treat diarrhea-induced dehydration has been widely promoted in many countries (Northrup and Hendrata, 1988). ORS may improve growth through two mechanisms. By preventing dehydration, ORS may reduce the associated anorexia and therefore result in enhanced nutrient intake. It appears, however, that the effects of ORS on growth are short term and that early feeding is more important (Santosham, 1987). Additionally, cereal-based ORS solutions have been shown to shorten the duration of diarrhea, which would be beneficial for child growth (International Child Health Foundation, 1987). When ORS is accompanied by immediate refeeding, its effect on weight gain is similar to that of cereal-based ORS (Kenya et al., 1989).

Dietary Management of Diarrhea

Strategies for promoting improved dietary management of diarrhea include continued feeding during diarrhea, enhanced feeding during convalescence, and improved general dietary practices (Brown and Bentley, 1988).

Continued Feeding during Diarrhea. It has been illustrated in rural Peru and Guatemala that caloric intakes decrease 10 to 20 percent during diarrhea (Mata, 1978; Esrey et al., 1989). Lesser decreases related to diarrhea have been shown when most caloric intake comes from breastmilk (Brown et al., 1985). As stated by Esrey and Bentley (1989), contrary to the common assumption that mothers "starve" their children during diarrhea, most mothers continue feeding but may alter the types and amounts of foods fed. Though mothers continue to offer foods, however, consumption is generally less than normal because the children lack appetite during illness. When the medical profession has intervened, food has been restricted in ill infants because of the misconception that there is a need to "rest the gut" during diarrhea. Households have often restricted breastmilk or food offered to sick children on the advice of physicians. Some ORT programs have attempted to reeducate both professionals and families about the need to continue feeding during diarrhea. The principal constraint, however, is the associated anorexia that limits the child's desire to eat.

The most common means of promoting dietary management of diarrhea has been through education to continue breastfeeding or continue feeding other foods. Even so, evaluations conducted on interactions between health center staff and mothers on feeding suggest that little information on feeding is given in ORT programs. For example, in the Philippines in one-third of rural health units in one province, only 39 percent mentioned the need for continued feeding, while 87 percent recommended the use of home ORS. In Niger, less than 1 percent of health workers provided information on feeding, while 23 percent discussed use of ORS (Stinson, 1989).

In Egypt, for example, rates of continued breastfeeding increased, following the Control of Diarrheal Diseases (CDD) program's campaign, from 68 percent in 1984 to 90 percent in 1986. In The Gambia, during the Control of Diarrheal Diseases campaign, rates of reported breastfeeding cessation during diarrhea decreased from one-third to 3 percent (UNICEF, 1987). The Honduras Mass Media and Health Practices Project had the goal of teaching mothers to prevent and treat acute diarrhea. The campaign included messages on the benefits of breastfeeding and the need to continue breastfeeding during diarrhea, but the rate of feeding during diarrhea did not change (Martorell et al., 1986).

A problem associated with messages to continue feeding is illustrated in one project in Egypt that added nutritional messages to the ORT program to enhance feeding. Messages to continue feeding were the major intervention even though only 10 percent reported stopping food during diarrhea. The recommendation was to continue feeding the normal diet so the intervention would be expected to have little impact on nutritional status because the normal diet would not allow for catch-up growth unless it consisted of more nutrient-dense foods (PRICOR, 1987).

As Griffiths et al. (1988) suggest, however, the simple messages stressed by CDD programs, such as to continue feeding during diarrhea, may be ineffective in changing behavior because communications research illustrates that specific instructions tailored to the situation are more likely to be heard and acted upon. Even when general messages are followed, they may not improve the diet because the normal diet is so low in nutrients, especially the diluted food commonly fed to a child with diarrhea.

Enhanced Feeding during Convalescence. The National Research Council (1985) suggests an intake of 125 percent above normal until preillness weight is attained and ideally until the child reaches normal nutritional status. Studies suggest that such increments in food intake do not commonly occur under normal household conditions. Thus a more appropriate intervention is to encourage households to feed children more food following illness, when anorexia is not a problem.

In rural longitudinal studies in Peru, diets of young children were found to be inadequate, meeting only about 85 percent of requirements, and reductions in dietary intake because of diarrhea were found to average an additional 10 percent decrease from normal intake. To counteract these poor dietary intakes, a nutrient-dense food was promoted during both diarrhea and convalescence. While the normal diet had a caloric density of about 85 kcal per 100 gm, the proposed weaning food that would be suitable during diarrhea contained 200 kcal per 100 gm. It was suggested that the feeding of the food be continued for at least several weeks following the diarrhea and longer if possible. There was no evidence of food withholding during diarrhea, although foods and liquids of lower energy density were offered more frequently. Energy intake was not increased during convalescence over that normally seen.

Results of the intervention in Peru illustrated that mothers generally required a face-to-face demonstration of the proposed food for use during and following diarrhea. Thus, even after an intense campaign with radio, clinic information, market demonstrations, and education in mothers' clubs, only 15 percent of mothers had ever prepared the food at home. Promotion of improved feeding following illness demands special emphasis and knowledge, and few ORT programs include any discussion of feeding, much less the level of intensity needed to change feeding patterns.

Improvements in General Feeding Practices. The third approach is to improve general feeding practices of young children so that diarrhea will not have such negative effects on nutritional status. Few diarrhea disease programs have attempted this approach, however. Recent data from Peru, Guatemala, and Colombia show that when a high-energy nutritionally balanced diet is fed to children, the adverse nutritional consequences of acute diarrhea can be prevented or reduced (Lutter et al., 1992). Becker, Black, and Brown (1989), using regression analyses of data from a longitudinal study in Bangladesh, estimated that if children had energy intakes at the recommended WHO level but diarrhea and fever at average levels for the population, their weight gain would be significantly greater than if both diarrhea and fever were eliminated. These results are supported by another study in Bangladesh that indicated that although *acute* diarrhea (that was treated with ORS) was associated with short-term losses in weight and reductions in linear growth, these deficits were no longer apparent after a few weeks. The authors suggest that "the effects of diarrhea on growth are transient and that efforts to control diarrhea are unlikely to improve children's nutritional status in the long term" (Briend et al., 1989, p.319). In contrast, malnutrition is associated with an increased risk of persistent diarrhea (Bhandari et al., 1989). Therefore, improvements in child nutritional status would aid the objectives of diarrheal control programs.

Previous efforts to treat diarrhea have thus not been associated with improvements in child growth. Preventive strategies recommended by the World Bank Health Sector Priorities Review, however, include promotion of breastfeeding and improved weaning, which would be likely to improve child growth (Martines et al., 1991).

Measles Immunization

Of the immunizable diseases, measles and pertussis exhibit the greatest nutritional consequences, though measles is associated with more deaths. There are about 880,000 deaths caused by measles annually (UNICEF, 1993b). Measles is associated with increased diarrhea and acute respiratory infection (ARI) among young children and has been correlated with increased rates of malnutrition. Pertussis results in about 360,000 deaths and probably contributes substantially to malnutrition because the severe coughing results in several weeks or months of reduced food consumption (Mata, 1978). There are less data on the impact of pertussis on nutrition than of measles.

Measles is associated with weight loss, especially in severely malnourished children. Over one-fourth of children with measles in Mata's (1978) study lost over 5 percent body weight. Because measles leads to diarrhea, acute lower respiratory infection, prolonged anorexia, and reduced food intake, it can have a major impact on child growth. Prevention of measles could therefore be expected to improve child growth.

In The Gambia, however, where promotion of immunization against measles was successful, no improvements in nutritional status of children were reported (Greenwood et al., 1987). Mortality rates remained high even though immunization coverage was high. Competing risks for other illnesses appear to override observable impacts of measles and other immunizations.

In Zaire, no differences were found in the anthropometric status of children receiving measles immunization from that of those not immunized. Mortality in the immunized group was lower until 22 months of age, when survivorship curves approached each other (Kasongo Project Team, 1981).

Holt et al. (1990), in a prospective study in Haiti, compared children who had received measles vaccination to children who had not, assessing survival after two and a half years when the children's median age was 39 months. Although they found lower mortality in the children who had been vaccinated, there was no statistically significant difference in nutritional status (controlling for age) between the two groups of children (Holt, 1987).

Thus, although measles immunization plays an important role in preventing morbidity and mortality, there is little evidence to suggest that it reduces child malnutrition.

Acute Respiratory Infections

Even more frequent than diarrhea are acute respiratory infections, of which there are about five to eight cases per child per year in the developing and developed worlds (Gadomski and Black, 1988). Acute lower respiratory infections (ALRI), more common in developing countries, account for about 3.6 million deaths among children less than five years of age (UNICEF, 1993b). Among infants, the incidence of pneumonia is about 20 to 40 percent, and among children aged one to four years it is 5 to 7 percent in developing countries, up to fifty times higher than in the United States (PRITECH, 1989). Mortality from ARI has been shown to be reduced by 50 to 60 percent using simple technologies (Sazawal and Black, 1992; Stansfield, 1987).

Control of ALRI consists of both curative and preventive actions. Curative measures include case management, which involves the appropriate use of antimicrobial agents when indicated, and supportive measures such as breastfeeding, frequent small feedings, and control of high fever. Prompt appropriate treatment is likely to shorten the severity, duration, and concomitant anorexia and metabolic losses of protein and fat and thus lessen the negative nutritional impact. Fever, often associated with ARI, causes an increase in the metabolic rate, and, because of anorexia and difficulty in breathing and swallowing, ARI is associated with reduced food intake.

Studies in The Gambia found that ALRI had a greater effect on growth per episode than diarrhea (15 gm per day deficit compared to 4 gm per day). Because of the greater prevalence of diarrhea, however, it caused larger total growth deficits (Rowland et al., 1988). These authors estimate that ALRI results in 25 percent of growth deficits and diarrhea in over half.

Preventive actions for ALRI are immunization, appropriate feeding practices (including breastfeeding and adequate vitamin A intake), improved environmental conditions (better housing and adequate ventilation), and prevention of low birth weight. Poor nutritional status is associated with an increased risk and severity of ALRI (Lehman et al., 1988; Berman and McIntosh, 1985). Nonbreastfed infants also have been reported to have higher mortality from ALRI than breastfed infants. Measles and pertussis are major causes of ARI. A study conducted in the Philippines observed that 48 percent of ARI cases were associated with measles (Tupasis et al., 1990). Malnourished infants are ten to twenty times as likely to contract pneumonia as normal weight children. Stansfield and Sheppard (1991) estimate that 70 to 90 percent of all pneumonia deaths occur among the malnourished. Measures that would control ARI (especially improved child feeding practices) are thus likely to have positive effects on growth. At the same time, practices that promote growth are likely to control ARI, particularly ALRI.

In addition to case management, promotion of breastfeeding and reducing child malnutrition are considered strategies to reduce mortality from ARI.

Improving Infant and Young Child Feeding

Appropriate feeding of infants and young children consists of exclusive breastfeeding for the first four to six months of life and the feeding of suitable complementary foods from then on. Breastfeeding has been shown to enhance nutritional status through its direct effect on nutrient intake and its ability to prevent diarrhea, acute respiratory infections, and other illnesses. Programs that have successfully promoted improved weaning foods have resulted in increased dietary intake and improved nutritional status.

Promotion of Breastfeeding

Few interventions have been shown to be as effective in preventing diarrhea among infants as breastfeeding. A case-control study in Brazil illustrated that the risk of mortality from diarrhea is twenty-five times higher in infants aged up to two months who are not breastfed than in infants who are exclusively breastfed (Victora et al., 1987). The risk of mortality from upper and lower respiratory infections and other infections was also found to be consistently higher among nonbreastfed infants than among exclusively breastfed infants.

The role of exclusive breastfeeding in preventing diarrheal morbidity has also been documented in an urban slum area of Lima, Peru. Infants under five months of age who received breastmilk plus other nonmilk liquids (teas, water), had a two times greater risk of diarrhea than infants who received only breastmilk. Infants who received no breastmilk had the highest rates of diarrhea (Brown et al., 1988).

In addition to these community-based studies, hospital-based studies in Indonesia (Lambert, 1988), Costa Rica (Mata et al., 1982), India (Anand, 1981), and the Philippines (Clavano, 1982) have compared the rates of diarrhea in neonatal wards. When breastfeeding was increased in hospitals where bottle-feeding had been the norm, rates of neonatal diarrhea consistently decreased.

Other studies have shown that the severity of illness is less for certain types of diarrhea when the infant is breastfed, even in the third year of life (Clemens et al., 1986; Briend et al., 1988). Breastfeeding is especially important during diarrhea because consumption of other foods is often reduced because of anorexia, as reported in Bangladesh, Peru, India, and Nigeria (Hoyle et al., 1980; Huffman et al., 1988; Bentley, 1988; Bentley, et al., 1988).

The benefits of exclusive breastfeeding for child nutritional status during the first few months of life have been shown in numerous studies (Rowland, 1986; Martines, 1988; Martorell and O'Gara, 1985). Continued breastfeeding, once other foods are introduced into the diet, is also a determinant of nutritional status. Brown et al. (1986) have shown the importance of breastfeeding to nutrient intake among children through the third year of life. In Bangladesh, breastmilk contributed over 60 percent of daily energy and vitamin A and nearly half of the protein intake for children over the age of two years. Briend et al. (1988) also found that among children twelve to thirty-six months those who were breastfed had larger arm circumferences than those who were not breastfed. Numerous other studies in developing countries document the benefits of breastfeeding on weight-for-age of young children (Almroth and Latham, 1982; Greiner and Latham, 1981; Kanaaneh, 1972; Lambert and Basford, 1977; Lebshtein and El Bahay, 1976).

The impact of breastfeeding on extending birth intervals and thereby enhancing child survival and child growth is well documented. It has been estimated that breastfeeding reduced fertility by 34 percent in five countries in Africa, 30 percent in twelve countries in Asia, and 16 percent in twelve countries in South America (Thapa et al., 1988). When birth intervals are increased, the preceding child has a greater chance of receiving better care and feeding from the mother, and the second child is more likely to be born at normal birth weight (Fleming, 1987).

UNICEF and WHO have focused programmatic activities on increasing breastfeeding rates through the Baby Friendly Hospital Initiative. A major aim of the program is to provide training of health professionals in breastfeeding promotion (UNICEF, 1993c). The International Conference of Nutrition held in Rome in 1992 emphasized the importance of promoting breastfeeding for child nutrition in its Plan of Action (ICN, 1992). Increases in breastfeeding are likely to benefit child nutrition both directly and by reducing diarrhea and ARI.

Promotion of Improved Weaning Practices

The weaning period, during which a child gradually becomes accustomed to adult food, is a vulnerable period in the life of infants in developing countries. At the time of weaning, the waning of maternal antibodies in the baby occurs at the same time that the child is losing the full benefit of the antibodies in the breastmilk, which in many cases is being replaced by an inferior diet. Breastmilk alone, however, generally cannot meet the nutrient demands of the infant older than four to six months. The diet fed to infants in many countries is of poor quality (often watery, starchy porridge), and adult diets that young children are expected to eat do not meet their needs. Resource constraints, customs, and lack of knowledge on the specific needs of growing children limit good weaning practices. In addition, traditional weaning foods in many settings have been found to be contaminated (Rowland et al., 1978; Black et al., 1983). Growth faltering and growth retardation are thus common at this time.

The lack of low-cost nutrient-dense foods that can be easily fed to young children has resulted in high malnutrition rates among young children. In developed countries, families have access to instant cereals (easily digested by older infants), animal products (such as cheese, yogurt, eggs, and meat, which provide a high proportion of calories from fat [calorically dense], protein, and other nutrients), automatic stoves, which enable foods to be cooked quickly at low cost, and refrigerators to store cooked food, all of which enable frequent feeding of high-quality foods for young children. In developing countries, however, cereals must be processed to be suitable for young children (at high cost or large time expenditures for mothers), calorically dense foods are costly or not available, cooking frequently during the day requires large amounts of time to gather large quantities of fuel needed to cook noninstant foods, and refrigeration is lacking, all of which impede proper feeding of young children.

Maternal education and time availability are important factors determining whether families are able to overcome these constraints. Households make decisions on the relative importance of how scarce family resources and time are spent. When understanding of the child's special nutrition needs is limited, these decisions may be detrimental to the child's growth.

Although improving the feeding of young children has been theoretically included as a component in child survival interventions, in fact little concentrated effort has been given to this important component. Emphasis in infant feeding has been on promotion of breastfeeding, rather than improved weaning practices. Improving these practices is one of the most effective ways to reduce child malnutrition, but few child survival activities have made it a priority. Improving young children's diets will also result in decreased morbidity and mortality from diarrhea and ARI, the two major causes of children's deaths.

Recent approaches to nutrition education have shown considerable promise for improving infant and child feeding as exemplified by projects in Indonesia and the Dominican Republic (see Chapter 4). Such activities need to become a central tenet of child survival activities to reduce child malnutrition.

Competing Risks of Death and the Impact of Combined Interventions

The assumption that child survival interventions, such as ORT and immunizations, result in major decreases in mortality (Hirshhorn, 1985) has been questioned (Costello, 1988; Kasongo Project Team, 1981). Mosley and Becker (1988) suggest that the overall impact of a specific intervention may be less than estimated because of competing risks of death. They also suggest that broadly based interventions that reduce the risk of several diseases at the same time may have a greater potential for reducing mortality. They emphasize the need not only to look at mortality outcomes but also at the impacts on the child's frailty. High rates of infection, even when treated, are shown to result in increased frailty, which they measure in the child's nutritional status. They emphasize that ORS is unlikely to affect frailty, but dietary management of diarrhea is apt to reduce it.

Through a mathematical model that includes estimates for competing risks of death and effects on frailty, they estimate that much greater reductions in mortality can be obtained by reducing the incidence of illness than by reducing the case fatality of illnesses. ORT obviously works in decreasing the case fatality, while breastfeeding promotion works both by decreasing the incidence of diarrhea and ARI and also directly reducing frailty.

Merson (1988) estimates that if CDD programs focus more on diarrhea prevention through attention to promoting breastfeeding, improving nutrition, and enhancing supply of clean water, sanitation, and personal hygiene, the result would be a 50 percent decrease in deaths from diarrhea. Data from Kerala and Sri Lanka suggest that medical services can reduce mortality from infectious diseases while morbidity remains high (Krishnan, 1985; Perera, 1985). Although immunization rates are high and rates of treatment of diarrheal cases with ORS greater than in many other countries, malnutrition remains high (DHS, 1988; Perera, 1985). As suggested by Joseph (1985), this may be a common pattern in developing countries where declines in mortality are achieved though little is done to reduce illness. High rates of morbidity among children can result in loss of income when parents remain at home to care for children, additional expenses for costs of treatment, reduced potential for children being able to learn when ill, and the suffering associated with illness.

Small-scale community studies in Guatemala (Mata, 1978) and Bangladesh (Black et al., 1983) also illustrate that elimination of certain diseases has little long-term effect on child growth. Studies such as Mata's that show that few preventive measures were taken but illnesses were treated, found continued losses in weight associated with infections. In Black's longitudinal studies in Bangladesh, immunizations against measles, pertussis, and other diseases were given, ORS provided for diarrheal cases, and treatment given for serious illnesses. This resulted in a child mortality rate of 18 per 1,000 children compared to 56 per 1,000 seen in the area surrounding the two villages. Levels of morbidity and malnutrition remained high, suggesting that replacement morbidity is not merely a hypothesis but rather a common occurrence. Thus if a child does not get measles or pertussis, it still remains at risk for lower respiratory infections and diarrhea that cause high morbidity and malnutrition.

In Honduras, it was reported that deaths from diarrhea declined substantially as a result of a mass media campaign to increase use of ORS, but the overall nutritional status of the children was lower at the end of the campaign than before it began (Sanghvi, 1985).

Given the multiplicity of factors that affect growth, it is not surprising that large-scale programs reported to have had favorable effects on growth have tended to have several components (Teller and Mora, 1988). Such integrated efforts in Narangwal, Tamil Nadu, and Iringa have always included improvements in child feeding as an important component.

Summary

Programs that have led to an increase in the incidence and duration of breastfeeding have resulted in improved nutritional status of infants and reductions in morbidity and mortality. Promotion of improved child feeding through appropriate weaning foods using carefully planned nutrition education also has had a beneficial effect on growth. Most of the activity on child survival, however, has been focused on oral rehydration therapy and extended programs of immunization.

- Oral rehydration therapy has dealt primarily with case management rather than prevention of diarrhea, and the available evidence suggests that ORT programs have had little impact on child growth.
- Although measles vaccination averts death, other factors such as poor diet and frequency of other infections seem to override the benefits of the immunization on the child's nutritional status.
- Improving young child feeding is the most direct child survival intervention to improve child malnutrition.
- Programs to reduce mortality from ARI are likely to improve child growth if they include promotion of improved infant and child feeding.

Until now, a major emphasis (by donors, countries, and even families) has been placed on health activities (either curative or preventive) or access to and use of family planning but little has been done to direct resources and political support for a program specifically to improve young child feeding. Poor children, even under conditions of low mortality (as in Kerala and Sri Lanka), have high rates of disease and live their young lives in varying states of malnutrition and thus are unable to live up to their potential in social, intellectual, and psychological development.

All the components of the child survival strategy are important for ensuring the well-being of the child. The evidence examined here shows that when major emphasis is placed on treatment of diarrhea and promotion of immunizations, deaths may be averted, but the surviving children often exist in a miserable state of frequent illnesses and malnutrition with barely enough energy to explore their immediate surroundings. Indeed, it may be argued that because a well-fed child has a much better chance of dealing with the assaults from the generally unhygienic environment found in most developing countries, the central focus of the "child survival revolution" should be the improvement of feeding of young children (and women to increase birth weights) in addition to interventions to control infections.

9

Water and Sanitation: Health and Nutrition Benefits to Children

Susan E. Burger and Steven A. Esrey

This chapter focuses on the two major pathways through which improvements in domestic water supplies, excreta disposal facilities, and hygiene education are thought to have the most direct potential to benefit the health and nutrition of children: (1) reductions in morbidity- and mortality-producing diseases such as diarrhea, and (2) reductions in water collection time with allocation of that time to child health and nutrition-enhancing activities.

Evaluations of water and sanitation projects have emphasized health impacts measured by reductions in diarrhea, improvements in anthropometric indexes of children, or reductions in total mortality; these effects are assumed to result from a reduction in the transmission of pathogens. This emphasis may be understandable in view of the high prevalence and severity of diarrhea among children under age 5 and its significant contribution to protein-energy malnutrition and death. Water and sanitation projects also have the potential to reduce exposure to pathogens that cause other diseases such as guinea worm, schistosomiasis, ascariasis, and trachoma. These diseases also afflict adults. Therefore, reductions in morbidity have the potential to benefit all members of households and communities, not just children.

The potential health benefits of water and sanitation actually extend

The authors wish to thank the Water and Sanitation for Health Project, the International Center for Research on Women, Katherine Tucker, Barry Popkin, and Joanne Leslie for documents provided and literature suggested, and the staff of the Interlibrary Loan Service at Cornell University for their efforts in tracking down difficult-to-find articles. They also wish to thank Harold Alderman, Per Pinstrup-Andersen, Sandy Cairncross, Jean-Pierre Hab-

153

far beyond those resulting from pathogen reduction alone. Accessible domestic water supplies have the potential to augment women's limited resources of time, energy, and income. Time saved by access to water that is closer to the home may be translated into more time spent on food production, income generation, self-improvement, and leisure, all of which may have an indirect impact on child health and nutrition. Allocation of time saved to child care activities such as feeding may have a direct impact on child health and nutrition. The energy saved may be particularly important during periods of low water availability and seasonal increases in agricultural work load, which often coincide with decreased food availability as well as energy stress such as pregnancy and lactation. Thus the easing of the energy-expenditure burden by more accessible water supplies might improve the nutritional status of the mother, the fetus, and the nursling. The increased available water could be used not only for hygienic purposes but also in home gardens, meal or beverage preparation, small animal husbandry, livestock production, and other water-requiring activities that increase food consumption or purchasing ability.

This chapter is limited to evidence for the two pathways described above through which improved water and sanitation may affect child health and nutrition. Each of the theoretical steps through which these pathways might confer benefits to children is examined separately because evidence for all of the intermediate steps is not available in just one study. If each separate step occurs as theorized, the pathway between the water and sanitation interventions and the health or nutrition outcome is considered to be plausible. For example, if evidence from several studies establishes that water supplies brought closer to the home reduce the time spent collecting water, the time saved is used to prepare more food, the preparation of more food results in greater energy intake by children, and that greater energy intake is associated with better growth, then it is plausible that water brought closer to homes improves child nutritional status through increased nutrient intake, not just by reduced disease.

In addition, studies that report the conditions under which single or combined water and sanitation interventions have the largest impact are included because such information may be useful for targeting, prioritizing, or combining interventions. Improvements in water supply may influence water quantity, water collection time, water quality, or some combination of the three. Distinctions between the impact of water quantity and quality are discussed in the section on pathogen reduction. Those

icht, Joanne Leslie, and David Pelletier for the thoughtful comments they provided while reviewing earlier drafts of this chapter. The authors take sole responsibility for any errors that remain.

Figure 9.1. Influence of water and sanitation on child health through decreased exposure to pathogens

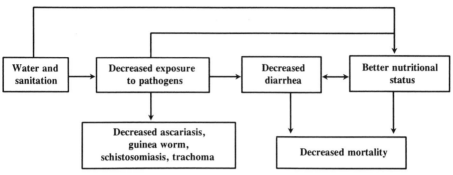

studies that report on distance traveled or time spent to collect water are discussed in the section on time savings.

Influence of Improved Water and Sanitation on Reductions in Pathogen Exposure and Disease

Evidence That Water and Sanitation Decrease Exposure to Pathogens

Water and sanitation interventions are thought to affect health primarily by reducing exposure to pathogens (Figure 9.1). Diminishing the ingestion of pathogens has the potential to prevent mortality and morbidity from diarrheal illness, an advantage not conferred by oral rehydration therapy, which only prevents the consequences of dehydrating diarrhea once it occurs. Furthermore, improvements in water and sanitation have the potential to reduce other diseases by intervening in their life cycle. Pathogens that lead to infection and disease may be transmitted by several routes including fecal-oral (e.g., all major diarrheal pathogens and *Ascaris*), fecal-cutaneous (e.g., hookworm and *Schistosomes*), cutaneous-oral (e.g., guinea worm), or cutaneous-cutaneous (e.g., trachoma and scabies). Some pathogens need intermediate hosts (e.g., guinea worms and *Schistosomes*) or a period outside the human host (e.g., *Ascaris* and hookworm) for transmission.

Thus ingestion of contaminated water (diarrheal disease agents and guinea worm), exposure to pathogens through poor personal and domestic hygiene (diarrheal disease agents, *Ascaris, Schistosomes,* and trachoma), or improper disposal of feces (diarrheal disease agents and intestinal para-

sites) can cause disease. Breaking these routes of transmission would reduce the incidence and severity of several diseases.

Decreased exposure to pathogens is inferred by use of latrines and
measured contamination levels on hands and drinking water with feces.
Community water supplies are often clean at the point of water collection
but become contaminated with feces between collection and ingestion
(Rajasekaran et al., 1977; Feachem et al., 1978; Shiffman et al., 1979;
Esrey, 1987). Thus improvements in the quality of drinking water may
be lost or diminished if the collection point is far from the point of ingestion or if ingestion is sufficiently delayed to allow contamination to occur.
Washing hands with or without soap also reduces contamination (Lowbury et al., 1964; Sprunt et al., 1973; Khan, 1982; Aung et al., 1986).
Finally, disposal of feces in properly constructed facilities should reduce
environmental contamination, but environmental contamination is difficult to measure. People live over a film of contamination, much of it
animal in origin.

Diarrheal and intestinal parasitic diseases can result in poor growth
through decreased absorption of nutrients and increased requirements,
thereby contributing to general protein-energy malnutrition (Martorell et
al., 1975; Cole and Parkin, 1977; Guerrant et al., 1983; Rowland et al.,
1988) as well as specific nutrient deficiencies such as vitamin A deficiency
from *Ascaris* and *Giardia* (Sivakumar and Reddy, 1975; Mahalanbis et
al., 1976, 1979) and iron deficiency from hookworm (Holland, 1987) and
Schistosomes (Stephenson, 1987). This situation may be exacerbated by
the reductions in energy intake that can accompany diarrhea (Mata et al.,
1977; Hoyle et al., 1980; Martorell et al., 1980; Molla et al., 1983; Esrey
et al., 1989).

The contribution of malnutrition as measured by anthropometry has
been found to be associated with a longer duration of subsequent diarrhea
(Black et al., 1984; Bairagi et al., 1987). Conflicting evidence exists, however, for the relationship between anthropometry and the subsequent incidence of diarrhea (Black et al., 1984; Bairagi et al., 1987; El Samani et
al., 1988; Sepúlveda et al., 1988). Regardless of the conflicting evidence
for nutritional status and subsequent diarrheal incidence or duration,
water and sanitation interventions may both reduce diarrhea and improve
nutritional status. Improvements in one are likely to reinforce improvements in the other.

Evidence of Improved Health and Nutritional Status
after Decreasing Pathogen Exposure

Decreased exposure to pathogens is inferred best by examining reductions in diseases. Systematic reviews (Esrey et al., 1985; Esrey and Ha-

Table 9.1. Expected reduction in morbidity and mortality from improved water and sanitation

Indicator of results	All studies			Better studies		
	No. of studies	Median (%)	Range (%)	No. of studies	Median (%)	Range (%)
Diarrhea						
morbidity	49	22	0–100	19	26	0–68
mortality	3	65	43–79	—	—	—
Ascariasis	11	28	0–83	4	29	15–83
Guinea worm	7	76	37–98	2	78	75–81
Hookworm	9	4	0–100	—	—	—
Schistosomiasis	4	73	59–87	3	77	59–87
Trachoma	13	50	0–91	7	27	0–79
Child mortality	9	60	0–82	6	55	20–82

Source: Esrey et al., 1991. By permission of the *Bulletin of the World Health Organization.*

bicht, 1985, 1986; Esrey et al., 1991) show that better water and sanitation is associated with decreased diarrheal morbidity, improved nutritional status, lower childhood mortality, and less morbidity from ascariasis, guinea worm, schistosomiasis, and trachoma. Evidence from human volunteer studies indicates a dose-response for diarrheal pathogens (Bille et al., 1964; Blaser and Newman, 1982; Dupont et al., 1971; Cash et al., 1974). Furthermore, the median reduction in diarrhea-specific and overall child mortality rates was found to be greater than the median reduction in morbidity rates following improvements in water and sanitation (Table 9.1). This suggests that as the dose of ingested pathogens is reduced, the severity of disease will decline first, followed by the incidence. Greater reductions in severity compared to prevalence or incidence have also been reported for *Ascaris* (Sahba and Arfaa, 1967; Arfaa et al., 1977), hookworm (Arfaa et al., 1977), and guinea worm (Tayeh and Cairncross, 1989), in which reductions in egg counts or worm load were larger than reductions in prevalence. For example, the magnitude of improvement in health outcome has been shown to increase from no sanitation, to latrines, to toilets (Anker and Knowles, 1980; Haines and Avery, 1982; Esrey, 1993). The evidence for a dose-response indicates that the level of a particular intervention should influence the degree of pathogen transmission and disease reduction.

The number of pathogens transmitted also depends upon the route(s) available and the opportunity for proliferation. Therefore, some interventions may reduce the transmission of pathogens by a greater number, and therefore reduce disease to a greater extent, than others. For instance, proper disposal of contaminated feces may reduce the number of pathogens being transmitted through several routes of exposure such as food, hands, and drinking water. Once in the environment, pathogens may not only survive and disperse but thrive in food or media that is ingested by young children (Barrell and Rowland, 1979; Esrey and Feachem, 1989; Imong et al., 1989). In addition to proper fecal disposal, increasing the quantity of water available may reduce the proliferation of pathogens in contaminated food if more water results in more frequent preparation and feeding, thereby reducing the opportunity for pathogens to multiply sufficiently to cause disease.

Results of studies that examine the health effect of water and sanitation can be extremely variable (Table 9.1). Impacts range from none to reductions in disease rates well over 50 percent for all health indicators so the average reductions in morbidity and mortality yield less information than understanding the conditions that produce the maximum beneficial impacts. Several reasons exist for this wide range of impacts, including the level and type of intervention, the degree of environmental contamination, and the extent to which the evaluation design and analyses account for sample biases and confounding. The actual success of an intervention depends largely on the degree to which pathogen exposure is reduced. Two questions arise from such an explanation: (1) Is the water or sanitation intervention targeted to eliminate the main route(s) of exposure to pathogens? (2) Is the water or sanitation intervention targeted to population groups whose practices are already reducing their exposure to pathogens? In other words, is the water or sanitation intervention designed to complement or compensate for other conditions that affect the transmission of pathogens? Water and sanitation interventions that complement pathogen-reducing factors would likely result in great improvements in health (Briscoe, 1984) when both are present. On the other hand, water and sanitation interventions that reduce pathogens in the same way as another particular pathogen-reducing factor would likely result in small or no improvements in health when the other factor is present but compensate for the absence of the factor with larger improvements in health.

The best way to examine whether water and sanitation complement or compensate for particular conditions is to evaluate the effects when an intervention occurs in the presence or absence of factors such as breastfeeding or of varying levels of factors such as education. The purpose of examining these varying conditions is to determine whether and where to target specific interventions, whether and in what order to introduce interventions, and whether and how to combine several interventions. Studies in which the effects of water and sanitation across different levels of socioeconomic, cultural, and environmental factors are reported are summarized in Table 9.2 and described below. Studies that compare the impact of combined interventions are also described.

Sanitation

Health impact studies that include analyses of improved excreta disposal among varying socioeconomic or environmental conditions were found for five countries: Malaysia, Fiji, Sri Lanka, Lesotho, and Malawi (see Table 9.2). Flush toilets existed in three locations and latrines in the other two. The other conditions present included breastfeeding and not breastfeeding, high and low income, high and low educational level, greater and lesser water quantity, and good and poor water quality. The analyses conducted in the studies below controlled for factors known to have the potential to confound the outcome of water and sanitation evaluations. This control renders the results more plausible.

Sanitation and Breastfeeding. In Malaysia, the presence of flush toilets was found to have the largest effect on mortality among nonbreastfed infants (Butz et al., 1984). In households with neither flush toilets nor piped water, nonbreastfed infants were five times more likely to die than breastfed infants, but in households with a flush toilet were only two and a half times more likely to die (Habicht et al., 1988). Thus presence of a flush toilet in the home reduced the relative risk of death for nonbreastfed compared to breastfed infants by twofold. Although flush toilets reduced the infant mortality rates among breastfed infants, the effect was much less. This suggests that breastfeeding acts independently of sanitation in reducing the transmission of pathogens and that breastfeeding and flush toilets are compensatory.

Sanitation and Income. In a native Fijian population, the presence of a flush toilet had its largest impact on anthropometry among preschool children in low-income households (Yee, 1984). The mean height-for-age of children in low-income households with a flush toilet was significantly higher than those with a pit toilet or no toilet at all, whereas the magnitude of the difference between those with and without flush toilets was much smaller among children in high-income households (Yee, 1984). A similar relationship was reported for weight-for-age (Yee, 1984). Households in rural areas had lower incomes compared to urban areas. Thus weight-for-age and height-for-age were greater among children in homes with flush toilets than without in rural but not in urban households (Yee, 1984). Because occupation was associated with income, the most marked difference in anthropometry between children in households with and without flush toilets occurred among those whose families earned income from farming, the occupation with the lowest average income (Yee, 1984). These findings suggest that improved sanitation will compensate for poverty and will have its greatest effect among low-income rural populations.

Sanitation and Education. In another analysis of the Malaysian data, the presence of flush toilets was found to have its largest effect on mortal-

Table 9.2. Conditions in which improvements in water and sanitation interventions may maximize child health benefits

Intervention	Joint effect of the intervention and the condition	Condition	Health benefit	Country/years of study (references)
I. Sanitation				
flush toilets	compensates for	not breastfeeding	< IMR	Malaysia/1976–1977 (Butz et al., 1984; Habicht et al., 1988)
	compensates for	low income	> W/A & H/A	Fiji/1981 (Yee, 1984)
	compensates for	illiteracy	< IMR	Malaysia/1976–1977 (Esrey and Habicht, 1988)
latrines	complements	literacy	< IMR	Sri Lanka/1975 (Meegema, 1980)
	complements	more water usage	> W & L gain	Lesotho/1984–1985 (Esrey et al., 1992)
	complements	less contaminated water	< diarrhea	Malawi/1985 (Young and Briscoe, 1987)
II. Water				
piped water	compensates for	not breastfeeding	< IMR	Malaysia/1976–1977 (Butz et al., 1984; Habicht et al.; 1988)
	compensates for	low income	< CMR	Brazil/1970–1976 (Merrick, 1985)
	compensates for	low income	> W/H	Fiji/1981 (Yee, 1984)
	complements	literacy	< IMR	Malaysia/1976–1977 (Esrey and Habicht, 1988)
	compensates for	low educational status	< CMR	Brazil/1970–1976 (Merrick, 1985)
more quantity	compensates for	large family size	< diarrhea	Haiti/1976–1977 (Thacker et al., 1980)
	complements	frequent maternal bathing	> W & L gain	Lesotho/1984–1985 (Esrey, 1987)
better quality	complements	high income	< diarrhea	Philippines/1977–1985 (Magnani et al., 1984)

Note: The table should be read as follows:

The intervention in column (1) complements or compensates for as indicated in column (2) for the condition (or intervention) in column (3) with the resulting health benefit in column (4). The first entry could be read as follows: flush toilets compensates for the lack of breastfeeding by reducing the infant mortality rate (Health benefit); < and > correspond to reduction or increases. IMR = infant mortality rate; CMR = child mortality rate; W/A = weight-for-age; H/A = height-for-age; W/H = weight-for-height; W + L gain = growth in weight and length.

ity among infants of illiterate mothers (Esrey and Habicht, 1988). Literacy was a more sensitive indicator of mortality than education. The magnitude of the effect for toilets was greater than for literacy when the effect of two was compared. Conversely, in Sri Lanka, the presence of a flush toilet had a larger (but not significant) impact on the mortality among infants of literate than illiterate mothers (Meegema, 1980). The analyses conducted with Malaysian data controlled for potentially confounding factors including breastfeeding, whereas the analyses reported in the Sri Lankan study did not. These contrasting results make it difficult to predict impacts from improved sanitation among populations with different educational levels. They also suggest that changes in hygiene behavior associated with improved sanitation will influence health impacts. Thus it is difficult to know if improved sanitation and knowledge of proper sanitation complement each other or each compensates for the lack of the other.

Sanitation and Water Quantity. In rural Lesotho, child growth was found to be greater among households that had both a latrine and increased their water usage than among those that only increased their water usage, only had a latrine, or neither. This was true whether or not improved water supplies had been installed in the village (Esrey et al., 1992). These results were more pronounced among infants than among older preschool children. Because proper excreta disposal complemented the use of adequate water, the two should be promoted together as an effective means of reducing pathogen exposure.

Sanitation and Water Quality. A study of the impact of sanitation and water quality was conducted in rural areas of Malawi (Young and Briscoe, 1987). The risk of diarrhea in children under five years of age was 20 percent less among those whose families had both a piped water system and a latrine than among those whose families had neither. Although these results were not statistically significant because of the small sample size, the trend was clear. There was little difference in the quantity of water used by those with and without a piped water supply, but the fecal coliform count was significantly lower both at the source and in the home for water collected from the piped water supply than from other sources (Young and Briscoe, 1987). These findings suggest that improved sanitation will enhance the effect of piped water in reducing exposure to pathogens, but this relationship needs to be replicated in other areas with larger samples. In addition, the effect of improved water quality and latrines together should be compared separately to the effect of improved water quality alone, to the effect of latrines alone, and to the effect of neither to determine whether the effect of both interventions together is greater than the separate effect of each.

Water

Studies that include analyses of the impact of improved water supplies by varying socioeconomic or environmental conditions were found for three countries: Malaysia, Fiji, and Brazil. None of these studies includes explicit evidence for whether households with piped water used a greater quantity or better quality of water than those without.

Water and Breastfeeding. Presence of piped water in Malaysia significantly reduced the mortality rates among nonbreastfed infants seven to twelve months of age (Butz et al., 1984). The lower risk of death cannot, however, be attributed to piped water alone because the vast majority of households in which piped water was present also had flush toilets. The magnitude of the impact of piped water among households with flush toilets was less than that of flush toilets alone (Habicht et al., 1988), possibly because many households with sanitation did not have piped water, whereas few households with piped water were without sanitation. Nevertheless, these findings suggest that, among breastfed infants, piped water will complement sanitation in reducing transmission of pathogens because an effect of piped water was found even when toilets were present.

Water and Income. In an urban area of Brazil, piped water in the home was associated with reduced mortality among preschool children (Merrick, 1985). The biggest reduction in child mortality occurred when piped water was available to low-income households (Merrick, 1985). As access to water increased over time, the significance of the association between income and reductions in child mortality disappeared (Merrick, 1985). This finding suggests that access to piped water reduced the differential impact of income on childhood mortality. A similar relationship between piped water and income was observed in Fiji for the impact on weight-for-height (wasting) among preschool children (Yee, 1984) suggesting that piped water can reduce exposure to pathogens to a greater extent among the poor than among the better-off. Whether the effect of piped water among low-income groups can be achieved without adequate sanitation is not known, but the results from the studies discussed above indicate that the addition of proper sanitation would maximize the health impact.

Water and Education. In Malaysia, the presence of piped water was found to reduce mortality among infants of literate mothers more than among infants of illiterate mothers (Esrey and Habicht, 1988). The analyses control for the effects of breastfeeding described above.

In contrast, analyses of data from urban Brazil show the opposite trend. The effect of piped water on mortality reduction was greater among children of less-educated mothers than among children of better-educated mothers (Merrick, 1985). These contrasting results make it difficult to predict impacts from improved water supplies among populations with different educational levels. The differences in conditions such as breastfeeding patterns (short duration in Brazil and longer in Malaysia) and age of the subjects in the two study populations could contribute to the discrepancy in results if maternal educational level has a different effect for different degrees of contamination or among different age groups. A more likely explanation may be differences in piped water. Improvements in water quality might have a different impact among children of mothers with different educational levels if education influenced either decontamination of impure water or protection of clean water from recontamination. Water quantity might have a better impact among children of better-educated mothers if education influenced the use of water for hygienic activities when sufficient water is available. The conflicting results make it difficult to know if improved water supplies and education are complementary or compensatory, particularly without identifying whether water quantity increased or water quality improved.

Water and Hygiene Education. Both hand pumps and hygiene education were introduced in a rural area of Bangladesh where levels of education were minimal. Unfortunately, both of these interventions infiltrated the nonintervention areas so it is difficult to determine the extent to which the interventions are responsible for the observed effects. In addition, there is no indication of whether the hand pumps improved water quality or quantity. The differences in the intervention and the nonintervention areas indicate that hygienic practices may complement the use of water from hand pumps. A larger decrease in diarrhea incidence was found among children of mothers who used hygienic practices compared to those who did not, and households in which at least one hygienic activity was practiced were more likely to be those in which several hygienic activities were practiced (Alam et al., 1989b). The incidence of diarrhea among children 6 to 23 months old in the intervention areas did not drop significantly until at least three of the four hygienic activities (use of hand pump water, no feces in yard, handwashing before serving food, and handwashing after defecation) were practiced together (Alam et al., 1989a). In the nonintervention areas, where fewer hand pumps were available, the incidence of diarrhea among six- to twenty-three-month-old children was higher, and hygienic practices had less of an impact than in the intervention areas.

Water Quality versus Quantity

Improved water supplies (i.e., more water or cleaner drinking water) may decrease exposure to pathogens. Previous reviews of water and sanitation interventions concluded that water quantity appeared to be more effective than water quality in contaminated environments and that water quality might not have an effect until most major routes of contamination were eliminated (Esrey and Habicht, 1986; Esrey et al., 1991). Studies that explicitly document whether improvement in the water supply was owing to water quality or quantity are discussed below.

Water Quantity and Crowding. During a drought-induced water shortage in urban areas of Haiti with high unemployment and low educational attainment, less water usage was associated with more illness and malnutrition in preschool children (Thacker et al., 1980). The effect of less water usage on rates of diarrhea and other illnesses was larger among children of families with more than four members than among children of smaller families. These findings suggest that the amount of water may be more critical for larger families, among whom person-to-person transmission is more likely, than for smaller families.

Water Quantity and Maternal Bathing. The combination of increased water usage with frequent maternal bathing, a proxy for better hygiene practices, was associated with better child growth in Lesotho (Esrey, 1987). Although the presence of either factor alone had a positive association with growth, only when both factors occurred together was the greatest growth evident. The same characteristics that lead to frequent maternal bathing may also lead to other hygienic behaviors that benefit child health. These findings suggest that if water is available and better hygiene is practiced, pathogen transmission can be reduced and health benefits can be achieved. Which behaviors are most responsible for the better growth of children cannot be determined from the data available.

Water Quality and Income Level. In urban areas of the Philippines, water quality was associated with low diarrhea rates only among children in high-income households (Magnani et al., 1984). Sanitation facilities and better hygiene practices were also associated with less diarrhea and better nutritional status, but these factors were controlled for in the analysis of water quality by income. If the quality of water was most beneficial to high-income households, it may be because pathogens are transmitted less frequently through routes other than drinking water in these households. When water quality is improved and transmission from other routes is already reduced by other means, then improving drinking water may effectively reduce transmission of pathogens. Conversely, if other routes of transmission are not broken, then improvements in drinking water may have little impact. These results suggest that improvements in drinking water quality complement improvements in sanitation and usage of more water but cannot compensate for the lack of either one.

General Trends
The above relationships indicate that improved sanitation has the largest impact in contaminated environments where breastfeeding is cur-

tailed and income is low. The effect of sanitation among breastfed infants is less, although still present. Sanitation appears to compensate for a low level of each factor. For instance, income-related discrepancies in child health indicators appear to diminish or even disappear when improved sanitation is introduced.

The effect of sanitation at different levels of education and literacy is less straightforward. Education may influence the degree of contamination before the introduction of the intervention, as well as the adoption of the intervention. This might explain why the better educated or literate benefited more in some studies and the less educated or illiterate benefited more in others. If better-educated mothers practice better hygiene than less-educated mothers, then children of less-educated mothers would live in a more contaminated environment and would stand to benefit more from improved sanitation than children of better-educated mothers. But if less-educated mothers are not as willing to use improved sanitary facilities, then the health and nutrition of their children will not improve. This may be one explanation for the discrepancy between the effects of education and sanitation in Malaysia and Sri Lanka. The literate in Malaysia may have practiced more hygienic methods of excreta disposal than the illiterate before the introduction of latrines, and the literate in Sri Lanka may have adopted the use of latrines more readily than the illiterate.

It appears that latrines and piped water together have a greater impact than either one alone. The effects of piped water interventions on improved health are more difficult to interpret than for sanitation because the effects could be caused by improved water quality, increased quantity, or both. The impact of improved water supplies in contaminated environments may be muted because, in many cases, proper sanitation does not exist, thereby permitting pathogen exposure to continue through other routes. These other routes may contribute substantially to pathogen exposure and disease. Nevertheless, piped water and sanitation benefit similar population groups. Piped water appears protective in areas of poverty and where breastfeeding is curtailed or not prevalent. Thus piped water can reduce the differences in health and nutrition between socioeconomic groups when installed in contaminated areas and in areas lacking other means to reduce pathogen transmission.

As with sanitation, the effect of piped water in areas where levels of education differ is not straightforward. Education could influence the degree of prior contamination, the use of the improved water supply, or the adoption of behaviors that maintain or enhance the improvements in the water supply. It is theoretically possible that improved water quality would benefit the less educated more than the better educated because the latter group already takes measures to decontaminate impure water.

If the better educated already know how to use more water for hygienic purposes when it is available, then increased quantity of water would do the reverse; it would benefit the better educated more than the less educated.

According to this line of reasoning, the larger effect of piped water among infants of the literate in Malaysia may have been due to more water, whereas the larger effect of piped water among children of the less educated in Brazil might have been due to better water. If the effect of piped water in Brazil among children of less-educated mothers was due to improved water quality, however, one would have expected to see a greater reduction in mortality among children of high-income households, congruent with the greater reduction in diarrhea among children of high-income households in the Philippines, where the improvement in water quality was measured. Instead, children of low-income households benefited more from piped water in Brazil.

It is also possible that improved water quality would benefit the better educated more than the less educated because the latter group takes measures to protect the improved drinking water from recontamination. This would be consistent with an improvement in water quality in Malaysia. If both water quality and water quantity improved together, positive effects among all children would be expected although the mechanism for better health may not be known. The effects of increased water quantity could be enhanced through better hygiene practices, but this may be confounded by increased time savings, which was not examined in any of these studies. Verification or refutation of these speculative explanations for the apparent connection between educational level and the impact of improved water supplies depends upon actual observation and quantification of hygienic behaviors, as well as identification of whether water quality or quantity improved.

Hygiene education appears to enhance the adoption of activities that improve the use and, hence, the impact of piped water. This seems to support the complementarity of improvements in water supply and hygienic behaviors but does not identify whether this is because of improved water quality or increased water quantity, and the specific hygiene practices are difficult to identify.

Although the separate effects of water quantity and quality are difficult to measure, the use of more water appears to have larger impacts than improvements in the quality of drinking water. The impact of increased water quantity may be greater in more contaminated environments, such as among children living in crowded households, than in less contaminated environments. Larger families could influence the need for more water and better hygiene because of increased exposure to pathogens through person-to-person contact, particularly if they have less housing space per child or if mothers or larger families have less time to spend per child. An increase in the quantity of water used may also partially or completely explain the larger effects of piped water among children of low-income households and among nonbreastfed infants, and a failure to increase water usage may explain the lack of positive results in other studies. The effect of water quantity on pathogen reduction may also depend on the adoption of hygienic activities permitted by the increased use of water. This theory is consistent with the findings in Lesotho. Thus, increasing water usage appears to compensate for the lack of some pathogen-reducing measures in highly contaminated environments but in conjunction with other pathogen-reducing measures that depend on sufficient water.

Improved water quality appears to complement other interventions, and the effects may be realized only in environments where contamination from other sources is low, as observed among children of high-income households in the Philippines. Contamination would likely be less among high-income households because these families have reduced their exposure to pathogens by better housing, sanitation, and hygienic practices. If improved water quality does not compensate for lack of pathogen reduction through other routes, then many water projects need to include improved sanitation and more water for better hygiene. Conclusive judgments of whether the largest impacts of piped water are due to water quality or quantity cannot be made until these differences are quantified and examined across different sites. Furthermore, hygienic behavior associated with these interventions needs to be understood.

Influence of Improved Water Supplies on Time Savings and Improved Child Health

In reviewing the role of women in water collection, van Wijk-Sijbesma (1985) concludes that water collection is probably one of the most time-consuming domestic chores. Although women occasionally get help from men and children in collecting water, nearly all the burden of this duty falls on women. If collection times were reduced by the provision of more readily accessible water supplies, then the potential to improve child health could be realized by converting this time into other beneficial activities (Figure 9.2).

Time saved from more readily accessible water could be spent on new activities, or the time spent on existing activities could be extended. In either case, child health could benefit by improving nutrient intake, de-

Figure 9.2. Influence of improved water supplies on child health through time savings

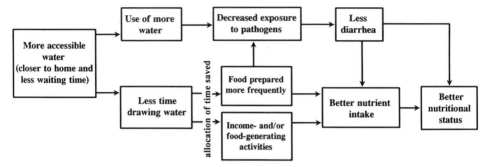

creasing the exposure to pathogens, or both. For instance, more frequent food preparation in an environment where refrigerators are a luxury may diminish food contamination, thereby reducing disease; and where bulky foods are common it may permit the child to eat more frequently, thereby increasing the total energy intake. This is just one of many time-consuming child care activities that may enhance child health and nutritional status.

Time Spent Collecting Water

The total time spent collecting water varies widely throughout the world, from virtually no time, where taps are in the home, to an estimated twelve hours per day (Russell, 1979). The time spent collecting water depends upon means of transportation, the terrain, the distance, the waiting time, the consumption rate, the number of consumers in the household, and the number of people available to collect water (Curtis, 1986). Seasonal and climatic changes can also substantially influence the time required for water collection. For example, in Ethiopia, round-trip collection time in the lowlands took thirty to sixty minutes in the rainy season but over three hours in the dry season; in the highlands, the median time per round trip was less than thirty minutes regardless of season (Kebede, 1978). In Nigeria, water collection times increased by nearly two hours from the wet to dry season (Akintola et al., 1980).

Evidence of Time Saved from Improvements in Water Supplies

The amount of time saved from collecting water from improved sources has been reported to range from zero to over an extreme of eleven hours in a rural village in the Sudan (Russell, 1979). Time savings in dry regions of Malawi, as a result of installation of gravity-piped water systems, was estimated to be more than thirty minutes per day (Warner et al., 1986). In the Peruvian Andes, installation of gravity-piped water systems with household connections resulted in time savings of about three hours per day (Haratani et al., 1981). In urban Philippines, the provision of piped water also reduced water collection times (Magnani et al., 1984).

Basing estimates on self-reported time savings may have biased these studies toward a higher than actual time savings, particularly if the respondents were aware of the purpose and wanted to fulfill the expectations of the interviewer. Actual time spent on water collection has been observed. In Lesotho, the difference in time between collecting water from improved sources and from unimproved sources was thirty minutes per woman per day in the lowlands and, in the highlands, where water was more readily available from springs, eighteen minutes per woman per day (Feachem et al., 1978). In Mozambique, comparison of time budgets from two villages, one in which a standpipe had been installed in the center of the village and one in which the standpipe was located in a neighboring village four kilometers away, indicate that in the village with the standpipe women spent about an hour and three quarters less per day collecting water (Cairncross and Cliff, 1987).

If recipients continue using traditional water supplies even when these are improved, there is no time savings. Traditional supplies might be preferred because factors such as the distance, reliability, waiting time at taps, adequacy for all the household needs, frequency of water collection trips, and willingness of other household members to assist in water collection have not improved or have worsened with the introduction of so-called improved water supplies. In Ethiopia, Kenya, Tanzania, and Zimbabwe, waiting time at an unreliable improved water supply canceled out any time saved in reduced travel (van Wijk-Sijbesma, 1985). Time may not be saved if water does not meet all the household needs, as illustrated in India, where an improved water supply was used only for drinking and cooking so trips to and from the traditional wells continued (van Wijk-Sijbesma, 1985). Improved water supplies no closer than traditional sources did not result in time savings in Malawi (Warner et al., 1986; Msukwa and Kandoole, 1981). If the distance from traditional sources constrains the total amount of water collected (White et al., 1972), even bringing the improved water sources closer may not result in greater time saved. When closer water supplies were provided in Kenya, women made more frequent trips to collect water without reducing the time spent collecting water (Whiting and Krystall, n.d.). Of course, more frequent trips to collect water results in increased use of water, which is in itself beneficial. Although time savings did not accrue to women in Kenya, Guatemala, and Mexico because assistance from other family members declined when improved water sources were introduced (van Wijk-Sijbesma, 1985), the increased time savings to other family members may have its own merit; for instance, young girls may spend more time attending school, baby-sitting, and assisting in food preparation.

Allocation of Time Savings from Improved Water Supplies

Time saved from bringing water supplies closer to people's homes has been reported to result in more time spent on food processing in Ghana (Harkness, 1983), in Mozambique (Cairncross and Cliff, 1987), in the Philippines (Magnani et al., 1984), and in the Sudan (Russell, 1979). The additional time spent on food-processing activities, such as grinding grains, may have increased the availability of food in the home, but such a result was not reported. In Ghana (Harkness, 1983) and Mozambique (Cairncross and Cliff, 1987), more time was spent cooking. Food-preparation activities, such as cooking, could increase the frequency of feeding or the amount eaten at each meal, but frequency and amounts were not measured in these studies. In the highlands of Peru, women reported using more water for food processing (Haratani et al., 1981). Because time saved can be allocated to more water collection, it is difficult to know if the increased time spent in food preparation was owing to time savings, more water, or some combination of the two.

The time savings resulting from more accessible water may lead to increased food-production or income-generating activities. The additional food produced from time savings can either be used for home consumption or sale. Because water use may increase from improvements in water supplies, it is often difficult to identify whether more time or more water or both is responsible for increases in these activities. Villagers reported that water and time gains were used for livestock watering or tending in Thailand (Dworkin et al., 1980), Peru (Haratani et al., 1981), and Malawi (Msukwa and Kandoole, 1981); for home gardening in Thailand (Dworkin et al., 1980), Peru (Haratani et al., 1981), Panama (Meehan et al., 1982), Malawi (Msukwa and Kandoole, 1981), and the Philippines (Magnani et al., 1984); and for agricultural work in Ghana (Harkness, 1983). In the Philippines, the installation of improved water supplies not only increased gardening for home consumption, but the water was also used for raising poultry and pigs (Magnani et al., 1984). In Sudan (Russell, 1979), beer brewing was increased. Village women brew and sell beer in villages (Esrey, personal observation), earning needed cash for families living on incomes that are marginal at best. Other increases in potentially income-generating activities included adobe making in Peru (Haratani et al., 1981) and brick making in Malawi (Msukwa and Kandoole, 1981). In the Philippines, the percentage of households that sold both prepared and unprepared food increased after the introduction of an improved water supply, and more households in areas where the water supply was improved sold prepared and unprepared food than did households in the control areas (Magnani et al., 1984). Teachers in Malawi (Msukwa and Kandoole, 1981) and villagers in Thailand (Dworkin et al., 1980) mentioned handicrafts, and women in Panama (Meehan et al., 1982) and Peru (Haratani et al., 1981) mentioned sewing and weaving as other benefits of improved water supplies.

Constraints to food-producing and income-generating activities include legislative restrictions against water usage for nondomestic purposes, lack of sufficient resources to exploit the time and income gains, and seasonal droughts. In Malawi, Panama, and Peru, official restrictions were placed on the uses of the improved water sources. Although one-fifth of the respondents in Malawi claimed no economic benefits from improved water supplies because decision makers prohibited the use of tap water for purposes other than drinking and cooking water, more respondents used the additional water available at the traditional sources for more purposes (Msukwa and Kandoole, 1981). In Panama and Peru, villagers reported that they used the additional water for nondomestic purposes despite the restrictions (Haratani et al., 1981; Meehan et al., 1982). Dry-season gardening, one anticipated benefit of an improved water supply project in Ghana, did not increase, possibly because no inputs, such as training, seeds, or fertilizer, were provided, nor were women encouraged to exploit this new resource (Harkness, 1983). In Burkina Faso, an integrated attempt to provide labor-saving devices, such as grinding mills, accessible wells, and carts, to increase the women's available time was hampered because the wells tended to dry up in the season when water was most difficult to obtain (McSweeney and Freedman, 1980).

Influence of Time Savings on Child Health

Child care activities that directly improve the health of children clearly require time. The amount of time spent on these activities is difficult to ascertain because it is often not counted as such when other activities are carried out simultaneously and is, therefore, underreported (Popkin and Doan, 1989; Leslie, 1989a). The benefit of allocating the time savings to different activities is likely to vary. For instance, the time spent breastfeeding or feeding children more frequently is likely to have more benefit than time spent sweeping the house. Thus it is important to determine how the time is allocated among the various activities that could be classified as child care. Empirical evidence for the amount of time spent on specific activities that are likely to result in health benefits to the child is almost nonexistent (Leslie, 1989a). Furthermore, alternative means for providing for a child may offset certain infrequently practiced activities. For instance, maternal employment in Panama was positively associated with higher calorie intake of children, despite the potentially detrimental effects of decreased time spent by mothers on the home production activities of cooking and serving food, child care, and housework (Tucker and Sanjur, 1988).

The evidence cited above suggests that time saved from water and sanitation has been allocated to activities that may improve child health and nutrition. Furthermore, the additional time and availability of water may increase commercial activities, such as preparing food for sale on the street, in markets, or in restaurants, as well as raising livestock or small animals for home consumption or sale. If the woman controls the increased purchasing power from these and other non-food-related commercial activities, even more food may be available to the child.

Conclusions and Recommendations

Water and sanitation interventions clearly improve child health and nutrition by decreasing exposure to pathogens. First, the severity of illness appears to decrease to a greater extent than the incidence rates of disease; the result has been found for diarrhea, ascariasis, and schistosomiasis. Second, rates of decline in diarrheal, infant, and total child mortality are larger than those for morbidity. Third, as the level of a particular intervention improves (i.e., from no sanitation to latrines to toilets) the magnitude of the impact on health also improves (Anker and Knowles, 1980; Haines and Avery, 1982; Esrey, 1993). Thus a dose-response relationship between the level of intervention and the severity of the health outcome is seen for pathogens that can be affected by water and sanitation interventions.

The wide range of impacts reported in the literature suggests that benefits following improvements in water and sanitation depend on the routes through which pathogens are transmitted in a community (Briscoe, 1984). Sanitation, water quality, water quantity, and hygiene affect different transmission routes. Thus water and sanitation interventions can either complement each other and existing efforts, such as education, or compensate for undesirable conditions, such as a lack of breastfeeding, to reduce pathogen transmission. This means that either a single intervention must be targeted to areas where it breaks the transmission of pathogens not dealt with by other means, or a package of interventions must be provided to a community to break transmission from several routes to achieve maximum health impacts.

Interventions can be prioritized as contamination in the environment is diminished. Highly contaminated environments require sanitation and water supplies, which appear to complement each other. In areas where breastfeeding rates and income levels are low or crowding is a problem, both improved sanitation and piped water will likely result in improved health. The relationship between these interventions and education is less straightforward. More information is needed on the differential impact of water quality and quantity among children of parents with different educational levels.

Improvements in water supply save women time in amounts that, like the degree of pathogen reduction, is specific to their socioeconomic, cultural, and environmental conditions. The amount of time saved as a result of more accessible water is likely to be greatest where traditional water is scarce, sources are distant, and travel is difficult. Evidence from several countries indicates that time spent on activities related to food production, processing, and preparation is increased after water is brought closer to the home. Further indirect evidence suggests that nutritional status of children can be improved following water supply interventions, even if disease is not reduced. In the Philippines (Magnani et al., 1984), Lesotho (Esrey, 1987), and Nigeria (Huttly et al., 1990) indicators of nutritional status were influenced by improvements in water supplies, but diarrhea was affected less or not at all.

In addition to improvements in food preparation and processing, women may also increase their income by devoting more time to learning and engaging in income-producing activities. Thus incomes may increase, and the increased purchasing power of women could lead to increased nutrient intake, not only of children but of mothers as well, if more food is bought and consumed.

The potential to use the saved time may be critical to other aspects of child care. For example, women may have more time to give oral rehydration therapy to dehydrated children, to take children to be immunized, to learn new recipes to increase nutrient density, or to participate in a growth-monitoring program. This aspect of time savings from water and sanitation interventions, in particular, needs to be carefully considered to optimize programs to improve child health and nutrition.

Although water and sanitation interventions clearly have numerous benefits and beneficiaries, a better understanding of many issues would improve the maximum impacts obtainable. Five general research areas, if better understood, would contribute to the ability to design such programs.

First, the conditions in which the benefits from improvements in water and sanitation could be maximized should be identified. The various factors that complement and compensate for improvements in sanitation, water quality, water quantity, and better hygiene should be identified. Identifying these factors will enable the initially costly investment to purchase new or improve existing water or sanitary facilities to be targeted to areas where the potential benefits would be greatest.

Second, the mechanisms by which increases in water quantity, improvements in water quality, and increased maternal time reduce pathogen transmission should be examined. Direct measurements are preferred to proxy indicators or estimations. Observations and measurements of specific hygiene practices should identify those practices that reduce transmission the most.

Third, time saving and its use should be investigated more rigorously. One, time should be quantified rather than estimated by travel distance. Two, the conditions that maximize time saving should be examined and quantified. Three, the activities that are undertaken by savings in time should be identified and quantified, and they should be operationalized according to functional categories of nutritional and health benefits rather than general child care activities. Four, the time costs of learning new activities beneficial to child health as well as the time costs of carrying out the activities should be quantified. Five, the decreases in travel time should be correlated with health benefits to determine the optimal location of water supplies. Six, the contribution of saving in time to food-producing and income-generating activities should be measured.

A fourth area of study is the poorly understood interaction between disease transmission, particularly diarrhea, and behavior. Therefore, several areas of study would ensure health benefits following the implementation of water and sanitation facilities. One, the lack of knowledge before implementation may constrain the use of facilities, but little is known about this preintervention knowledge. Two, the influence of knowledge on changes in hygiene practices when new facilities are introduced should be determined. Three, the influence of knowledge on adoption and use of new facilities should be understood. Four, the influence of different levels of knowledge of proper hygiene on disease transmission and behavioral changes should be determined.

Fifth, the links between water and sanitation on the acceptance and use of other interventions is not well appreciated and is poorly understood. These links should be investigated. One, the influence of recent water and sanitation interventions on the acceptance of immunizations, oral rehydration, and growth-monitoring activities should be studied. This acceptance may be through reductions in time to collect water or general acceptance of new interventions. Conversely, the influence of other sectors (e.g., agricultural extension and vitamin A–rich gardens) on the acceptance and use of water and sanitation facilities should also be investigated.

10

Family Planning as a Promoter of Child Survival and Growth

John G. Haaga

Among the strongest justifications for promoting use of contraceptives is concern for the health of women and their children (however many). Even those who consider Malthusian arguments exaggerated or irrelevant to their immediate concerns can still support family planning as a health program that is particularly important for poor countries and for poor people in rich countries.

A report of the National Academy of Sciences Committee on Population has explored the connections between contraception and women's and children's health (Committee on Population, 1989). These include direct causal connections, such as the role of contraceptive use in reducing the numbers and proportions of high-risk pregnancies, and indirect pathways, for example, reducing the numbers of unwanted children and the numbers of siblings competing for severely limited family resources. The report establishes the case that children are more likely to survive and to thrive in families that can control their fertility.

The first two sections of this chapter summarize and assess the evidence that associations between demographic factors, notably birth spacing and high parity, and child health, are causal. The third section discusses the evidence that family planning programs actually bring about changes in these demographic factors. Finally, priorities for basic and applied research on these issues and ways in which research and information systems

I would like to thank Julie DaVanzo, Harold Alderman, Sandra Huffman, Reynaldo Martorell, David Pelletier, and Per Pinstrup-Andersen. Errors that remain are not to be charged to their accounts.

can help make family planning programs more effective in promoting child survival and growth are discussed.

Effects of Birth Spacing and Child Survival and Child Growth

Research on fertility and infant mortality in developing countries was given a notable boost in the 1970s and 1980s by the World Fertility Survey (WFS) program, which produced comparable, high-quality demographic data from large samples of women in forty-two developing countries. Because the WFS included pregnancy histories, data on infant and child deaths could be linked to data on the timing of pregnancies. As Samuel Preston saw it, "Certainly the most surprising and probably the most important new finding from the WFS concerns the exceptionally high mortality rates among children born after a short birth interval" (Preston, 1985, p. 266). More recently, data from the Demographic and Health Surveys (DHS) have expanded both the number of countries and the possibilities for linkage of health and fertility information.

Of course, this finding was not entirely new. Previous reports had linked increased risk of infant mortality to the length of both preceding and succeeding birth intervals (Omran et al., 1976). But the WFS studies (and others of newly available retrospective survey data) showed that the association of birth interval length with mortality was robust across a wide variety of settings. Nor could the association be explained away by sample selectivity or other methodological problems of the sort that had made it difficult to assess earlier results.

Evidence

Figure 10.1 shows in summary form the bivariate association of preceding birth interval length with infant mortality rates (IMR) in the WFS data sets. (The IMR for children born less than twenty-four months after their preceding sibling is calculated only for pairs in which the first child survived to at least twenty-four months to mitigate the effects of some possibly confounding variables.) Infants born within two years of a previous pregnancy outcome had higher rates of mortality, in thirteen low-mortality, fourteen medium-mortality, and thirteen high-mortality countries.

The excess risk associated with a short preceding birth interval persisted from early infancy through childhood. Hobcraft (1987), taking into account maternal education and some other socioeconomic factors in a comparative analysis of WFS data, found a relative risk of 1.8 for infant

Figure 10.1. Infant mortality by preceding birth interval, WFS Surveys, 1970s

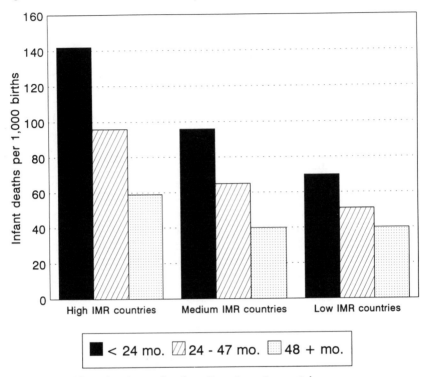

Source: World Fertility Survey data from Rutstein, 1984a, 1984b.

deaths and 1.3 for deaths in childhood after infancy for those born less than two years after the preceding birth, compared to those born after an interval of two to four years.

This excess risk of death is in part related to an association of short intervals with premature birth.[1] Short preceding intervals are also associated with intrauterine growth retardation (IUGR) independent of the length of gestation or other possible confounding factors such as maternal weight (Gribble, 1993). Both prematurity and IUGR are manifest in low birth weight, which in turn is associated with diminished immunocompe-

[1] The association between short interbirth intervals and infant deaths is in part an artifact because pregnancies ending in a premature delivery (for whatever reason) are overrepresented in the category of short interbirth intervals. But the association of short intervals with increased risk of death persists, even when gestational duration is controlled (Miller et al., 1992).

Figure 10.2. Prevalence of stunting by preceding birth interval, DHS, 1980s

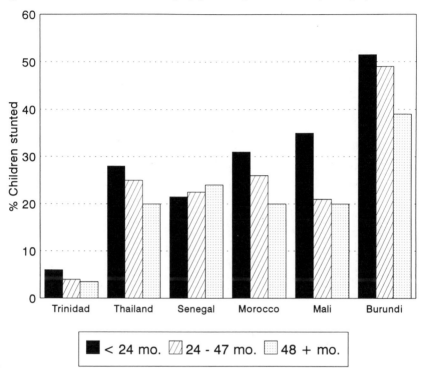

Source: Institute for Resource Development, DHS Reports, 1980, 1989. The data were developed by Macro International, Inc., with funding from the United States Agency for International Development.

tence and poor growth in childhood.[2] Thus child health is likely to be compromised even for the survivors born after short intervals.

This failure of short-interval babies to catch up in growth can be seen in data relating birth intervals to indicators of children's nutritional status. Figure 10.2 shows the bivariate relationship between preceding birth interval and low height-for-age of children aged six to thirty-six months in six countries participating in the DHS program. The overall proportions of children considered stunted (that is, two or more standard deviation scores below the mean height of children of the same age in the reference

[2] Infants born with low weight because of prematurity have higher rates of neonatal mortality than those carried to term whose low weight is due to IUGR (Haas et al., 1987), but most studies in developing countries of the effects of short intervals, maternal age, and birth order do not distinguish between the two because of the difficulty of measuring gestational age.

population) ranged from 5 percent in Trinidad and Tobago to 48 percent in Burundi. Despite this great range in the overall prevalence, in every country except Senegal, children born less than two years after the preceding pregnancy had a higher prevalence of stunting than those born after a gap of twenty-four to forty-eight months. Boerma and Bicego (1992) found in multivariate analyses of DHS data from seventeen countries that children born after short intervals are about 20 percent more likely to be stunted than those born two or more years after the previous child.

Mechanisms

Several mechanisms can account for the bad outcomes of pregnancies that too closely follow a previous pregnancy. One involves the need for some recuperation time, for restoration of reproductive tissues following parturition, and for the rebuilding of nutritional stores depleted by pregnancy (and even more by lactation). An analysis of data from a prospective field study in Guatemala and of recall data from Malaysia showed that short recuperative intervals before the index child's conception were associated with low weight gain during pregnancy and low birth weight when the outcome of the previous pregnancy and maternal characteristics were taken into account (Pebley and DaVanzo, 1988). A study of a hospital-based sample in northeastern Brazil showed that infants born after a short pregnancy-to-next-conception interval had higher rates of IUGR (though not, as in some other studies, premature delivery), controlling for many other factors affecting birth weight independent of the interval. The relationship became insignificant when the mother's prepregnancy weight was included in regressions, suggesting that the mechanism for the association was indeed the lack of time for the mother to rebuild nutritional stores after the previous delivery (Ferraz et al., 1988). Merchant and Martorell (1988) discuss the problems of both theory and measurement that have bedeviled research on maternal depletion. They conclude that "under some conditions the nutritional demands of reproductive cycling negatively affect maternal nutritional status" (p. 362).[3]

An earlier multivariate analysis of the same Guatemalan data used by Pebley and DaVanzo showed that infants conceived less than twelve months after the birth of their next oldest living sibling gained 380 grams less during the first year of life, on average, than those conceived after a longer interval (Clark, 1981).

Another mechanism that could account for continued deprivation of the child born before a short interval is the effect on the mother's lacta-

---

[3] The maternal depletion hypothesis is further discussed by Leslie in Chapter 7.

tion. Either the new pregnancy interferes directly with lactation and thus lowers the intake of breastmilk by the suckling infant, or maternal behavior intervenes, for example, if the infant is abruptly weaned as soon as the new pregnancy is recognized. This factor in the etiology of protein-energy malnutrition has been recognized in the nutrition literature for over fifty years; Cicely Williams gave the name "kwashiorkor," meaning "displaced from the breast" in the Ga language of West Africa, to a severe form of PEM.

Besides inadequate maternofetal nutrition, there are other possible explanations for the association of short preceding intervals and poor infant health. Infectious diseases cause most of the mortality and morbidity of infants and young children in poor populations so it is useful to examine possible effects on the incidence or severity of common infections.

The problem of short intervals in the postnatal period could be that infants reach the vulnerable age during which weaning foods are introduced and maternally acquired immunities disappear at a time when the next older sibling is a toddler. Toddlers are prey to infectious diseases, notably diarrheal diseases and measles, that they can pass on to younger siblings. As one example, the feces of very young children, who have little or no control over their defecation, may be handled differently than the feces of older children and adults, and thus an infant comes into more contact with fecally transmitted pathogens if there is an older sibling less than three years old. Black and his colleagues pointed out that "in many communities, even where basic sanitation facilities exist and adults use them, young children are often permitted to defecate indiscriminately. Because diarrhea attack rates are highest among children, it is defecation in this age group that deserves most attention" (Black et al., 1983, p. 299). A study of cholera transmission in Bangladesh has shown a greater likelihood of infection in families with suckling infants apparently because of careless handling of young children's feces (Riley et al., 1987). There is some evidence from Africa that closely spaced children are more likely to catch measles from each other and more likely to die as a result than children two or three years apart in age (Aaby et al., 1983).

Children born either before or after a short interval could be at higher risk simply because families in which birth intervals are short tend to have many young children. Many siblings could mean both competition for scarce resources that promote survival (food, preventive and curative medical care, the attention of adults) and increased opportunities for transmission of infections through both of the main routes (airborne and fecal-oral). Short intervals in this sense would be a marker for many dependent children and crowding; unfortunately, these effects (which could have different implications for health and family planning programs) are not distinguishable in many studies.

Children born before a short interval are also at increased risk of death. Hobcraft (1987) found an average relative risk of 2.2 for childhood deaths for those whose mothers gave birth again within a year. Koenig et al. (1990) found that the excess risk of a short succeeding interval was highest for the neonatal period. Here the mechanisms are less well understood, and the direction of causation is more difficult to sort out. Short succeeding intervals may be caused by the weakness or death of the first child, rather than the other way around (Koenig et al., 1990). A slow-growing child may not suck strongly and frequently, thereby reducing the effect of lactation on postpartum amenorrhea and hastening the return of fecundity. Or the early death of the first child of a pair may lead to an early succeeding pregnancy, either because breastfeeding (and therefore amenorrhea) is abruptly terminated or because of a conscious effort by parents to replace the lost child. Finally, the effects of a short succeeding interval can easily be confounded with those of a short preceding interval; the two go together in the families at greatest risk, those in which women are having babies too fast relative to their physiologic and economic ability to nurture them. Several studies have taken the effects of breastfeeding and prior losses into account in various ways and generally found that there is still a significant effect of short succeeding intervals, increasing the risk of infant deaths (Palloni and Millman, 1986; Pebley and Stupp, 1986; Retherford, et al., 1989).

Yet another reason for the association of short intervals with child survival and growth does not involve any direct causal connection between the two. Women with access to means of spacing births (and motivation to use them) may be more likely than other women to know how to promote their children's health and to have access to means for doing so, such as medical care. For example, a study in rural Mexico has shown the important links between family planning and maternal and child health services; if women make their way into one set of services they are more likely to be referred to the other (Potter et al., 1987). Women who have achieved control over one aspect of their reproductive lives (the timing of pregnancies) for a variety of reasons, such as influence over their husbands and family resources, social support, and motivation, also tend to have some control over other aspects of their reproductive lives, including the raising of healthy children (Potter, 1989). Lengthening intervals between births would not by itself improve the survival chances and health prospects of the children involved.

Despite the inadequate knowledge about the reasons for the strong association of short pregnancy intervals with poor infant and child health, the evidence suggests that the former cause the latter to a significant degree. The association of short intervals with poor health can be ascribed only partly to causation in the reverse direction, to the effects of poorly measured confounding variables, or to errors in the measurement of birth and death dates. There is evidence supporting both direct physiologic mechanisms, by which short preceding intervals lead to poor prenatal growth and development, and indirect social mechanisms that put multiple young children in poor families at risk in postnatal life.[4]

Effects of Maternal Age and Parity on Child Growth and Survival

Young Maternal Age and First Parity

The WFS studies showed a very consistent pattern of excess risk of infant mortality for children born to young mothers. The ratio of infant mortality rates for children of mothers less than twenty years old to the rates for children of women in their twenties is virtually constant across both high-and low-mortality countries (Figure 10.3). By contrast, the WFS studies did not find much excess risk of infant mortality for first births, and the risk was concentrated in countries with very high mortality. This finding is something of a puzzle because there is more evidence for biological mechanisms that put first births at risk than for mechanisms that affect children of young mothers per se. In the United States most of the excess risk to infants of teenaged mothers is due to prenatal causes (notably inadequate health care) and postnatal causes, such as infections and trauma, which mediate the influence of economic and social deprivation (McAnarney, 1987). A study of children of poor teenagers in the United States showed an effect on child growth that continued past infancy (Cherry et al., 1987).

A reason commonly given for the deficit in birth weight and length of infants born to young mothers is that girls grow in height for four or more years after menarche, and any pregnancy during those years will produce competition between fetal nutrition and the linear growth of the mother (Committee on Nutritional Status during Pregnancy and Lactation, 1970; Naeye, 1981). In poorly nourished populations, menarche occurs at later ages, and linear growth lasts longer (Riley et al., 1989). Thus, in poor populations, the period during which a pregnancy would coincide with linear growth of the mother would last on average until higher chronological ages than in rich countries.

---

[4] For further discussion of the physiologic mechanisms, see Haaga (1989), and for further discussion of both the social mechanisms and some of the problems of confounding, see Potter (1988).

Figure 10.3. Infant mortality by mother's age, WFS Surveys, 1970s

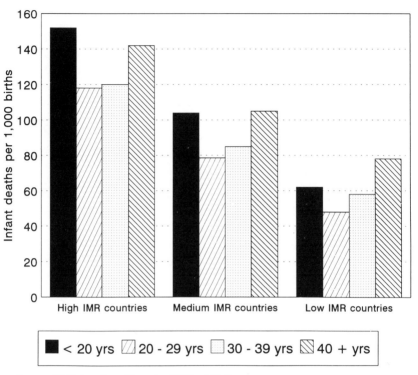

Source: WFS data from Rutstein, 1984a, 1984b.

It is unlikely that this mechanism is a simple matter of an insufficient overall supply of macronutrients. The energy cost of linear growth is small in percentage terms, and linear growth (at younger ages) is usually interrupted when other demands are placed on the organism. The fetus appears to be buffered against extreme shortages of macronutrients. The absolute energy cost of a pregnancy is surprisingly low (Briend, 1985). It is more likely that adolescent women, especially very young adolescents, are somehow less capable of transferring nutrients efficiently to the fetus.

Some mechanisms through which first births are at increased risk are well-known and have been demonstrated in both high-and low-mortality settings. Women during their first pregnancy are more likely to suffer from pregnancy-induced hypertension (PIH), which in its severe form (eclampsia) is life-threatening to both mother and baby. PIH is associated with premature delivery and placental abruption, and both are associated with low birth weight. Infants born to women diagnosed as having the less severe forms of PIH have elevated risk of perinatal death—double that of non-PIH babies, even in samples of women giving birth at teaching hospitals in the United States (Davies and Dunlop, 1983). The precise etiology of PIH is not known, but it is thought to be a reaction of the maternal circulatory system to the placenta because it never occurs among nonpregnant women and is especially associated with first pregnancies.

Some studies of hospital-based samples in Africa have shown an interactive association of PIH with maternal age and primiparity; very young women pregnant for the first time were more likely than older primiparas to be diagnosed with the severe forms of PIH (Harrison, 1985; Crowther, 1986; Ojo and Oronsaye, 1988). This evidence suggests that delaying first births would be beneficial.

Maternal infections pose a risk to the fetus, and young mothers are often more likely than older mothers to have sexually transmitted diseases and other infections. Efiong and Banjoka (1975), for example, found a higher prevalence of syphilis in very young mothers than in older mothers in urban Nigeria. A prospective study in Sierra Leone found that pregnant women under age twenty were more likely than older pregnant women to have both urinary and genital tract infections (WHO Family Health Division, 1981). The incidence of gonorrhea, syphilis, and chlamydia infections in developing countries is high and probably rising, and the effects on infant health can be significant (de Schryver and Meheus, 1989). Here the policy implication is probably the need to improve adolescent health services in general, including family planning, with an emphasis on contraceptive methods that inhibit the spread of infections.

Malaria is a major public health problem in the tropics, and it may explain some of the excess risk associated with first pregnancies in the areas where it is endemic. Infants born to African women with parasitized placentas averaged 50 grams lighter at birth than infants born to women whose placentas were free of the malaria plasmodium. Women pregnant for the first time are almost twice as likely as higher-parity women to be infested with malaria (Bray and Anderson, 1979). Congenital malaria is rare in areas of endemicity, but maternal malaria may put infants, particularly firstborn infants, at risk of morbidity and death as a result of low birth weights and depressed immunocompetence.

Besides these fairly direct physiologic mechanisms, there are socially mediated mechanisms that can account for associations of both young motherhood and primiparity with poor health of the infant in poor and rich countries alike. Young mothers and first-time mothers are often at a disadvantage because of their poverty and lack of knowledge about, and access to, health facilities. The proportions of illegitimate and unwanted births may be higher among young mothers; the lack of social sanction and parental readiness for childbearing and child rearing may lead to failure to acknowledge pregnancy early and seek adequate care. Even when the pregnancy is wanted, first children often arrive at a stage when young couples are economically struggling. (Hoorweg and Niemeijer, 1989, discuss the consequences of this for child feeding and nutrition in rural Kenya.) This effect may be stronger where newly married women are cut off from their own relatives and where young couples set up on their own, rather than retaining close economic links with their families of origin.

Several studies have shown that young women and first-time mothers receive little prenatal care, and their infants are less likely to be immunized than those of women in their twenties and thirties. Harrison (1985) and his colleagues in northern Nigeria, for example, reported that primiparas do not seek medical care, if they seek it at all, until a much later stage of pregnancy than multiparas; some would be taken to the hospital only in the later stages of an obstructed delivery or in PIH-induced convulsions. Such disparities in access to, and use of, curative and preventive care would put teenaged and first-time mothers and their infants at even greater risk.

Finally, some association between young maternal age and low birth weight and infant mortality may simply be an artifact of short gestational age. If two women conceive at the same age, the one who gives birth prematurely will have the lower maternal age at birth; the corollary is that births at any exact maternal age in the lower end of the distribution include higher proportions of premature births than the next higher age. Santow and Bracher (1989) used simulations to show that this effect could account for a surprisingly large age difference in fetal loss ratios even if true underlying risks were the same across ages.

Of the physiologic mechanisms discussed above, the strongest evidence concerns the link between primiparity and PIH and resultant poor outcomes of pregnancy. The behavioral mechanisms are less clear-cut and in all likelihood vary greatly in importance among and within societies. Because many of these deaths could be prevented by better outreach for prenatal care, or by enabling women to delay unwanted births until they are "ready to be mothers" (as socially defined), these mechanisms have great significance for policy.

Older Mothers

Many studies have found higher rates of infant mortality among children of older mothers, even controlling for parity. Fortney and her colleagues (1983) found an excess risk of neonatal mortality in every parity category for women over age thirty-five, compared to women aged twenty to thirty-four, in hospital samples in Mexico and Egypt. In the WFS studies, the bivariate association between maternal age and infant mortality generally followed the expected U-shape; in the lowest-mortality countries, the IMR for children of women over forty years old was higher than that for children of teenagers.

Infants born to older mothers have been found to have increased rates of both low birth weight and very high birth weight; the former are likely because of increased risk of PIH, the latter, increased risk of gestational diabetes for older women (Hansen, 1986).

First births to older women are at especially high risk of chromosomal abnormalities, such as that leading to Down's syndrome (Hook, 1985). Chromosomal abnormalities account for only a portion of child morbidity and mortality in poor countries, however. In poor, high-fertility countries, a more likely explanation for the excess risk associated with births to "elderly primigravidae" is that such women have had previous miscarriages, stillbirths, or chronic disease (Ojo and Oronsaye, 1988).

High-Parity Births

The WFS studies generally showed higher rates of both infant and child mortality for children born at parities seven and above. This association was stronger in the high-mortality, which also tend to be high-fertility, countries than in the low-mortality, low-fertility countries (Figure 10.4). In the prospective Narangwal study in the rural Punjab, children who died were twice as likely as children who survived to have been born at seventh or higher order (Kielmann et al., 1983, p. 199). Multivariate analyses of data from developing countries show conflicting results, but several, including Pebley and Stupp (1986) using data from Guatemala, show higher risks of infant mortality for infants born at higher orders, even when other risk factors (such as birth interval length and family incomes) are controlled.

The mechanisms through which high parity[5] affects infant and child health include some prenatal and obstetric factors. For example, "grand multiparas" (women who have had many previous pregnancies—the exact definition varies among studies) have been found to have a higher incidence of iron-deficiency anemia than women at lower parities (Kessel et al., 1985). Maternal anemia, in turn, is associated with premature delivery and low birth weight.

---

[5] Parity, as usually defined, includes pregnancies that did not end in a live birth, whereas birth order counts only previous live births to the same woman. Data are more often

Figure 10.4. Infant mortality by birth order, WFS Surveys, 1970s

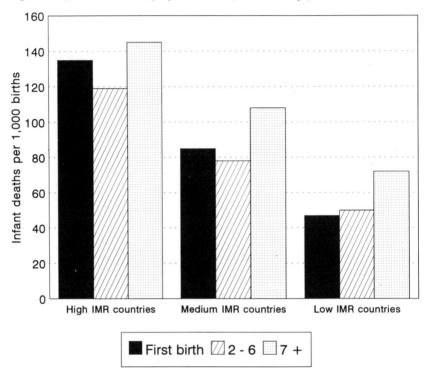

Source: WFS data from Rutstein, 1984a, 1984b.

Women at very high parities (and older women) also have a higher incidence of malpresentations, which pose a risk of asphyxia to the newborn; this may be owing to weakened uterine muscles and incompetent cervix caused by the exertion of many previous pregnancies and deliveries (Seeds, 1986).

In rich, low-fertility countries, where frequent pregnancies constitute deviant behavior, much of the association between high parity and poor pregnancy outcomes such as low birth weight disappears when prior poor outcomes are controlled. In large part, the risk associated with high parity in these settings is risk of recurrence of previous complications of pregnancy (Powell-Griner, 1987).

More important in poor countries, in all likelihood, are postnatal influ-

---

available for birth order only. Even when miscarriages, abortions, and stillbirths are included in pregnancy histories, they are usually seriously undercounted.

ences on growth and development. Because of the inverse association of education and socioeconomic status with fertility, women who reach high parities include a disproportionate number of the poor. Later-born children in poor families, almost by definition, have more competitors for scarce family resources, including food, the time and attention of adults, and money required to obtain adequate preventive and curative health care. Infants born at high parity are less likely to have been wanted, which may consciously or unconsciously affect parents' willingness (as well as their ability) to make the investments necessary for their optimal health.

Effects of Family Planning Programs on Contraceptive Use and Birth Intervals, Maternal Age, and Parity

To argue that family planning programs are a worthwhile investment in improving child health, it is not enough to show that demographic factors affect child health. One must also argue that family planning programs cause greater contraceptive use and lower fertility than would have been the case without the programs and then show that greater contraceptive use leads to changes in demographic and social factors in directions that promote child health.

It is always difficult to prove a proposition about what would have happened in the absence of a strong family planning effort by a government. The fertility transition in Europe, for example, took place without modern contraceptives and without much encouragement by governments, occasionally with discouragement. Many quasi-experimental studies in developing countries, however, have shown that particular program designs and resource intensity are associated with increased contraceptive use and fertility decline. An especially useful quasi-experiment in Matlab Thana, Bangladesh, showed that appropriate design of the family planning program can induce contraceptive use, even in an unpromising setting where none of the "demand side" factors seem conducive to change (Koenig et al., 1992; Phillips et al., 1988).

Observational studies relating program inputs to contraceptive use are tricky: public programs may respond with resources to areas where strong demand for their services exists independently. Conversely, as may be the case in Indonesia, program managers may devote extra effort to areas known to be "problem areas" for the family planning program (Lerman et al., 1989).

But cross-national and long-term evidence suggests that there is indeed an effect of program effort independent of demand-side factors. A series of studies, using ever-improving data on program effort, has shown con-

Table 10.1. Percentages of births at risk, by contraceptive prevalence

	Contraceptive prevalence		
	Low (0–10% of MWRA)	Middle (10–40% of MWRA)	High (40–60% of MWRA)
Percentage of births to			
Teenage mother	20	14	12
First order	18	22	28
Order 7 +	21	15	13
Less than 2 years after preceding birth	24	30	36

Source: Bongaarts, 1987, using results from 39 WFS surveys.
Modified with the permission of the Population Council, from John Bongaarts, "Does Family Planning Reduce Infant Mortality Rates?," *Population and Development Review* 13 (2) (June 1987): 323–334.

sistently that program effort is associated with contraceptive use, largely through increasing the number of methods available (Mauldin and Ross, 1991). The evidence justifies Mauldin's conclusion that "large-scale family planning programs, when well managed, have a substantial effect on fertility independent of the influence of socioeconomic factors" (Mauldin, 1983, p. 289).

Cross-sectional evidence from the WFS on the second part of this causal chain, linking contraceptive use to changes in the demographic factors, has been summarized by Bongaarts (1987). Table 10.1 shows unweighted averages of the percentages of births to mothers less than twenty years old, that were first or seventh or higher parities, and that occurred after intervals of twenty-four months or less in three groups of WFS countries, ranked by the percentage of married women of reproductive age (MWRA) using modern contraceptives at the time of the surveys. The percentages of births to teenaged mothers and the percentages of high-order births were lower in the countries with high prevalence of contraceptive use. The percentage of first-order births was somewhat higher in the high-prevalence countries, which is an arithmetic necessity caused by the decline at higher orders. Most significant is the higher percentage of short intervals in the countries with high contraceptive prevalence. This last, especially, is an unexpected result, discussed in more detail in the following sections.

Birth Intervals

Contraceptive use is not synonymous with birth spacing. The aggregate cross-sectional results shown in Table 10.1—higher proportions of short intervals in the countries where modern contraceptives are more common—mask considerable variation across countries and conflicting trends in recent decades. In some Latin American and Caribbean countries where fertility rates were falling, there was indeed a significant decline in the proportion of short intervals during the 1970s and 1980s (Committee on Population, 1989, pp. 82–86). By contrast, the proportions of short intervals rose rapidly in Taiwan and Senegal (the latter being the only African country for which data from two times were available—ibid., Table 6.5).

To investigate the reasons for the lack of a simple causal connection between increased contraceptive use and the proportion of short intervals, it is useful to examine the intermediate variables through which public programs can affect the length of interpregnancy intervals. Bongaarts (1982) proposed a useful method for accounting for differences in fertility rates using a list of seven mutually exclusive variables: (1) proportions married; (2) contraceptive use and effectiveness; (3) prevalence of induced abortion; (4) duration of postpartum infecundity; (5) fecundity (or frequency of intercourse); (6) spontaneous intrauterine mortality; and (7) prevalence of permanent sterility. Of these, the first four account for most variation across countries and over time in total fertility rates. The proportion of pregnancy intervals that are perilously short will be reduced as contraceptive use increases only if there are no countervailing changes in the other intermediate variables affecting the duration of pregnancy intervals.

The duration of postpartum infecundity, which is affected by the duration and intensity of breastfeeding, is most likely the variable on this list that has offset the effect of increased use of contraceptives on interval length in many countries. This can be seen indirectly in the cross-sectional evidence. Figure 10.5 shows a negative association between the median duration of breastfeeding and the percentage of MWRA using modern contraceptives in twenty-seven WFS countries.

Such a negative association can also be seen in the few studies, mainly in Asia, that have examined changes over time within single countries. DaVanzo and Starbird (1990), for example, have shown with recall data from Malaysia that decreases in breastfeeding almost exactly offset the effects of increased contraceptive use among urban dwellers and members of the Chinese minority. The negative association between breastfeeding and contraceptive use cannot simply be explained as spurious, caused by common association of both breastfeeding and use of modern contraceptives with some third factor. Such a negative association persisted in multivariate analyses with controls for a variety of other socioeconomic and health-related variables (see DaVanzo and Starbird, 1990, and review by Millman, 1985).

Figure 10.5. Use of modern contraception and duration of breastfeeding

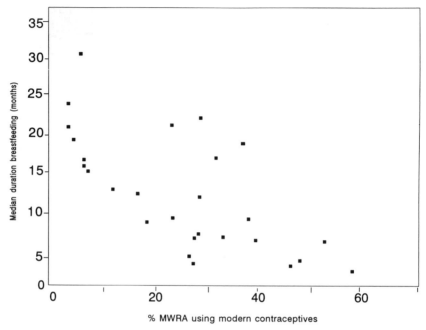

Source: World Fertility Surveys.

One possibility is that hormonal methods (the most common being contraceptive pills and, more recently, injections and implants) interfere physiologically with lactation. This problem was probably more significant with the first generation of high-dose, mixed-hormone oral contraceptives. But even contraceptive pills with low dosages of estrogen have been found to reduce milk volume (WHO/NRC, 1983, p. 373). An expert committee of the World Health Organization and the United States National Research Council has recommended that programs promote non-hormonal contraceptive methods only for the first four to six months postpartum; should lactating women still desire hormonal methods, progestogen-only methods should be used (ibid., p. 380).

Women may stop breastfeeding soon after giving birth (for any reason), then observe an early return of their menses and begin to use contraceptives because of their desire to space pregnancies. In this case, the availability of modern contraceptives does not cause the decline of breastfeeding. Rather, modern contraceptives mitigate one of the potential harmful consequences of the decline of breastfeeding, the loss of protection against a rapid succession of pregnancies. On the other hand, women may know about the contraceptive effect of breastfeeding and decide that modern

Table 10.2. Proportion of women who want to give birth within specified times, by time since last pregnancy outcome, Malaysia, 1984

Months since last pregnancy outcome	Percentage of women who want to give birth		
	During next year	12–23 months from now	24 + months from now
0–5	10.0	11.0	79.0
6–11	10.0	10.0	80.0
12–17	15.0	13.0	72.0
18 +	37.0	15.0	48.0

Source: National Population and Family Development Board, 1984/85 Malaysian Population and Family Survey, unpublished data.

Note: Limited to women who want at least one more child, not currently pregnant.

contraceptives can serve as an acceptable substitute. Or they may believe (or be told by family planning program staff) that breastfeeding is incompatible with contraceptive use and cut short their breastfeeding deliberately to be able to begin or to resume use of contraceptives. Insofar as either of these theories is accurate, the availability of modern contraceptives is contributing to the decline in breastfeeding. Gomez and Potter (1989) showed that in rural Mexico, the decision to stop breastfeeding early was likely to be followed quickly by the adoption of a modern contraceptive and vice versa, which strengthens the case for a conscious trade between the two practices by women who have recently given birth. There were also indications that family planning workers were advising women to wean their infants so they could start using oral contraceptives.

Besides breastfeeding and the duration of postpartum amenorrhea, frequency of intercourse is another of the intermediate variables that could change to counteract the effect of contraception on birth intervals. Caldwell and Raven (1977), for example, showed that a rapid increase in contraceptive use in one Nigerian city had little impact on fertility because contraceptive use mainly substituted for the traditional abstinence following a birth. Abstinence has been studied far less than breastfeeding, in part because of the difficulty of collecting good data.

There is very little research on what women in poor countries know and believe about the value of child spacing. The Burundi DHS included a question, addressed separately to women and their husbands, on the ideal interval between births. For both sexes, the modal choice was thirty-six to forty-seven months. Women tended to choose longer intervals, but only 2.2 percent of men and 1.2 percent of women thought that an interval less than twenty-four months was best.

Results from a 1988 survey in Malaysia give further evidence on the

Table 10.3. Contraceptive use by time since last pregnancy outcome, Malaysia, 1984

Months since last pregnancy outcome	Proportion of those whose menstruation has resumed who are using modern contraceptives (includes pill)	Proportion of those whose menstruation has resumed who are using pill
0–5	0.38	0.18
6–11	0.42	0.24
12–17	0.44	0.27
18–29	0.40	0.20
30+	0.33	0.09
Total	0.36	0.14

Source: National Population and Family Development Board, 1984/85 Malaysian Population and Family Survey, unpublished data.

"latent demand" for birth spacing (Table 10.2). The great majority of women who had recently given birth and who wanted another child said they wanted to have their next child more than two years after the interview date. By contrast, of those who wanted another child and had not given birth for at least eighteen months, a majority wanted to give birth within the next two years.

But these data also show that despite the widespread preference for gaps of at least two years between births, most women at risk of a closely spaced birth do not use effective contraception (Table 10.3). Of the at-risk women, those whose menstruation had resumed since their last pregnancy outcome, 38 percent of those whose most recent pregnancy ended less than six months before the interview were using effective contraception, compared to 42 percent of those whose most recent pregnancy had ended six to twelve months before the interview date. This difference was attributable to the lower proportions of women using the pill among those whose pregnancies had ended most recently. This was not because of a lack of knowledge of effective means of contraception: virtually all respondents were familiar with at least one effective method. These data, from a country with an active family planning program and a fairly high (36 percent of MWRA) prevalence of modern contraception, illustrate a general problem: to increase their impact on child health, family planning programs need to do a better job of reaching postpartum women who have resumed menstruation.

Maternal Age Distribution

When fertility limitation becomes more common and is more effective, not only overall rates but the age pattern of fertility changes. Births to

Table 10.4. Use of modern contraceptives by woman's age, 1980s

Ages	Senegal	Liberia	Morocco	Trinidad and Tobago
15–19	0.4	2.0	14.0	30.0
20–24	1.0	5.0	23.0	45.0
25–29	2.0	7.0	29.0	48.0
30–34	5.0	6.0	36.0	48.0
35–39	4.0	5.0	33.0	48.0
40–44	1.0	6.0	32.0	43.0
45–49	2.0	7.0	22.0	30.0
All ages	2.0	6.0	29.0	44.0

Source: Institute for Resource Development, published reports in DHS series.

older women[6] and high-parity births are reduced more than proportionally (Knodel, 1977). For somewhat different reasons, the proportion of births to very young mothers often declines faster than overall fertility as well.

Little of the decline in births to teenage mothers (shown in Table 10.1) can be ascribed to the direct efforts of family planning programs. Most of it is owing to the rising age of first marriage that has occurred, especially in East Asia, as a concomitant of social change and economic growth. Table 10.4 shows the proportions of married women using modern contraceptives in four countries that have recently published results of DHS surveys. Two have the very low contraceptive prevalence typical of sub-Saharan African countries; Morocco is a medium-prevalence country; and Trinidad has high prevalence. In each country, married women below age twenty are less likely to use modern contraceptives than are older married women. Contraceptive use is especially low in the interval between marriage (or the beginning of cohabitation) and the first birth. This probably shows that most contraceptive use is for limiting family size after couples have had the number of children they desire, rather than for postponing the first birth or spacing births. Younger women may also lack information and the sense of self-efficacy, which come with experience, that they need to take control of their reproductive lives.

At older maternal ages, the effect of family planning programs is more mixed. In countries where modern contraception has not been long established, a characteristic age distribution for modern contraceptive use is the inverted U—older women belong to the cohorts born before girls' education was common, and they married and began raising children

---

[6] In some rich countries at very low levels of fertility, delayed childbearing has become common and the proportion of births to older mothers is increasing.

before fertility control was much discussed or approved. Rates of contraceptive use are lower for women in their forties than for women in their thirties in three of the four countries shown as examples.[7] This pattern may change as the "traditionalist" cohorts are replaced at these ages by cohorts of women more familiar with modern methods.

The overall effect of rising age at first marriage and increased use of effective contraception by older women is a compression of the childbearing years into the twenties and thirties. This should have the effect of reducing infant mortality rates and improving the health of surviving children because these are usually the socially optimal maternal ages for childbearing and child rearing, unless birth intervals are also shortened.

Information and Research Needs

Family planning programs have always put forward as an important rationale their effects on maternal and child health. Almost all the literature on evaluation of family planning programs, though, is concerned with the effects on fertility (for example, United Nations, 1979). The editors of a collection of papers on cost-effectiveness and cost-benefit analyses of family planning programs did point out that "beneficial effects on the health of women and children are legitimately viewed as additional outputs" (Sirageldin et al., 1983, p. xviii). But the methods of measuring program outputs they discussed mostly entailed conversion of service statistics into estimates of couple-years of protection and ultimately into estimates of births averted. The impact of contraceptive use on health depends in large part on the age and parity of women using contraceptives and the timing of use after pregnancy outcomes, which are not directly reflected in these summary measures.

Likewise, methods of setting targets for family planning programs emphasize effects on fertility, with no attention to effects on child health. If the health rationale for family planning is taken seriously, then it should be reflected in methods for evaluating or simulating program impact, in the setting of targets and incentives for staff, and even in propaganda. This would require an emphasis on potential high-risk pregnancies averted, rather than only on births averted or acceptors.

Taucher (1982) pointed out that the health rationale is especially important in Latin America, where contraception just for the purpose of limiting family size contravenes religious teaching and traditions. In Chile,

---

[7] Part of the age difference could be accounted for by women in their forties being postmenopausal or otherwise not truly at risk of conception, though the denominators for the rates shown exclude women who reported that they were no longer fertile.

between 1965 and 1972, the infant mortality rate declined from 107 to 64 per 1,000 live births. Of the total decline, 13 percent could be attributed to the decrease in the proportion of births at high risk because of maternal age and parity. Hobcraft (1987) estimated that infant and second-year mortality rates could decline by almost half for second and higher-order children if all births took place at intervals of two or more years after the preceding birth and before the next birth to the same mother. As Hobcraft acknowledged, such estimates give an upper bound on the true direct impact because some part of the excess risk associated now with these births results from social and biological confounding factors that would not necessarily change when the demographic factors change.

To achieve the potential, though, would require special efforts to reach high-risk women. Family planning programs do not have as successful a record in promoting use of contraceptives for birth spacing as they do in promoting contraceptive use by couples who intend to have no more children.

An emphasis on averting high-risk pregnancies could have implications for the method mix promoted by family planning programs. The temporary methods are relevant for averting teenage pregnancies and closely spaced pregnancies. Sterilization is aimed almost entirely at only one category of high-risk pregnancies, the very high-parity ones. In the world, as a whole, about 340 million of some 850 million married couples of reproductive age used modern contraception. Of these, nearly half (about 155 million couples) rely on sterilization, which is not appropriate to very young women or to couples desiring to space their births (Mauldin and Segal, 1988).

For program managers, increasing the effectiveness of family planning programs for child survival would require market research among high-risk populations currently underrepresented among the acceptors. What do the potential customers know and believe about the value of birth spacing? How can programs reach young women in particular? Earlier generations of knowledge, attitude, and practice surveys focused primarily on desired family sizes and willingness to limit family size; far less has been done on women's (and still less on men's) knowledge and motivations to postpone first births and space later births.

An important concern is the degree to which family planning is somehow interfering with the process of lactation. One form of feedback that is seldom available deals with what the family planning staff (and private providers) are actually telling people about ways of managing contraception in the early postpartum period (as opposed to what is in the training manuals or the official guidelines of family planning agencies). Observations and interviews of both staff and patients could provide more information about what messages are being conveyed, and these could well show a need for corrective action to reduce any collateral damage done by contraceptive promotion to breastfeeding promotion.

Child survival programs, as they are now promoted by international agencies and governments, require the active cooperation of the child's caretakers to have an effect—mothers breastfeed and make the weaning decisions; mothers (usually) are responsible for keeping track of the immunization schedule, for learning how to treat diarrhea at home, for monitoring child growth and intervening when growth falters. All of these stand a greater chance of success when mothers are not too young to take on their demanding role, not trying to cope too soon with too many young children, and not trying to support too many children altogether. In this sense, family planning can be seen as the piece of a child survival strategy that makes the other pieces possible.

II

Feeding Programs and Food-Related Income Transfers

Beatrice Lorge Rogers

This chapter evaluates the relative effectiveness and cost of two related classes of nutrition intervention: direct feeding and food-related income transfers. Recent reviews have synthesized much available information on these programs (Anderson et al., 1981; M. Anderson, 1986, 1989; Beaton and Ghassemi, 1982; Ghassemi, 1989; Pinstrup-Andersen, 1988a; Alderman, 1991; Mateus, 1983), and the evidence is clear. It is simply not possible, or reasonable, to characterize one program type as preferable to another on the basis of its effectiveness, cost, or efficiency in the use of resources. Each individual program is unique in its design, its environmental context, and the problem it is designed to address; these factors together determine a program's effectiveness and cost.

This chapter, therefore, addresses the following questions:

(1) What should be the bases for selecting one type of program intervention over another?
(2) What specific program design characteristics are associated with increased effectiveness, reduced program cost, or both?
(3) What information is needed to select and design an appropriate intervention, and how can it be obtained?

Clearly, because no generalizations are possible a priori regarding the

I would like to thank Harold Alderman, David Pelletier, Ellen Kramer, Mary Ann Anderson, and Per Pinstrup-Andersen for helpful comments on an earlier draft.

choice of intervention approach, local, situation-specific information is absolutely critical to the process of intervention selection and design.

Program Definitions

Direct feeding, food supplementation, food stamps, and subsidies represent a diverse group of programs, and they address somewhat different aspects of the nutrition problem. The common element in both feeding programs and food-related transfers is that they transfer resources to target households, thereby raising the households' real income. Within these two program types are enormous variations in design and implementation. These variations are more important in determining a program's cost and effectiveness than the program's underlying concept.

Feeding Programs

Direct feeding involves the provision of prepared food to target individuals, usually malnourished infants or children and occasionally pregnant or lactating women. Direct feeding requires that the food be consumed by the recipient on site. On-site feeding includes both the provision of food supplements to preschool children at feeding centers and full feeding of children on an in-patient basis at nutrition rehabilitation centers.

The definition of food supplementation overlaps with that of direct feeding. Supplementary feeding can consist of prepared food to be consumed on site or a food package intended for a particular target individual within the household but given to any member to take home. Weaning foods, nutritionally dense foods intended to supplement breastmilk during the weaning period, represent one category of supplementary feeding. All feeding programs provide a food ration to a target individual within a household, with the explicit intention of reducing or eliminating the nutrient gap between the person's actual food consumption and presumed nutritional needs.

Food-Related Transfers

Food-related income transfers differ from feeding programs in that they are directed at the household as a unit, although the targeting mechanism may use a particular individual as an entry point. For example, nutritional status of children was used as the criterion for households to receive food stamps in the Colombian program (Ochoa, 1983; Pinstrup-Andersen, 1984). Food-related income transfers include food stamps, which entitle the holder to a discount on selected food items purchased at private-sector retail outlets, and food price subsidies, which lower the prices of selected foods below free market levels. These programs are intended to raise the household's access to food in the market, thus to increase the household's food supply, with the intention of raising the food consumption levels of vulnerable individuals to meet their nutrient needs.

Criteria for Evaluating Cost and Effectiveness

Measure of Effect

To determine the program that can most effectively address malnutrition, it is necessary to establish specific objectives. Most nutrition interventions are evaluated in terms of their effects on children's achieved growth: height and weight adjusted for age (Anderson et al., 1981). Focusing exclusively on nutritional status of a target child, however, completely devalues any effects of the program on the nutritional welfare of other household members, as well as nonnutritional welfare effects of the increased level of household resources resulting from an intervention. This is unreasonable. Households with malnourished children are likely to have severe resource constraints so that increased consumption of nonfood goods, made possible by the implicit income transfer in the food, can significantly improve welfare. Such households are also likely to contain other members not in the target group identified by the program who are also at high risk of malnutrition. Reviews of food-related income transfers have pointed to the presumed value of raising household income, even if anthropometric or dietary changes resulting from the programs could not be measured (Pinstrup-Andersen and Alderman, 1988).

Another problem with using changes in anthropometric status as the criterion for evaluation of a program's effectiveness is that other important possible effects of improved nutrition, including physical activity levels and cognitive skills, are often excluded from these definitions (Ghassemi, 1989). Severely growth-retarded children respond to increased food intake with improved growth. Moderately malnourished children, however, respond to improved dietary intake with increased physical activity, greater resistance to disease, and possibly improved cognitive development (Beaton et al., 1990). These outcomes are less frequently measured in program evaluations than is growth, in part because they are more difficult to assess.

Measures of program effectiveness that focus on the transfer of resources rather than on the nutritional outcome correct for the intervening variables that are unrelated to the program, which can prevent increased household resources from being translated into dietary improvement or dietary improvement from resulting in improvements in health and growth (Ghassemi, 1989). For that very reason, however, they fail to measure success at achieving the underlying goal of improved nutrition and health. For example, the substantial food consumption increments attributable to the Egyptian food subsidy system did not result in commensurate improvements in health measures such as infant mortality because of poor environmental sanitation and hygiene and poor health practices (Alderman and von Braun, 1984, 1986). The programs were highly effective by one criterion, yet they failed in meeting another.

Cost

Estimation of program cost raises a host of problems even before the issue of cross-program comparability is confronted. First, direct costs are only one component of program costs. Alternative use of program resources is virtually never considered in program cost analyses (Alderman, 1991). Furthermore, many programs contribute to economic distortions that impose unpredictable indirect costs, which may also affect program participants. For example, Scobie (1983) argues that deficit financing of the Egyptian subsidy system is related to the rate of inflation, which of course affects the real income level of the entire population. Scobie also demonstrates second-order effects through the demand for imports. He suggests that reducing the subsidies would directly reduce Egyptian food imports, permitting the import of more capital goods and raw materials, which would contribute to economic growth and presumably therefore to employment and income. These complex effects are surely an element of program cost that are rarely accounted for in program evaluations.

The cost of a program is determined by local prices so that extrapolation of one program's costs to other settings is not justified. Programs that use volunteer labor (such as Iringa in Tanzania) show misleadingly low personnel costs. Food aid may reduce the fiscal cost of the food component. In programs that offer a wide range of services other than feeding, costs may be lower because administration and infrastructure costs are divided among several distinct programs that operate together.

Cost-Effectiveness

Another issue is whether costs should be considered in terms of all recipients, needy (target group) recipients, or recipients in whom a measurable improvement is observed. For example, Anderson et al. (1981) report costs for four feeding programs ranging from $13.55 to $94.54 per year per child. Aside from the difficulty of measuring total program cost, the figures show how different conclusions can be reached depending on the reference group used. The costs per needy child as measured by caloric deficit ranged from $14.89 to $112.21, but per child with malnutrition as indicated by anthropometric status the range was $45 to $290. When the ration provided was adjusted for substitution, the cost per net gain of 300 calories per day per target child showed a similar range but was distributed quite differently. For example, the Colombian take-home program cost $260 per malnourished child, but only $90 per 300 calorie gain in intake, because substitution was low and sharing was minimal. The dry take-home ration in the Dominican Republic cost $66 per malnourished child, but $241 per 300 calorie gain because of high leakage to the nontarget group. This shows that not only do the costs of a single type of program vary widely from one location to another, but their relative cost changes, depending on the environment, the program's design, and the measure used.

A program can be extremely cost-effective and still very costly if the malnourished population is large and the need is great. The more widespread and severe a nation's malnutrition problem is, the more cost-effective but also the more costly a program will be; the larger the target group is as a proportion of the total population, the easier it is to ensure that any intervention reaches at least some of its members. Where malnutrition is rare, more intensive and more costly efforts are needed to reach each affected member. Also, the underlying causes of malnutrition may be more complex and difficult to address in an environment where extreme poverty and poor sanitation are not the norm.

One reason for the very mixed results of nutrition program evaluations is the complex interactions among program components. For example, nutrition education coupled with a food supplement or subsidy may be more effective than either alone (Anderson et al, 1981; Garcia and Pinstrup-Andersen, 1987; Brown et al., 1993). Thus the measurement of both cost and cost-effectiveness of just the food component is difficult.

Furthermore, programs affecting food consumption and nutrition are undertaken for a variety of reasons. Food price subsidies in particular were, in many cases, originally implemented for economic and political reasons that did not include the alleviation of poverty-induced malnutrition. Nutritional benefits of such programs may be seen as secondary, the primary purposes being urban provisioning, the maintenance of low wages, or political stability.

Issues in the Selection and Design of Appropriate Programs

A program should be matched not only to the underlying causes of malnutrition but also to the capacity of the country to undertake it. In this regard, cash, food, human resources, and physical infrastructure are important. There is a political and social dimension to the choice as well. Exclusion of low-income households from a nutritionally targeted program may be politically unacceptable. This was the case of the Integrated Child Development Service feeding program in India (Berg, 1981). Government employees, though not nutritionally at risk, may be a major constituency for a food price subsidy program, as in Egypt, for example. In such cases, nutritional impact and cost-effectiveness may not be the most important considerations operating in the design of an intervention.

Matching the Program to the Causes of the Problem

Understanding the causes of malnutrition in a given setting is absolutely critical to selecting effective interventions. For example, determining the relationship between household dietary adequacy and children's dietary intake would suggest whether behavioral factors or an absolute income-related food supply constraint was at the root of an observed nutrition problem. Where household calorie availability is more than adequate, nutrition education may be sufficient. Where resources are an absolute constraint, some form of resource transfer is required. The appropriate intervention is quite different in each case.

Households consuming the least expensive acceptable diet and still obtaining less than 80 to 90 percent of recommended levels of calories and protein are likely to have a relatively high marginal propensity to consume these nutrients (Lipton, 1983; Alderman, 1986; Ravallion, 1992). Lipton (1983) identifies the "ultrapoor" as the group that consumes less than 80 percent of recommended calories while spending more than 80 percent of its income on food. For this group, he argues, income transfers translate directly into increased dietary adequacy. Income transfer mechanisms alone may not be as appropriate a nutrition strategy where such a binding constraint on consumption does not exist. For example, as discussed in Chapter 4, a growth-monitoring and nutrition education project in the Dominican Republic achieved growth and health benefits comparable to those of food supplementation programs in other countries. By contrast, a nutrition education intervention in the Philippines was found to be ineffective without a resource transfer (although it did increase the impact of the transfer) because food availability at the household level was a binding constraint (Garcia and Pinstrup-Andersen, 1987).

Caution is needed, however, in making assumptions about households' ability to change their food consumption patterns. For example, in urban Mali, even poor households consume half their cereal calories from rice, which is almost twice as expensive per kilo as the alternative (millet). This pattern seems economically irrational on the surface. Accounting for the higher time costs of processing the grain before preparation, the cash costs of milling, and the lower bulk of millet as cooked, however, the relative prices of the two grains are about equal (Rogers and Lowdermilk, 1988). Similar patterns of consumption in urban Burkina Faso, where poor consumers also purchase significant quantities of rice at apparently higher prices, has been attributed to the increasing time costs of processing coarse grain as women enter the paid labor force (Reardon, et al., 1988). These cases underline the importance of understanding the determinants of existing consumption patterns in each locale.

Patterns of Resource Allocation within the Household

A household is an economic system consisting of individuals with differing needs and wants. Welfare as perceived by one member may be quite different from that of another. The household's priorities for the allocation of resources are established through a combination of processes, undoubtedly including varying degrees of mutual agreement (Becker, 1991); bargaining based on social and economic power (Folbre, 1986; Jones, 1983); and implicit contracts among members (Folbre, 1989). Each household has its own rules for allocating consumption goods among its members. Simply providing an additional resource does not affect the household's internally established allocation rules. If it has the power to do so, the household, in response to a resource transfer from the outside, will reallocate its other resources so that the overall pattern conforms to the intrahousehold allocation rules already established (Rogers, 1990; Rosenzweig, 1990).

Substitution of program resources such that the net transfer to the target child is less than planned indicates that the household's allocation rules do not match those of the transfer program. One approach to this issue of substitution is to provide a large enough transfer that the household's allocation rules will result in a significant benefit to the target child. An alternative is to alter the household's existing priorities so that they match more closely those of the program. Some studies provide suggestive evidence that education programs can alter some household feeding practices (Zeitlin and Formación, 1981). The record of supplementary feeding programs, however, shows relatively high levels of substitution and leakage, even in programs that include growth monitoring and health care and thus provide at least the opportunity for maternal education.

The potential for altering intrahousehold allocation patterns by means of education is even more limited in most food subsidy programs. A major advantage of such programs is that they can be administered through the market, minimizing the need to set up the costly person-to-person distribution systems that would make direct education feasible.

Household allocation rules are specific to each cultural setting. Understanding these rules and their determinants is central to effective program design. For example, it is important to know how readily transfers of food or purchasing power to the household are translated into improvements in dietary intake of the target child. Malnutrition of vulnerable individuals within households whose food availability is adequate has been documented in a variety of settings. In such cases, efforts to alter a household's allocation rules may have significant nutritional payoffs. But this is not true if intrahousehold allocation is already equitable and the problem lies elsewhere. Lipton (1983) reviews a wide range of studies indicating that women and children receive equitable shares of household food in most cases and suggests that preschool children suffer greater prevalence of malnutrition because of their vulnerability to diarrheal disease, not because of inadequate food intake. He cites Chaudhury (1984) to argue that households must be severely calorie deficient, below 60 percent of recommended levels, before they selectively deprive certain members of food. These results appear to contradict other studies from other regions of the world but indicate the importance of situation-specific information in program design.

An understanding of intrahousehold processes is important not only for analyzing the causes of a nutrition problem but also for predicting the effectiveness of alternative solutions. The effect of a resource transfer program, for example, depends in part on who controls the resource (whether food, food stamps, or cash). It is widely reported that women have a higher preference than do men for spending on food and other basic household needs (Blumberg, 1988; Lipton, 1983). Whether because of gender-related preferences or other reasons, there is evidence that resources associated with food may be disproportionately devoted to increasing food consumption.

For example, Senauer and Young (1986) report that the income transfer embodied in food stamps in the United States was more likely to increase food expenditures than an equivalent cash transfer. This was true even for food stamps representing less than the household was already spending on food (that is, for inframarginal transfers), although economic theory would argue that such transfers should be fully fungible with household resources and so should be used no differently than cash.

The time use of household members is another aspect of internal household dynamics central to program design because interventions must be designed to accommodate available time of participants.

Of course, behavioral constraints such as seclusion of women or the strong association of some tasks with a particular age or sex group must also be considered in program design.

Prevalence and Severity of the Problem

Resource transfer programs show greater effectiveness when they are targeted to those most severely affected. This is the reason that food supplements targeted to children in growth failure in the Tamil Nadu program were, on average, more effective than those distributed to all economically needy children in the ICDS (Berg, 1987a). In fact, the effect of the ICDS on each child suffering from malnutrition was comparable, though costs were higher because of leakage. A complicating factor in this comparison, however, is that a school feeding program implemented in Tamil Nadu shortly after the Tamil Nadu Integrated Nutrition Program (TINP) was started also contributed to the measured improvement in preschool children's nutritional status because of substitution within households having both preschool and school children, though its costs were not taken into account.

Similarly, Anderson (1989) reviews evidence that food supplements directed to pregnant women are effective in improving birth outcome and raising birth weight if they are provided to women who are thin, who show poor weight gain in pregnancy, and whose calorie intake is quite deficient (Lechtig and Klein, 1981; Rush, 1982; Herrera et al., 1980). Anderson suggests that there is a dietary threshold below which supplements to pregnant women result in significant improvements in birth weight.

Food subsidy programs similarly show greater effects in settings where dietary intake is inadequate to begin with. In the United States, food stamps have been shown to increase food expenditures significantly (see Fraker, 1990; and the studies reviewed therein), but the effect on caloric and protein adequacy has been negligible because inadequacy is infrequent (West and Price, 1976; Whitfield, 1982). In Sri Lanka, where caloric intake in the low-income population is marginal, reduction of the food subsidy significantly reduced food intake and was even associated with increased infant mortality (Edirisinghe, 1987).

Resource Base

Selection of an appropriate program must also consider the country's resources. For example, adding a supplementary feeding component to a widely used and widely available system of primary health care centers will entail much lower costs[1] than establishing a new network of food distribution/health care centers. The availability of a network at ration shops to administer food price subsidies and the long history of experience on the part of the shop owners represent a valuable resource in the countries of the Indian subcontinent, which would be very costly to replicate in countries without this experience.

One important advantage of most food price interventions, compared with either feeding programs or food stamps, is that they are administered through the market system. They can therefore reach more people in more widely dispersed areas, with much lighter demand on physical infrastructure and personnel. Of course, even the private-sector marketing system is often limited in reaching remote areas. Targeting such programs is more difficult, but wider coverage can be achieved more quickly than would be the case where new distribution centers need to be established and personnel trained.

Food stamps, though they use the private sector retail system for food distribution, require an efficient and reliable banking system for redemption of the stamps, as well as the faith of food marketers in the continued commitment of the government to the program. Without this confidence, food stamps will not be accepted in lieu of cash. Food stamp programs also require a system for determining eligibility, which must make use of literate and numerate program staff, often a scarce resource in poor countries.

Feeding programs are necessarily local, not national, because of the need for frequent, regular, face-to-face contact between program participants and administrators to distribute food and other services. Thus one reason for selecting price policy as opposed to feeding or food stamp programs would be the urgency of reaching as widely dispersed a population as possible and the lack of availability of resources and personnel to implement the more intensive interventions.

Scale of the Program

Cost-effectiveness is determined in part by the scale of a program. Experimental programs often demonstrate high levels of effectiveness (Ghassemi, 1989), which are not always replicable on a large scale.

One reason for this difference between experimental and scaled-up programs is the intense supervision normally given to experiments. Careful attention is given to methods of implementation and evaluation, and the

---

[1] It should not be assumed, however, that the additional work of food distribution can be absorbed by existing staff without reducing their effectiveness in other activities; additional staff would usually be needed.

input of staff time and resources is closely monitored. It is difficult to maintain this high level of commitment when a program, experimentally proven effective, is undertaken on a much wider scale. New, experimental programs often attract very highly qualified and personally committed staff. Expanded programs may not always attract personnel of the same caliber. In the scaling-up process, attention should be given to developing a system that does not depend on extraordinary levels of personal commitment (long hours and difficult conditions, for example) and does not require unrealistic levels of training and competence.

As a program is expanded, it may be implemented in places where it is less appropriate to the specific nutrition situation. Plans to expand any program should include an assessment of whether it needs to be modified in any way to meet the local context.

It is frequently argued that community participation in program design is critical to successful implementation (Anderson et al., 1981), but this process naturally slows the scaling-up process. This must be a consideration in the choice of implementation approaches.

Alternative Program Designs

The different resource-transfer programs have varying degrees of effectiveness in alleviating malnutrition for the following reasons:

(1) Design and implementation of the program are at least as important as the underlying concept.
(2) The program must be matched to the underlying cause of the problem it is designed to address.
(3) Effectiveness will be greatest where the problem is most severe and widespread. This is a function of the problem, not the program.

The variations within each category of nutrition intervention are easily as great as the differences among them. It is these specific program characteristics, interacting with the environmental context, that determine the effectiveness and the appropriateness of a particular program.

Targeting

While feeding programs and food-related income transfers differ in the type of targeting most commonly used, the degree of targeting is a program characteristic which is independent of the specific program type.

Types of Targeting. Feeding programs are frequently targeted on the basis of nutritional status as measured by growth (weight and height for age or weight gain over time). Many feeding programs require face-to-face contact between program staff and beneficiaries so that the marginal cost of screening by anthropometry is lower than it would be otherwise. Food-related transfers may be targeted based on the same nutritional criteria (for example, the United States Special Supplemental Feeding Program for Women, Infants, and Children and Colombia's food stamp program). Many subsidy schemes operate through the open market, however, requiring minimal contact between beneficiaries and the program administration. Using intensive criteria such as growth screening in such programs would be costly. Subsidy schemes are more often explicitly targeted based on probabilistic criteria such as household income. They may be targeted as well by selecting for subsidization less-preferred foods, which are chosen disproportionately by the poor. Self-selection as a means of targeting has been tried in direct feeding programs as well, though it requires identification of a suitable food. Chile's Complementary Feeding Program provided acidified milk to children to reduce sharing of the food with other household members. It was estimated that 80 percent of the calories from this food went to the target child (Harbert and Scandizzo, 1982).

Although many food price subsidy programs are untargeted, Alderman (1991) points out that all such schemes are, intentionally or not, targeted in the sense that the benefits are unevenly distributed. Targeting of any nutrition program—restricting the transfer of resources to those in nutritional need—can help reduce the cost of nutrition programs and increase cost-effectiveness (Rogers, 1988; Alderman, 1991; Ghassemi, 1989; Timmer et al., 1983). But there is always a trade-off between the degree of targeting and coverage of the population affected by malnutrition or inadequate diet. Narrow targeting criteria and rigorous enforcement reduce errors of inclusion, that is, of serving the non-needy, but increase errors of exclusion, that is, of failing to reach all intended beneficiaries. This means that narrow targeting improves cost-effectiveness and reduces cost but at the same time is likely to reduce the overall impact. For example, use of an income criterion reduced the number of relatively well-off households receiving food stamps in the Sri Lanka program, but it also eliminated a significant proportion of the needy, especially the Tamil tea estate workers, whose cash income was easily documented (Edirisinghe, 1987).

Furthermore, targeting reduces the political constituency of the program. Although popular support may be high for a program widely perceived as serving the very needy, a subsidy may receive still stronger support if a large proportion of the population directly benefits from it. Resistance to cutting such relatively untargeted programs is likely to be strong, as has been clearly shown by the public demonstrations against subsidy reductions in Egypt, Morocco, and Tunisia, among others.

The appropriate basis for targeting is a controversial point, which raises the question of whether nutrition interventions are best perceived as curative or preventive in nature. Preventive programs provide resources to high-risk households or individuals, those with low income, few assets, vulnerable age or physiological status, high-risk household composition (including large numbers of closely spaced children and often female headship). Because many high-risk households somehow manage to avoid malnutrition (Zeitlin et al., 1990), it is axiomatic that targeting based on risk will result in a high rate of errors of inclusion.

Programs targeted on the basis of poor nutritional status or inadequate growth reach only those children already suffering from some degree of malnutrition. Such targeting clearly improves cost-effectiveness by including only children (or children and pregnant women) who demonstrably need the program. The obvious disadvantage of this rehabilitative approach to targeting is that some long-term irreversible damage to health and development may have already taken place before a child becomes eligible to receive services. Furthermore, targeting on the basis of current nutritional status or growth may exclude households whose members are at high risk, and thus the opportunity to prevent malnutrition and growth failure is lost. Even if malnutrition rather than poverty itself is the criterion for targeting of social welfare programs, prevention rather than cure is still the optimal goal.

The objective of targeting is to reduce leakage of program benefits so as to reduce cost and improve cost-effectiveness. But targeting itself entails costs, which will be high wherever face-to-face contact with recipients is required for determining eligibility. Intervention targeting based on household income, for example, requires a staff of literate, numerate workers to determine eligibility. Staff salaries are not the only cost of such administrative targeting; in many countries, the availability of such skilled personnel is extremely limited, and they could be more productive in alternative jobs in the economy. Targeting based on nutritional status also requires relatively intensive, face-to-face interaction between the program and its participants. Such targeting also changes the intervention in the sense that growth monitoring itself, irrespective of any resource transfer, has been shown in some cases to be an effective educational tool contributing to improved child nutrition (see Chapter 4 and Rohde et al., 1975).

Leakage and Substitution

Excluding the non-needy from a resource-transfer program reduces one type of leakage, but leakage also occurs when nutritionally needy households or individuals receive the resource transfer but use it to substitute for food already consumed, rather than as a net increment to food consumption (Anderson et al., 1981).

Feeding programs differ from food-related income transfers in the degree to which the resources transferred by the program are fungible with the rest of the household's income and resources. Fungible resources simply increase the household's total real income and are used according to the consumption or investment priorities already established within the household. Fully fungible resources are used no differently from an equivalent-value cash transfer.

Food stamps valid for the purchase of any food, such as those in the United States Food Stamp Program, are of course nearly equivalent to cash (MacDonald, 1977; Fraker, 1990), while those that can be used only for certain selected foods (such as those used in the United States WIC program [Rush et al., 1988a, 1988b] and in the Philippines [Garcia, 1988; Garcia and Pinstrup-Andersen, 1987] and Colombian [Ochoa, 1983; Pinstrup-Andersen, 1984] programs, for example) are less so. Supplementary food is more difficult to use as cash because of transaction costs of selling or exchanging it. Such food is more easily converted to uses other than increased consumption by the target child if it is provided as a take-home ration than if it is given on site, where consumption by the target child is assured. Food supplements are more fungible with other household resources if they are nonperishable and easily marketable.

Still, it is a mistake to assume that on-site feeding automatically guarantees that the entire food supplement goes to increasing consumption by the target child. Substitution of on-site feeding for food that otherwise would have been consumed at home has been thoroughly documented (Anderson et al., 1981; Beaton and Ghassemi, 1982). Leakages of on-site feeding, that is, the difference between the calorie content of the ration and the net increase in calorie intake by the target child, has been estimated in several studies to range between 37 and 53 percent of the calories provided (Anderson et al., 1981). By comparison, leakage in several take-home programs was higher, ranging from 46 to 82 percent of the ration calories (Anderson et al., 1981). This suggests that on-site feeding tends to have less substitution, although the variation among programs of one type is as great as the variation between types of program.

This leakage is not necessarily a lost benefit. It must be assumed that the supplementary food was either consumed by other household members, possibly also nutritionally deficient, or traded for other goods that may contribute to the household's welfare.

Food-related transfers generally involve even higher levels of leakage, if leakage is understood to be the difference between the increase in calorie consumption made possible by the transfer (caloric value of the transfer if used to purchase the cheapest available calories) and the net increase in calories consumed as a result of the program. The usual basis for assessing the contribution of income transfers to caloric intake is the income elasticity of demand, which measures the percentage change in food consumption resulting from 1 percent change in income. A food-related transfer in an amount less than the amount already devoted to food (or to the particular food[s] in question), that is, an inframarginal subsidy or transfer, is assumed to have the same effect as an equivalent cash transfer (Reutlinger and Selowsky, 1976a, 1976b).

From a review of a wide variety of studies, Alderman concluded that among low-income consumers the income elasticity of demand for food is between 0.6 and 0.8. That is, a 10 percent income transfer will increase food expenditures between 6 and 8 percent. The income elasticity of demand for calories is about half that so the net increase in calorie intake for such an income transfer would be from 3 to 4 percent (Alderman, 1986).[2] The absolute size of the calorie increase depends on the initial level. Households with deficient levels of food consumption show much greater responsiveness to rising incomes (Ravallion, 1992).

Complementary Services

Another important dimension along which feeding programs and food-related income transfers vary is the degree to which complementary services are provided as part of the program and what these services are. Food stamp programs offer a potential entry point for nutrition education, growth monitoring, and immunization if they are used in the context of the primary health care system, as was Colombia's program. Many programs, however, such as those in Sri Lanka and the United States, use household income as the basis for targeting and are administered independently of the health network. Feeding programs are commonly administered in conjunction with a wide range of health and nutrition services (see Anderson et al., 1981; Austin et al., 1981; Ghassemi, 1989). In some cases, the food is used explicitly as an incentive to bring mothers and children into the primary health center so that the health intervention takes precedence over the feeding program. The greater nutritional effec-

---

[2] Recent empirical evidence discussed in Chapter 3 indicates that although households do adjust to changes in incomes by altering their nutrient intakes, there has been a tendency in the literature to overestimate these adjustments.

tiveness of such integrated programs, compared with feeding programs alone, is well documented (Austin et al., 1981; Berg, 1987a).

Size of the Transfer

One reason for the very mixed record of supplementary feeding programs, in spite of clear evidence that a food supplement under the right circumstances can have a significant positive effect on growth, is that in most cases insufficient additional food reached the target child. Possible explanations are (1) irregular participation or irregular delivery of the food; (2) leakage resulting from sharing with other household members or sale of food; (3) substitution of program for household food; (4) insufficient food provided to close the nutrient gap of the target child; (5) insufficient calorie density so that the target child cannot consume enough to close the calorie gap. Adequate ration size can address all these possibilities except the last. If the transfer is large enough, leakage to other household members is accommodated, and enough additional food still reaches the target child to affect growth. This may appear costly, but it may still be the most cost-effective possibility, given the difficulty of manipulating household consumption decisions (Berg, 1981).

In the Philippine food stamp experiment, the transfer was large enough so that measurable improvement was observed in the growth of the target children, even though they received a proportionately smaller share of the benefit than adults (Garcia and Pinstrup-Andersen, 1987). The success of the United States WIC program in raising birth weights and improving child growth has also been attributed to the generous size of the food supplement, which accommodates substantial leakage (Rush et al., 1988b).

Nutrition rehabilitation centers typically provide complete feeding of the malnourished child. This approach is costly, however, and the net additional quantity of food may be only a small percentage of the food provided by the program.

Many of the same considerations apply to food stamps and food price subsidies. An estimate of the size of income transfer needed to achieve a given level of increase in calorie (or protein) intake can be made by computing the income elasticity of demand for calories (or protein) in the target population, remembering that the target population ordinarily has incomes well below average.

Price subsidies are more complicated. A subsidy on the price of a given food affects food consumption in two ways: it reduces the price of the food relative to the prices of other goods, and it increases the purchasing power of the household. The effect of a price subsidy on consumption of the subsidized food can be measured by the price elasticity of demand for that food, provided the subsidy is not limited to inframarginal rations. The impact on total energy and nutrient consumption must also consider the adjustments in the consumption of other foods.

A milk subsidy in Mexico did not increase calorie or protein consumption among recipients because households substituted the milk for other foods, but it did increase calcium intake because the milk was substituted for foods with lower calcium content (Kennedy, 1988). In some feeding programs, the substitution effect was so great that the net change in consumption was negative (Anderson, 1986). In the Dominican Republic, low-income consumers responded to a subsidy on chicken by reducing their consumption of rice, beans, oil, and plantain, which reduced both calorie and protein consumption in spite of the increase in chicken consumed (Rogers and Swindale, 1988).

Timing and Duration

Some timing questions are specific to each type of program, and others are common to both. Questions for feeding programs concern the time of day, the time of year (if seasonal malnutrition is an issue), for how long, and at what age or physiological stage (e.g., pregnancy, lactation) feeding should be offered.

Some evidence suggests that on-site feeding is less likely to substitute for family food if it is provided as between-meal snacks than if it is given at mealtimes (Ghassemi, 1989; Balderston et al., 1981). One program that showed measurable effects on adult nutritional status provided the supplement ad libitum throughout the day, at the convenience of participants (cited in Hamilton et al., 1984). Providing food only seasonally might improve the program's cost-effectiveness. One supplementary feeding program in The Gambia found a significant improvement in pregnancy weight gain and birth weight during the harvest, rainy, "hungry season," but no significant effect during the dry season, when food was plentiful in the market (Prentice et al., 1987). A disadvantage of seasonal feeding is that fixed costs for staff and buildings may continue all year even if the cost of food does not.

Several studies cited in Anderson (1989) suggest that nutritional supplementation affects birth outcome only during the last trimester of pregnancy, when the fetus is gaining weight most rapidly (see, for example, Mora et al., 1979). In her own study in India, however, Anderson (1989) found a significantly greater effect of supplementation—twice the effect on infant weight—if it was started in the second rather than the third trimester. She cites mixed evidence regarding the effects of maternal supplementation during lactation. It appears from her thorough review that supplementation started in pregnancy may marginally improve lactational performance and thus infant nutritional status if continued into lactation, but supplementation only during lactation appears to have no positive effect on lactation or child growth, though it may have the negative effect of reducing interpregnancy interval (Anderson, 1989).

It is widely agreed that the age at which children most need food supplements is from six months to two or three years (Anderson et al., 1981). This is a vulnerable age because breastmilk ceases to be nutritionally adequate for children between the ages of four and six months, and in many cultures infants over six months are provided either no weaning food or foods that are not sufficiently calorie-dense for adequate growth. Because of the small stomach capacity of children of this age, feedings more frequent than family meals are needed for adequate intake. Above age two or three children are better able to compete for family food, and they are able to eat more at a sitting so they can get sufficient calories from relatively bulky staples such as rice and cassava. Many supplementary feeding programs do a poor job of reaching children under two (Anderson et al., 1981), which may be one reason for their poor record of success.

The timing questions for food-related income transfers are similar to those for feeding programs. The convenience of beneficiaries applying for the program or making use of distribution outlets must be considered. Seasonal provision of stamps or price subsidies is clearly an option. If private-sector channels are used to distribute subsidized food, the problem of facilities lying idle in the off-season does not arise because presumably they would continue to operate with or without subsidized food. But seasonal subsidies risk reducing the incentive for the private sector to expand storage and distribution infrastructure by reducing the potential return to such investment.

The frequency of food (or income) distribution also affects the degree of the program's effectiveness. Small, frequently distributed rations are more likely to add to consumption than equivalent rations distributed less frequently and in larger quantities (Hamilton et al., 1984), just as regular, frequent wages are more directly related to food consumption than seasonal, lump-sum payments. Frequent distribution of small quantities also increases the time cost of participation, however, other things equal. Feeding programs should have anthropometric exit as well as entry criteria to prevent continued feeding after adequate growth has been achieved. In administratively targeted subsidies or food stamps, as well, explicit entry and exit criteria and periodic eligibility reviews are critical to cost-effectiveness.

Cost of Participation

Cash. Some programs discussed in this chapter require a cash outlay from recipients. Food stamp programs, for example, often provide a discount on particular foods; the foods are not free of charge. This was the case in the Philippine program, for example. Until 1979, the United States Food Stamp Program required participants to pay a percentage of the value of the food stamps received. This cost was a barrier to participation by the neediest households, which became evident when elimination of the purchase requirement brought almost 4 million new participants into the program (USDA, 1988).

Similarly, consumer food price subsidies typically require people to purchase the subsidized food for cash in order to take advantage of the price reduction. In Sri Lanka, the ration program (before it was eliminated in favor of food stamps) provided free rice in addition to the subsidized grain, but most subsidy programs require a cash purchase. The price of the subsidized food can be a barrier to participation, especially if unsubsidized foods on the market are cheaper. For example, benefits from the wheat subsidy in Brazil went disproportionately to the wealthy rather than the poor because rice, though unsubsidized, was a cheaper substitute (Williamson-Gray, 1982).

If a minimum quantity must be purchased to take advantage of a subsidy, or if the participants are permitted to make only one subsidized purchase in a given time period, the lump-sum cash requirements may prevent the neediest people from obtaining the full benefit of the subsidy. In Pakistan, the lowest decile of the population obtained less of the subsidized wheat ration than the second decile, presumably because of cash constraints (Alderman, 1988). In contrast to food-related income transfers, direct and take-home feeding are more commonly provided free. Some programs charge a token amount to ensure commitment on the part of the participants. This token amount can be a significant source of financing for programs. For example, a number of African programs operated by Catholic Relief Services alone have at least partially financed the provision of primary health care services with the money received for supplementary food (Pinstrup-Andersen, personal communication, 1990). It is a question of judgment and local conditions whether the token charge represents a serious disincentive to participation of the neediest households.

Time. Even when the resources in a transfer program are provided without charge, participation entails real costs. Some of these may be cash costs, such as for transportation to the feeding or food distribution centers. The most significant cost of participation, however, is time, including the time required to travel to and from the center, time spent waiting for service, and time spent actually participating in infant feeding. The alternative uses of the participant's time determine the time cost of participation. The time cost is the reason that in programs of every type (feeding programs as well as food stamps and subsidies) participation rates are inversely related to distance (Anderson et al., 1981). Time spent waiting for service is also a barrier to participation. Alderman (1987b) found that the time cost of waiting in line to purchase subsidized foods in Egypt resulted in an inequitable distribution of benefits not matched to economic need.

In some intervention designs, high time costs are unavoidable. A direct feeding program in Kinshasa originally required mothers to attend a feeding center every day to receive health and nutrition training while their preschool children were being fed a supplement. This requirement was modified to once a week because the women reported that they could not feed the rest of their families if they could not spend their full day in market work (Drosin, 1989). Because education was considered essential to the intervention, the program designers were not willing to drop the attendance requirement entirely. This desperately poor population must make a trade-off, however, between the benefit of maternal education and the nutritional value of the food she could have purchased had she been able to work during the time she received nutrition education.

Whether a household chooses to take advantage of a resource transfer will depend not only on the real cost (time, cash, other) but on the balance between that cost and the perceived value of the benefit received. If a large ration or allotment of food, or one of high value, is provided, high costs are less likely to be a barrier.

Summary and Conclusions

Feeding programs and food-related income transfers are two categories of nutrition intervention that raise households' real income as a way of improving the dietary adequacy and nutritional status of their members.

Each category is extremely variable in the size of the resource transfer, the degree of targeting to the needy population, and the additional services or benefits offered as part of the program. In addition, each of these types of programs has been implemented in widely varying settings in terms of the severity of the nutrition problem, how widespread it is in the population, and what are its underlying causes. Each type of program has been clearly demonstrated to be effective in reducing malnutrition and dietary inadequacy if it is designed appropriately and matches the cause of the malnutrition problem, but similar programs in other settings have produced no measurable results.

The clear lesson of experience with these interventions is that each situation is unique. Programs must be based on local information about the nature of the problem and the feasibility of alternative solutions. The solution must be carefully designed to meet the needs of the target population and to accommodate the resource constraints of the country. This means that a local primary data-collection effort, including research at the household level, is an unavoidable element of effective program design.

Some factors that enhance the effectiveness and efficiency of a program are (1) the degree of targeting to those most in need; (2) coverage of the most vulnerable population (pregnant and lactating women and children under age two); (3) sufficient size of the benefit; (4) reduction of barriers to participation, especially those of time and money; and (5) careful matching of the program to the causes of malnutrition in addition to household food availability. The cost of program is not the same as its cost-effectiveness. The prevalence and severity of the nutrition problem may be so great as to render a very efficient program costly. In such cases, programs must scale down their objectives, in particular, by careful targeting to accommodate resource constraints.

Much has been learned in the past twenty years about the conditions for success in alleviating malnutrition. As our understanding of the underlying issues becomes more sophisticated, the need for careful fine-tuning of programs to match their unique settings becomes more apparent. Specific local information on the nature of the problem to be addressed and its environment is central to the success of nutrition interventions.

12

Agriculture and Nutrition

Saba Mebrahtu, David Pelletier,
and Per Pinstrup-Andersen

Efforts to assure good nutrition for a population naturally focus on agriculture. Furthermore, in most developing countries that have severe nutrition problems, a large share of the at-risk population is associated or perceived to be associated with agriculture as members of families of small farmers or landless agricultural workers.

Although nutritional goals are often implicit, the explicit goals of externally induced changes in the agricultural sector are more likely to be enhanced production, incomes, or foreign exchange earnings. This focus raises three questions of relevance for nutrition. First, would better nutritional effects result from changes in the agricultural sector if nutritional goals were made explicit? Second, are explicit nutrition goals compatible with the goals more commonly pursued? And third, what are the trade-offs between the two sets of goals?

In other words, as friends of nutrition, need we worry about lost opportunities for assuring good nutrition because nutrition goals are not made explicit at the time of designing and implementing changes in the agricultural sector? Or can the pursuit of the usual goals of agricultural change be expected also to fulfill nutritional objectives?

Several answers have been attempted. The international agricultural research centers (IARCs) (Pinstrup-Andersen, et al., 1984), the World Bank (Pinstrup-Andersen, 1981), the Food and Agricultural Organization (FAO) (FAO, 1984; Nygaard and Pellett, 1986), and the United Nations Subcommittee on Nutrition (ACC/SCN) have been particularly active in this

Assistance by Rajul Pandya-Lorch in the revision of this chapter is gratefully acknowledged.

regard. Many other organizations have also been working to enhance the nutrition effects of agricultural changes.

Research and project assessments have been undertaken on the subject, and attempts have been made to develop ex ante and ex post project assessment methods. The main purpose of this chapter is to provide a synthesis of what is known about the nutrition effects of selected agricultural changes, including agricultural research and technological change, commercialization of agricultural production, rural development, and agricultural pricing and marketing, and from that synthesis to provide an answer to the above questions.

Unfortunately, much past research on the subject has been based on a very simplistic perception of the relationships between agricultural changes and nutrition and has therefore failed to identify the appropriate nutrition effects. Such research will be discussed only in passing because it generally confuses rather than enlightens. Emphasis instead will be on recent research based on more solid theory and concepts. To assist in providing a more realistic framework for synthesis and future analysis, the chapter begins with a presentation of a framework believed to identify the most important pathways through which agricultural changes may affect nutrition.

Agricultural Change and Nutrition: A Proposed Conceptual Framework

Figure 12.1 provides an overview of the major links between agricultural changes and human nutrition, as perceived by the authors. Some important links and feedbacks, such as the impact on birth weight, operating through changes in the nutritional status of pregnant women and through their agricultural work, are excluded for the sake of clarity. The immediate effects, which are often the explicit goals of externally induced changes in the agricultural sector, include changes in agricultural production, resource productivity, input use, and output utilization. Production changes may include changes in the output mix, production risks and fluctuations, and changes in the nutrient composition of individual commodities. Resource productivity changes may refer to land (e.g., increased crop yields per hectare), labor, or other agricultural resources (e.g., milk or meat yield per animal per unit of time). Changes in input use refer to fertilizers, pesticides, water, land, and other inputs. Output utilization refers to the use made of the commodities produced, for example, home consumption or sale.

Agricultural changes may affect food consumption and nutrition

Figure 12.1. Overview of major links between agriculture and nutrition

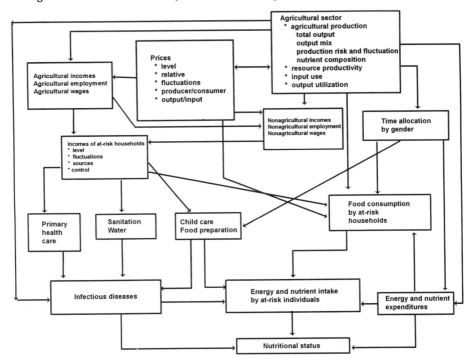

through six major pathways: (1) incomes of households with at-risk members (level, fluctuations, sources, and control), which, in turn affect child care, food preparation, and, in the longer run, sanitation, access to water, and use of primary health care; (2) food prices (absolute, relative, and fluctuations); (3) time allocation, especially of women, which, in turn, influences child care, food preparation, and energy and nutrient expenditures; (4) energy and nutrient expenditures; (5) exposure to diseases caused by changes in sanitation, access to water, and living conditions associated with input use, technical change, resettlement, and other rural projects; and (6) changes in the nutrient composition of individual foods (evidence regarding the last pathway requires further analysis). Most available information concerns those effects operating through incomes of households with members at risk of malnutrition (agricultural as well as nonagricultural households) and the prices they have to pay for food. Changes in prices received by farm families are important as well through their effects on income.

It is critical to note that changes in the quantity of food produced will affect nutrition primarily through changes in incomes and prices, especially those affecting households with at-risk members.[1] But the average levels of incomes and prices need not change to incur nutrition effects; changes in cash flows, other income and price fluctuations, relative prices, income control, and income sources may also affect nutrition.

On the basis of the above framework, available evidence regarding the nutrition effects of each of the four types of agricultural change mentioned above—agricultural research and technological change, commercialization of agriculture, rural development, and agricultural pricing and marketing policies—will be synthesized in the following sections.

The Nutrition Effects of Agricultural Changes: The Evidence

Agricultural Research and Technological Change

Although few studies have been done on the nutrition effects of agricultural research and technological change, a large body of evidence about the effects on some of the key variables in the pathways mentioned above provides strong indications of the nutrition effects. For example, if there is clear evidence that agricultural research has increased incomes of a certain group of households and evidence from other sources demonstrates a strong positive nutrition effect of such income changes, it is reasonable to conclude that agricultural research has had a positive impact on nutrition unless other changes, such as changing income control or changing prices, were brought about simultaneously. In such cases, the effect of each of the changes should be assessed separately.

Production, Incomes, and Prices. Modern crop varieties resulting from agricultural research, together with expanded use of modern inputs, clearly have had a dramatic impact on aggregate food supplies in many developing countries of Asia and Latin America (Pinstrup-Andersen, 1982; Pinstrup-Andersen and Hazell, 1985). Progress has been much slower in sub-Saharan Africa, with a few exceptions such as maize in Kenya, Zambia, and Zimbabwe (Lipton and Longhurst, 1989; Rajpurohit, 1983). Similarly, irrigation technology has been a key factor in increased agricultural production in developing countries; an estimated 60 percent of all grain produced in developing countries comes from irrigated land. Irrigation has had a much more significant impact on Asian than on African agricultural production.

[1] Recent econometric estimates based on cross-sectional data have identified a positive correlation between production and on-farm consumption of a particular commodity, after controlling for the effects of price and income differences (Alderman, 1990). This correlation may be due to perceived or real differences in transaction costs between produced and purchased quantities, but more research is needed to test the hypothesis that there is an effect over and beyond that working through incomes and prices.

These expansions in production have been brought about primarily through increasing yields per unit of land and are often associated with lower production cost per unit of output and with reduced production risk. As a result, incomes of producers have increased, in some cases rather dramatically (von Braun et al., 1989b; Pinstrup-Andersen, 1982; Goldman and Overholt, 1981; Goldman and Squire, 1978; IRRI, 1978; Kikuchi et al., 1977; Rao, 1975).

Very little research has been done on the effects on household nutrition of agricultural research and development of modern crop varieties. Adoption of high-quality protein maize as a substitute for local maize in children's diet in Guatemala improved the nutritional status of children under two years of age (research by Valverde and others, discussed in Tripp, 1984). In Kenya, however, cultivation of hybrid maize had no positive effects on income, food security, or nutrition because lack of supporting appropriate inputs resulted in poor yield response (Lele, 1989).[2]

Modern varieties of wheat and rice have resulted in increased labor requirements of the magnitudes of 20 to 40 percent (Barker and Herdt, 1984; Jayasuriya and Shand, 1986; Bray, 1986). Although this has resulted in increased employment and incomes to hired labor, rural real-wage rates have often not increased (Jayasuriya and Shand, 1986; Leaf, 1983; Blyn, 1983; Lal, 1976) primarily because of population growth and labor migration into regions where technological change has taken place (Lipton and Longhurst, 1989). Labor-saving mechanization, however, has also responded to temporary labor shortages, upward pressures on wages, and government subsidies to import labor-saving machinery. There is recent evidence that labor use in crop production is diminishing (Binswanger and von Braun, 1991).

Two major at-risk groups of households—small-scale farmers controlling resources suitable for the new technology and landless agricultural workers in the regions where technological change has occurred—have shared in the income benefits. The adoption rate of improved crop varieties and the associated increases in profit per unit of land have been at least as high among smaller, low-income farmers as among the larger

---

[2] This does not invalidate the suggestion that emphasis should be on the development of lower-cost technologies that are sensitive to the low economic resource base of the poor farmer. Such an emphasis would help alleviate problems associated with institutional arrangements and local power structures resulting in differential access to technology and modern inputs. IITA's development of valley-bottom irrigation and ICRISAT's micro-watershed development have proven successful in this regard (Lipton and Longhurst, 1989). Other efforts biased toward low-income farmers include low-cost methods of irrigation through off-season conservation (Lipton, 1978), appropriate new systems of foot pumps (Biggs et al., 1977), bamboo tube wells (Clay, 1974), and crop varieties with improved yields at low levels of use of purchased inputs.

ones, except during the initial period of the "green revolution" (Herdt and Capule, 1983; Pinstrup-Andersen and Hazell, 1985; Lipton and Longhurst, 1989).

Except for studies in the North Arcot region of India (Pinstrup-Andersen and Jaramillo, 1989; Hazell, 1987), where increased incomes from technological change resulted in diet variations and large increases in food and nonfood consumption among small farmers, little research has been done on how increased incomes from technological change have influenced food consumption and nutrition. Studies of agricultural commercialization, however, discussed in the next section, show a strong positive effect of income increases on food consumption among small farmers. In some cases, a positive effect on nutrition was also detected. From this evidence it can be inferred that because of the income gains, household food consumption and probably the nutritional status of the two groups identified above are better than they would have been in the absence of the agricultural research and technological change. Whether different research activity or technological change could have resulted in even better nutrition for these groups cannot be assessed on the basis of available information.

In some countries, notably India, considerable labor migration from regions that experienced little or no technological change to regions that did has resulted in a sharing of income benefits across regions, but technological change has tended to worsen regional income distribution (Pinstrup-Andersen, 1982). Farmers who do not have access to the resources necessary to capture benefits from new technology, primarily irrigation, are relatively worse off. Whether they are absolutely worse off depends on whether technological change has resulted in increasing prices for the goods and services they buy or decreasing prices for the goods they sell.

In a closed economy with no government intervention in the price formation for food, technological change resulting in expanded supply causes decreases in food prices, to the consumers' benefit, but the prices of agricultural inputs, which form part of the technological change package, will increase, as will the prices for other goods, including consumption goods, demanded by the farmers experiencing gains from technological change. Under this scenario, producers who cannot benefit from new technology will be worse off both absolutely and relative to adopters, as exemplified by developments in India (Pinstrup-Andersen, 1982). Foreign trade and government intervention also exert important influences on food prices. Therefore, although prices of wheat and rice are undoubtedly lower in many Asian and some Latin American countries than they would have been in the absence of the technological change that occurred in these two commodities since the 1970s, it is difficult to establish a clear causal link for a particular time period.

Price decreases have been advantageous for consumers, particularly low-income consumers who spend a large share of their income on food. No estimates of the actual impact of technological change on low-income consumers through price effects are available, but apparent large price effects in some countries, such as India at times, are likely to have added significantly to real incomes and food consumption of poor consumers.

Time Allocation and Gender Issues. Current understanding of gender-specific effects of technological change in agriculture is very deficient, although there are indications that women and men often are affected differently and play a different role in effective use of technology. It is clear that women do a large share of agricultural work in most developing countries, especially those in Africa (Chapter 7; Olawoye, 1985; Longe, 1985; Dixon, 1982; Mueller, 1979; McSweeney, 1979; Clark, 1975; Boserup, 1970; Leslie, 1989b).

In some countries, some crops are traditionally considered women's crops (Nweke and Winch, 1980; Boserup, 1970), while in other countries such as The Gambia, "the concept of women's crops and men's crops is not very useful in this context, where divisions of labor by sex and by crop have been shown to be less rigid than often proposed" (von Braun and Webb, 1989, p. 531). The nutrition implications resulting from gender specificity in crops are not clear, partly because the roles of men and women are not clear-cut. In some cases, women provide most or all of the work needed to grow the so-called women's crops. Yet in many cases, some of the work, such as land preparation, is done by men. Similarly, women commonly work on the so-called men's crops. Therefore, it is difficult to delineate the gender-specific effects.

Agricultural research and technological change affect individual and household nutrition via effects on incomes, intrahousehold allocation of labor, and time allocation to nurturing activities and child care (Kennedy and Bouis, 1993). It is not clear that incomes generated by women's crops are necessarily controlled by women, although the probability is higher than it is for men's crops (Loose, 1980). The question of gender-specific control of income within the household is important for nutrition primarily if incomes controlled by women are spent differently than incomes controlled by men. As further discussed in Chapter 7, there is growing evidence that women's income is more likely than men's to be spent on food, notably in Africa (Guyer, 1980; Haddad and Hoddinott, 1991). Research from Malawi indicates that in female-headed households where women have greater decision-making powers, mothers allocate a larger share of household food to preschool-aged children (Kennedy and Peters,

1992). But the evidence is as yet weak and conflicting; for example, Jones and his colleagues (1987) found no such difference in Cameroon. Much of the available evidence is not based on solid research and should be considered hypotheses pending further research.

Some evidence suggests that technological change based on improved crop varieties in some African countries has benefited men more than women (Tinker, 1979; von Braun and Webb, 1989), either because the technology was for crops traditionally controlled by men, or because men took over the control of women's crops when new technology became available, as happened, for example, in The Gambia after the introduction of new rice-production technology (von Braun and Webb, 1989).

Adoption of new technology may influence the intrahousehold allocation of labor to production and processing activities. In some cases, adoption of new technology seems to result in increased unpaid agricultural work for women (Spencer and Byerlee, 1976; Dey, 1985) while their access to the resources needed for higher productivity in the crops for which they are responsible is reduced (Jiggins, 1986; Jones et al., 1987). This is not always the case, however; in Sierra Leone, demand for men's time increased by about 80 percent, but that for women remained unchanged, when new rice technology was introduced (Spencer and Byerlee, 1976). Technological change aimed at reducing the labor demand for weeding and postharvest processing has had negative effects on wage-earning women from poor landless households (Greeley and Begum, 1983; Binswanger and Shetty, 1977). Although the income effects are negative, the impact on the demand for women's time is positive, reducing energy expenditures and leaving more time for child care or other nutrition-related activities. This potential conflict between reductions in the demand for women's time and their income earning is of critical importance in all agricultural development efforts, including technological change. One solution is to develop technology and supporting policies that increase labor productivity for women in paid as well as unpaid work.

Time allocation studies indicate that women in developing countries work longer hours than men and have less leisure time (Juster and Stafford, 1991). Agricultural research or technological change that reallocates women's time away from child care or nurturing activities can adversely affect individual or household nutrition (Kennedy and Bouis, 1993; Paolisso et al., 1989).

Nutritional Quality. Historically, nutritional concerns among agricultural researchers have been focused on changing the nutrient composition of individual commodities. Attempts to increase the quantity and improve the quality of protein in cereals were particularly widespread, but increasing the content of vitamin A and other nutrients has also been identified as a goal of agricultural research.

Efforts to improve the amino acid composition of maize protein by increasing the content of the most limiting essential amino acids, lysin, tryptophan, and methionine, which were initially successful in the United States, were continued at CIMMYT (CIMMYT, 1983, 1984) and national agricultural research institutions in several developing countries. The main motivating force behind this research was the perception that the nutritional problem in the developing countries was primarily lack of protein or certain essential amino acids. This perception changed during the mid-1970s as it became clear that widespread energy deficiencies existed alongside protein deficiencies and that enhanced protein consumption alone was in many cases an expensive way of enhancing energy consumption. Therefore, the perception of the nature of the nutrition problem was changed to a combined protein-energy deficiency, and the solution was perceived to be to increase the consumption of the current diet with minor adjustments as needed in specific cases. The change in perception among nutritionists all but removed the nutrition justification for research to improve the quality of protein in cereals (Ryan et al., 1974), while emphasizing the importance of incomes and food prices. Yet recent research indicates that the magnitude of the problem of micronutrient deficiencies is so large that long-term sustained improvements in micronutrient status can be achieved only through more food consumption and higher-quality diets, which calls for greater and more varied food production (IFPRI, 1993).

Agricultural research to enhance the content of other nutrients in crops has not been widespread, and promising links between production, food technology, and consumption to diet quality and nutritional improvement have been neglected. It must be stressed that because of the expected cost, probability of success, and conflicts with other research goals, it is important that the appropriateness of such research be assessed within the context of a typical diet of the target group and alternative opportunities for dietary changes to meet the same goal. For example, in maize-based diets, for which lack of certain essential amino acids is the most limiting constraint to good nutrition, dietary changes toward a proper combination of ordinary maize and beans would solve the problem just as well, and probably at much lower costs, as improved maize. The nutrient content of the diet may in some contexts be of greater importance than the content of an individual food commodity.

Although the quality-protein issue may be of merely historical interest, agricultural research managers today face similar decisions with respect to other nutrients and food characteristics with nutrition relevance, including the content of vitamin A and energy density in cereals. Both extensive vitamin A deficiencies and the problem of low density of weaning foods can be addressed by changes in diets and related household behavior. Alternatively, they can be tackled through agricultural research. Biotechnology in plant (and animal) breeding has tremendous potential for increasing food supplies and the micronutrient contents of diets. The decision as to whether agricultural research resources should be focused on micronutrient and other nutrition problems must be based on solid assessments of costs and benefits associated with the various options within and outside agriculture. Failure to undertake such assessments could result in very costly misallocation of resources. For instance, despite the proven effectiveness of quality-protein maize in children's nutritional status in Guatemala, farmers did not widely adopt the improved seed initially because they preferred the taste of the local maize (research by Valverde and others, discussed in Tripp, 1984) and more recently because of lack of demand differentiation.

In this context, it is important to note that there are other activities such as home gardening, crop diversification, and use of crop by-products that also have important implications for supply of key micronutrients. Studies in Indonesia show that home gardening is most effective in preventing xerophthalmia in very poor households (IFPRI, 1993). Yet many of these activities, especially home gardening, have not been well conceived or properly executed, and there is much room for improvement.

Energy Expenditures. Evidence on the nutrition effects of technological change in agriculture via labor demand and energy expenditures is scanty. An often-quoted study for northeastern Brazil (Gross and Underwood, 1971) found a negative relationship between the introduction of sisal agriculture and child nutrition because of its high energy demand among adult men, which in turn increased the competition for energy within the household and resulted in reduced energy consumption by children. This and similar studies (Taussig, 1978a, 1978b; Nietschmann, 1973) are plagued by methodological problems inherent in conceptualizing and measuring individual food intake. The results should be interpreted with caution.

Some limited information is available about energy expenditures for an array of agricultural and nonagricultural activities for men and women (Pollitt and Amante, 1984; Durnin and Passmore, 1967). This information can be important for planning agricultural research and rural development, but it is insufficient for reducing energy expenditures among the most vulnerable groups—women and children.

Health Risks. The nature of the technological change can influence the health environment and, thereby, the population's nutritional status. For instance, gravity-flow irrigation systems can increase health risks, such as malaria in Asia and Africa and schistosomiasis in Africa (Chambers and Morris, 1973; WHO, 1980). In Sudan's Gezira Irrigation Scheme, for instance, 30 to 60 percent of the resident population was infected with schistosomiasis after fifteen years of operation, whereas before the project began there had been no cases (FAO, 1987). In Turkey, poor water control in a major irrigation project, combined with substantial in-migration from a malaria-endemic area, led to a massive outbreak of malaria—from 49 to 115,000 cases (Gratz, 1987). The magnitude of the health risks from irrigation are not yet fully known, but standard guidelines to reduce health hazards in irrigation projects have been developed (FAO, 1987; Lipton and de Kadt, 1987; Tiffen, 1989).

Interestingly, in areas already prone to malaria, irrigation does not seem to increase the prevalence of malaria cases. In fact, a study of The Gambia shows that participants in irrigation schemes had a lower prevalence of malaria than observed in nonirrigated areas, partly because the higher incomes that resulted from irrigation enabled these households to purchase treatment (reported in von Braun, 1991).

Other health risks from technological change include water contamination by chemical fertilizers and pesticides. Accurate data on pesticide poisoning and related health risks are scarce, but the few studies that are available on the effects of pesticides on human health and nutrition suggest that the use of pesticides has adverse effects on health, which can overwhelm the positive effects on production (Antle and Pingali, 1992; Marquez et al., 1992).

Commercialization of Agriculture

Past studies of the nutrition effects of cash cropping have been reviewed by Fleuret and Fleuret (1980); von Braun and Kennedy (1986); Longhurst (1981); Maxwell and Fernando (1989); Dewey (1989); and Brun, Geissler, and Kennedy (1990). No conclusive finding that cash cropping was either bad or good for nutrition emerged from these reviews. Many of the studies reviewed showed no significant nutrition effects, many others showed negative nutrition effects, and a few claimed positive nutrition effects of cash cropping. Von Braun and Kennedy (1986) concluded that the results of the studies they reviewed were mixed and no apparent trend in the nutritional effects of cash cropping was discernible. Maxwell and Fernando (1989) generally concur with the conclusions of these other reviews, finding that "the naive view that cash cropping necessarily competes with food production and worsens food security is wrong: cash cropping can be associated with increases in the production and availability of food at both household and national levels" (p. 1692). They further conclude that "the greatest effect of cash cropping on nutrition may be through the impetus it gives to social differentiation" (p. 1692).

Unfortunately, many of the studies reviewed suffer from serious methodological flaws, and it is unclear whether the identified effects are caused by cash cropping or some confounding variables. Few of the studies were successful in elucidating and quantifying the processes through which commercialization of agriculture affects household behavior, food consumption, and nutrition, and many were based on simplistic views of the relationships between agriculture and nutrition. Therefore, the results of past research have only limited usefulness in formulating policy (Pinstrup-Andersen, 1985a; von Braun and Kennedy, 1986).

The International Food Policy Research Institute's (IFPRI) household-based studies represent the first consolidated attempt to account for the major ways that commercialization of agriculture may affect nutrition. The studies were conducted in The Gambia (rice), Guatemala (export vegetables), Kenya (sugarcane), the Philippines (sugarcane), and Rwanda (export vegetables). Most of the discussion in this section is based on the results of this work (von Braun et al., 1989b; Webb, 1989; von Braun et al., 1989a; Kennedy and Cogill, 1987, 1988; Rubin, 1988; Bouis and Haddad, 1990a, 1990b; von Braun et al., 1991; von Braun and Kennedy, forthcoming).

Food Production, Prices, and Incomes. The extent of competition and complementarity between food and nonfood crops (allocation of land, labor, and capital) has been the subject of ongoing discussions. Some authors (Dewey, 1979, 1981; Lappe and Collins, 1977; Hughes and Hunter, 1970) have argued that at the national level, food imports do not compensate for food lost because of export crop production, hence adversely affecting aggregate food supplies and driving up food prices, with negative implications for human nutrition. As pointed out by Pinstrup-Andersen (1985a), however, the extent to which foreign exchange—whether generated by agricultural export or otherwise—will be used for food import depends on various factors, including internal food demand, the development strategy, government policies, and the demand for foreign exchange from other sources. These factors transcend the issue of commercialization per se.

At the household level, the IFPRI studies showed that farm households often expand staple food production along with cash crop production (von Braun et al., 1988; von Braun and Kennedy, forthcoming). This finding coincides with those from aggregate data showing positive correlation between cash and food crop production trends (von Braun and Kennedy, 1986). In Guatemala, despite a substantial reallocation of land to the new cash crops, more intensive crop production practices overcompensated for the adverse effects and left export crop producers with higher yields and higher total supply of subsistence crops (von Braun et al., 1989a). In Kenya, the absolute area planted in food crops was almost identical for sugar and nonsugar producers (Kennedy and Cogill, 1987). The case studies indicated that farmers generally attempted to maintain or even increase their food production in the context of commercialization of agriculture, partly as a response to market and production risks.

Despite the higher profits from cash crop production shown in all the IFPRI studies, all farmers participating in the scheme maintained staple food production for home consumption. This response by farmers relates to differential selling and buying prices for the staples needed for own consumption (Bouis and Haddad, 1990a) as well as to price risks and fluctuations. The latter may be viewed as a food security insurance.

The impact of government market interventions on the price of cash crops or food crops is an important consideration in establishing price linkages. In three of the IFPRI studies (The Gambia, Philippines, and Kenya), the new cash crops were substantially protected by government price and trade policy, and domestic prices for these crops exceeded international ones. Without such price supports, sugarcane production in the Philippines and Kenya may not have been competitive with maize, and labor productivity in fully water-controlled rice in The Gambia would have come close to that in upland cereal production (von Braun et al., 1989b). Government policy actions did not always benefit the farmers producing cash crops; in Guatemala, for instance, exchange rate regulations effectively taxed production of export vegetables (von Braun et al., 1989a).

Total per capita farm income in all of the IFPRI case studies was highest for cash crop producers, and incomes increased with commercialization. But the income effect was lower than expected because considerable substitution occurred between on-farm and off-farm work, as well as between crops, resulting in a larger change in agricultural income than in total income. Cash crop producers had 17 to 25 percent higher total income, while the shift to cash crops doubled returns per day to family labor in every case except Rwanda (von Braun et al., 1988). In general, commercialization of agriculture generated additional employment (except in the Philippines) or increased labor productivity in agriculture (von Braun et al., 1988). In general, women were found to work less on the more commercialized crops than men and to work much more on the subsistence crops, except in Guatemala.

Some authors (Valverde 1977; Taussig, 1978b; George, 1977) have argued that commercialization of agriculture aggravates income distribution among farmers through drastic changes in the distribution of land and land tenure relations, hence jeopardizing the nutritional welfare of the near-landless and landless population groups. Land consolidation on some farms and corresponding loss of access to land among lower-income households and even displacement of marginal producers were found to be associated with expanded sugar production in the Philippines (Bouis and Haddad, 1990b). The IFPRI studies revealed that the smallest farm households participate less than proportionally in the commercialization schemes (except in The Gambia), thereby possibly affecting relative income distribution among farmers. When the small farmers did participate, they tended to allocate more of their resources to the new cash crops. Thus the effort to integrate the smallest farms into the schemes should be enhanced by program design and management, especially where access to projects is rationed (von Braun et al., 1988).

Although von Braun, Kennedy, and Bouis (1988) report generally positive impacts of commercialization on incomes, they did identify household groups that lost. For example, in The Gambia, pastoralists lost grazing grounds in the area that was taken over by the fully water-controlled rice scheme. Furthermore, female farmers lost out to male farmers. In Guatemala, increased returns to land because of export vegetable production may have put upward pressure on land rental values, thus increasing the cost of food security for those households that obtain most of their cash income from off the farm and who desire to maintain a certain level of "food insurance" on the basis of their own production on rented land. In Kenya, some households were displaced by the sugar factory and own substantially less land than before the commercialization scheme was set up. About 13 percent of the relocated sample is classified as landless. Some farm households were displaced by tea factories in the scheme area in Rwanda. Seventy-two percent of the surveyed households reported having smaller farms than before, although the relocated households were not found to consume less food (energy) on an adult equivalent basis than other sample households. In the Philippines, some farmers were displaced and lost access to land. These tendencies toward economic displacement during commercialization suggest that measures are needed either to compensate losers or to generate alternative employment. Special attention must be paid to those households that lose not only relatively but also absolutely, so that they face nutrition and food security risks.

Time Allocation and Gender Issues. Earlier reports (Tinker, 1979) that women participate in commercialization schemes to a much lesser extent than men, thus affecting their control over income from commercialization of agriculture (Guyer, 1980; Tripp, 1982), were confirmed in IFPRI's case studies. In general, women's work in cash crops and direct control over income from the new cash crops and crop technologies is much less than men's. Women did not play a significant role as decision makers and operators of the more commercialized crop production line in any of the schemes, even when typical women's crops were promoted (rice in The Gambia) or the agricultural production environment was largely female-dominated (potato with modern inputs in Rwanda). In terms of direct labor inputs, the cash crops and cash-intensive new technologies largely became men's crops (von Braun et al., 1988).

There was a large variation in how cash cropping affects, directly or indirectly, women's time-use patterns in the five IFPRI studies, making generalizations difficult. In Kenya, women were found to spend equal amounts of time on farming, animal care, or child care in both sugar- and nonsugar-producing households and to spend virtually no time on production of sugar (Kennedy and Cogill, 1988). In Guatemala, by contrast, von Braun, Kennedy, and Bouis (1988) indicate that the introduction of the new export crops increased women's participation in agriculture by 78 percent compared to 33 percent for men, although in absolute terms men provided more additional work per season (21 days) than women (15 days). Children's incremental labor input was also significant, with 15 more days of work per household. Increased participation in cash crop production in Guatemala required women to reduce time spent in nonagricultural income-generating activities such as marketing, their traditional income sources. Men continued to make the major decisions in agriculture and to control the income generated. In The Gambia, although changes in production systems induced by the commercialization scheme led to an absolute increase in the burden of communal agricultural work for both men and women, the increase was relatively more for women than men (von Braun and Webb, 1989). As in the Guatemala study, however, men's labor in communal agriculture for the common food stock remained higher than women's.

Food Consumption and Nutrition. There is little evidence from recent studies that commercialization per se alters food expenditure and consumption patterns in a way that is detrimental to nutrition (von Braun et al., 1988). Commercialization has generally led to increased incomes, which, in turn, have led to generally higher calorie intakes. It was generally found that with rising income the relative proportion of income spent on food decreases, but the absolute food expenditures as well as food consumption increases. As incomes increase, more expensive sources of calories are being consumed, which may improve diet quality and increase the intake of micronutrients (von Braun and Kennedy, forthcoming).

Table 12.1 summarizes findings on the nutrition effects, in terms of

Table 12.1. Prevalence of malnutrition, stunting, and wasting among preschoolers: Participant/nonparticipant households

Country	% preschool.<90% height/age		% preschool.<80% weight/age		% preschool.<80% weight/height	
	Part.	Nonpart.	Part.	Nonpart.	Part.	Nonpart.
The Gambia	9.4	17.4	27.5	27.0	29.0	28.7
Guatemala	66.7	72.8	47.2	49.8	6.3	6.9
Kenya	24.3	25.3	20.1	23.3	12.3	16.3
Phillippines	32.2	36.3	45.7	51.8	22.4	27.1
Rwanda	18.6	24.0	11.3	11.5	4.5	3.9

Source: von Braun, Kennedy, and Bouis, 1988.

prevalence of stunting (less than 90 percent height-for-age), wasting (less than 80 percent weight-for-height), and weight-for-age (less than 80 percent) from the five IFPRI studies. Although the prevalence of malnutrition was found to be lower among cash-crop-producing households in all five study sites for most indicators, the difference between cash crop producers and food producers was not always statistically significant. Height-for-age was found to be consistently better for participants than for nonparticipants. Because this is a measure of longer-term nutritional status, it may be hypothesized that the difference reflects differences between the two groups of households before the cash cropping projects began.

No significant differences were observed in the incidence of illness among preschoolers in participant and nonparticipant households in commercialization schemes, except in Guatemala, where the children of the cooperative members of the smallholder export vegetables scheme had a lower incidence of illness than the children of noncooperative members. This difference was attributed partly to the package of social and health services provided by the cooperative.

Malnutrition remains high among cash-crop-producing families. The effect of increased income on the nutritional status of preschool children, though generally positive, was less than expected, probably because of the existence of poor sanitary conditions, poor quality of water, lack of access to primary health care, poor knowledge of nutrition-related issues in the households, and other causes of malnutrition not directly and immediately influenced by higher household incomes and food consumption. In the longer run, income gains are likely to influence some or all of these factors. In addition, income-generating activities, including cash cropping, should include efforts to assure the supply of primary health care and nutrition education and support of community-level changes in sanitation and water quality.

Rural Development

Initial efforts to include nutrition concerns in rural development projects took place in the context of large integrated projects, consisting largely of infrastructural development, extension of green revolution technologies into rural areas, and provision of social services. Unfortunately, there have been few careful evaluations of such projects (DeWalt, 1989; Martin, 1982), particularly with regard to the various project- and non-project-specific intermediate factors and human nutrition (Pinstrup-Andersen, 1981). Therefore, information on the nutritional effects of rural development projects is limited to a few small-scale studies (Kennedy and Pinstrup-Andersen, 1983).

Rural projects influence nutrition by affecting food availability, prices, and household income, but these effects are confounded by contextual factors, such as government price interventions, local market infrastructure, and whether the projects include households at risk of malnutrition (Pinstrup-Andersen, 1981). Much of the evidence of the adverse effect on nutrition of rural development projects on rural poor producers and consumers through prices involves local consumer food price increases caused by market inefficiencies, and government price interventions (e.g., price ceilings on producer prices), which prevented achievement of anticipated real income growth from expanded agricultural outputs (Pines, 1983).

Agricultural and rural development projects also affect income through employment and wage labor. The effect on composition and total demand for labor varies with crop and innovation, as shown by several researchers (Goldman and Squire, 1978; Partridge and Brown, 1980; Dewey, 1979, 1981; Hernandez, 1974). Some projects displaced women from the agricultural labor force, thus affecting their income and income control (Palmer, 1979). More important, intrahousehold distribution and control of income can have substantial effects on nutrition. These and other social factors, often neglected by rural development planners, could be part of the translation of income increments into improved nutrition and could be essential to the sequence leading from agricultural innovation to better nutrition (Goldman and Overholt, 1981; Pines, 1983).

Agricultural output goals have not been achieved in many rural development projects; the evidence suggests that farmers prefer to maintain subsistence food production and food supply (Lele, 1975; Cernea, 1979; Calkins and Sisler, 1978; Funnell, 1982; Deboeck and Rubin, 1980; Hoben, 1979; Teitelbaum, 1977), partly as a risk insurance strategy. This illustrates some of the early obstacles in the translation of agricultural innovations to improved nutrition (Pines, 1983).

The nutritional consequences of agricultural and rural development projects are heavily influenced by the contexts in which they occur. The complex social process of agricultural development and resulting nutritional changes require analysis that explores carefully the interrelationship of economic and social variables (Pines, 1983).

Agricultural Pricing and Marketing Policies

General macroeconomic and sectoral policies define the context within which agriculture operates and determine its impact on income, prices, and, consequently, nutrition. Distorted macro policies, such as overvalued exchange rates or subsidized interest, penalize agricultural growth (Timmer et al., 1983) and can adversely affect nutrition because they prevent long-term economic growth and make painful adjustment measures all but necessary (Kennedy and Bouis, 1993). This section, while stressing that general agricultural and economic policies can have important consequences for nutrition, focuses on food price interventions, which are among the most potent short-run policy instruments available to governments to influence consumer welfare, producer income, and the economy of rural areas (Meier, 1983; Tolley et al., 1982).

The impact of changes in food prices differs among groups of low-income people, and the immediate impact may differ significantly from that in the longer run (Pinstrup-Andersen, 1987). The most obvious distinction is whether or not the poor depend on food production for their income.

Because price elasticities for staple foods tend to be relatively large in absolute values among the poor (see Alderman, 1986, 1991; Pinstrup-Andersen, 1985b), a major source of nutritional vulnerability is a sudden increase in the price of the basic foods purchased by the poor. Mellor (1978) suggests that in India the poorest 20 percent of the rural population would lose from increased food prices because they are net buyers of food. Similarly, in Thailand (Trairatvorakul, 1984), the rural poor did not benefit greatly from increased rice prices. Even though many of the rural poor were rice producers, their marketable surplus was often small, and a large proportion were net buyers of rice.

A decrease of 10 percent in food prices is likely to result in an increase of 6 to 8 percent in the real incomes of the poorest decile of urban consumers in many developing countries, while the increase may be only 1 to 3 percent among the richest decile (Pinstrup-Andersen, 1988b). Positive effects of food price decreases would be captured by many of the rural poor who are net buyers of food. Recent evidence from many African countries suggests that a relatively large and increasing proportion of the rural poor are net food buyers (Pinstrup-Andersen, 1989). In many countries, however, a large share of the households at nutritional risk earn some or all of their income from the production and sale of food. The impact of food price decreases on these households would be negative.

The extent to which the benefits or costs from food price changes are captured by consumers rather than passed on in the form of lower or higher wages varies among countries, and empirical evidence is scarce (Pinstrup-Andersen, 1987).

The importance of increased prices to expand food supplies has been exaggerated in many developing countries (Pinstrup-Andersen, 1988b). In general, raising farm prices is by itself a poor instrument for increasing food production in developing countries (Mellor and Ahmed, 1988). Even where higher food prices do lead to substantial expansion in food production, the consumption and nutrition of people, especially the poor, do not necessarily improve. In India, higher food prices did induce greater production, a notable production success, but the added production did little to improve the food intake of the bottom 40 percent of the population thought to suffer caloric deficits because the higher prices used to stimulate production further reduced access to food by the poor (Reutlinger and van Holst Pellekan, 1986). Similarly, large price increases for maize in Malawi during the early 1980s resulted in a large production expansion, excess stocks, and reduced access to maize by poor consumers (Pinstrup-Andersen, 1989).

By the same token, producers and farm laborers can be drastically affected by low producer prices. Usoro (1972) found that in southeastern Nigeria, a relatively low producer price of an export crop (palm oil) led to a decline of male labor in palm production. The relative income of men from palm production dropped from 80 percent in 1952–53 to 39.6 percent in 1971, forcing male rural laborers to engage in other income-generating activities, such as trading, or to migrate to urban areas. On the average, annual per capita income in the study communities declined by about 50 percent from 1952–53 to 1971.

Thus it is important to manage short-run policy in such a way as to protect long-run investments in the rural sector, while guaranteeing the welfare levels of the most vulnerable in urban and rural areas. A more desirable strategy for expanding food supplies and increasing farm incomes includes a combination of new production technologies—improved seed varieties, greater use of fertilizers and irrigation, appropriate mechanization—as well as improved infrastructure and marketing, which together reduce costs per unit produced and marketed, increase productivity, and expand output (Pinstrup-Andersen, 1989). Such a strategy permits farm incomes to increase and consumer prices to decrease. Food price policy alone cannot solve the problem of food insecurity and malnutrition of the poor any more than it can solve the problem of agricultural productivity. For both problems, agricultural development is needed (Timmer, 1988a, 1988b).

Summary and Conclusions

Agriculture and human nutrition are linked, but the links are much less direct than often assumed. Although obviously food must be produced to be consumed, changes in overall national food production are usually not a good proxy for changes in human nutrition in a particular country. Similarly, except for pure subsistence farms, changes in food production on a particular farm may not result in changes of similar magnitudes in the nutritional status of the farm family. There are several reasons for this. National food production is available to individuals according to their ability to get access to it, not according to their nutritional needs. Therefore, changes in national food production or supply may have little or no impact on a food-deficient household's or individual's ability to acquire food. Similarly, the nutritionally at-risk population's ability to acquire food may change without any change in food supply. Only when changes in food supply and in the ability to get access to food are closely correlated—for example, when expanded food production results in either higher incomes for food-deficient households, lower food prices for food-deficient consumers, or both—are changes in food production likely to be closely correlated with changes in nutrition. Such correlations may still be weak, partly because improved access to food may be used instead to acquire nonfoods; additional food may not be given to the household members who need it the most; and sufficient food consumption, though necessary, is not sufficient to assure good nutrition. Infectious diseases may prohibit improved food intake from resulting in better nutrition.

Thus changes in agriculture are important for nutrition in much the same way that changes in other sectors are: through changes in real incomes and in income fluctuations for food-deficient households. In addition, agriculture may influence nutrition in other ways. The price of food is of critical nutritional importance for food-deficient households that produce as well as for those that consume. The price is, in turn, influenced by efficiency in food production and distribution, production and distribution costs, and government policy. The nutrient composition of a particular food commodity may be manipulated to alleviate specific nutrient deficiencies such as vitamin A deficiencies, and, as illustrated in Figure 12.1, other variables may be influenced by changes in agriculture in such a way as to have nutritional implications.

Agricultural research and the resulting improved technology, together with expanded use of modern inputs, have made a very significant contribution to total food production in most Asian, many Latin American, and a few African countries since the late 1960s. In many cases, improved technology has led to decreased production costs per unit, increased farm incomes, and lower consumer food prices. Furthermore, increased demand for labor has resulted in higher incomes for agricultural workers either through more employment at the existing wages or higher wage rates. Thus, to the extent that participating farmers, workers, and consumers were food deficient, agricultural research is likely to have improved nutrition by strengthening their access to food.

Expansions in food supply resulting from technological change have countered rapidly increasing demand for food from population growth and income increases. The net result of these opposing developments has been that poor people's food consumption is almost unchanged (Lipton and Longhurst, 1989). Most urban and rural poor are probably better off with the technological changes that occurred than without (Pinstrup-Andersen and Hazell, 1985).

As in the case of technological change, commercialization of agriculture usually increases incomes and access to food of participating farmers. Whether this translates into improved nutrition depends on the extent to which the participating farm families suffer from food deficiencies and the prevalence of infectious diseases. Shifts from subsistence or semi-subsistence farming to full participation in the exchange economy entail risks, however, including nutritional risks, which small farmers may be ill equipped to handle. Price fluctuations are of particular concern, although other risks, including those associated with possible contractual arrangements among partners of unequal bargaining power and the production of a new crop, may be important. Public policy may reduce or increase such risks.

Thus the resulting impact on nutrition is a function not only of whether the participating farmers are food deficient and the nature of the commercialization process per se but also of the nature of the related government policy and marketing structure. It is clear from recent studies that commercialization or cash cropping, as it is often called, is neither inherently good nor inherently bad for nutrition. The effect depends on the socioeconomic and policy environment within which it takes place. To enhance positive and avoid negative nutrition effects, emphasis should be placed on assuring an appropriate economic and policy environment for commercialization to take place while promoting improved sanitation, primary health care, and nutrition education in low-income rural areas, where income constraints to good nutrition are becoming less binding.

Although rural development projects often are focused on improving the welfare of the rural poor, few such projects have included improved nutrition as an explicit objective. Furthermore, few such projects have been evaluated for their impact on nutrition and the available evidence is very limited. The conceptual links between rural development and nutrition are known, but more empirical information is needed to assist in the design of projects with appropriate nutrition effects.

Food price policy may be effective in transferring income between the agricultural sector and the rest of the economy. The nutritional effects of such transfers are not obvious. Households that buy more food than they sell, such as urban and many rural households, will be negatively affected in the short run by food price increases. In the somewhat longer run, wages are likely to adjust to compensate for at least some of the loss. Many households at nutritional risk are not employed in the formal sector but instead earn whatever little income they can from informal activities. The extent to which these households are compensated is less clear. Food producers who sell part or all of their production would gain from price increases, and the magnitude of the gain will be in proportion to the amount sold. Thus to the extent that such producer families are at nutritional risk, the nutritional effect is expected to be positive. Furthermore, the time lag between changes in food price policies and the nutrition effect is usually much shorter than the time lag associated with changes in agricultural research and land tenure. But farm families with malnourished members are unlikely to sell large quantities so price increases are generally a very inefficient tool for redistribution of income in favor of the poor because the large share of the transfers will originate with low-income consumers and be captured by large producers.

This does not imply that food prices should be kept artificially low to the producers. Such attempts will result in efficiency losses in the economy and reduced production of the foods for which prices are kept low. There are better policy measures for dealing with rural poverty and malnutrition than artificially high food prices. Such measures include support of small-scale rural enterprises and targeted transfers as well as unit-cost-saving technological changes and improvements in rural infrastructure, marketing, and more efficient input use. These measures would make more food available at lower rather than higher prices, thus facilitating access to food by nutritionally at-risk consumers and producers alike.

Although this chapter has focused exclusively on how agriculture and agricultural changes can improve or hurt human nutrition, it must be noted that human nutrition, in turn, is an input into agriculture (Kennedy and Bouis, 1993) and can influence outcomes of agricultural changes. Malnutrition has negative effects on labor productivity, cognitive development, and health and thereby on the capacity to participate actively and to the fullest extent in the economy. Studies show that improved consumption is linked to improved productivity (Sahn and Alderman, 1988; Strauss, 1986), and better nutritional status is linked to improved productivity (Deolalikar, 1988; Haddad and Bouis, 1990). Agricultural activities that promote nutrition, directly or indirectly, will lead to improved agricultural and economic growth.

In conclusion, changes in the agricultural sector are important for human nutrition, not just because more or less food is produced but because these changes may enhance or reduce access to food by households and individuals at nutritional risk. The impact on such access depends on the nature and implementation of the changes. If nutritional concerns are explicitly considered and the relevant information is available, the nutritional impact of agricultural changes will most likely be enhanced.

13

Community Participation in Food and Nutrition Programs: An Analysis of Recent Governmental Experiences

Roger Shrimpton

Popular participation as an essential element of sustainable development is gaining widespread acceptance, especially in the area of food and nutrition. The difficulty of reaching the most deprived segments of society by traditional development methods has contributed to the emergence of participatory methodologies. Participation here implies a strengthening of the power of the underprivileged. Its three main elements have been defined as the sharing of power and scarce resources, deliberate efforts by social groups to control their own destinies and improve their living conditions, and opening up of opportunities from below (Dillon and Steifel, 1987; Ghai, 1988). At the Alma Ata conference on primary health care (PHC), community participation (CP) was accepted as the basis of the strategy to achieve health for all by the year 2000, and one of the eight priority areas for action identified was food and nutrition (WHO, 1978). Active community involvement in the initiation, design, and operation of nutrition programs is considered to be a critical determinant of the long-term success of nutrition intervention strategies (Austin and Zeitlin, 1981; Underwood, 1983).

Participatory development has proved difficult to achieve through government extension agencies. CP was considered to be one of the most essential elements of health projects found to be effective in reducing infant mortality (Gwatkin et al., 1980). But these projects were all small-scale private volunteer organization (PVO) experiences, and their success has been considered a result of charismatic leadership and impossible to duplicate in large governmental programs (Gwatkin et al., 1980; Faruqee and Johnson, 1982). Analysis of experiences in rural development programs have shown that government bureaucracies are generally too inflexible and centralized to provide the sort of support that participatory approaches to development require (Korten, 1980). The influence of the dominant classes in political and state bureaucratic apparatuses, as well as at the local level, can impede CP even when central political will exists (Pyle, 1981a, 1981b; Jobert, 1985).

Evidence is accumulating that government food and nutrition programs can be successfully developed using participatory approaches. Well-targeted food supplements in well-managed projects can have significant effects on nutritional status (Habicht and Butz, 1983), in contrast to the findings of a review of a large number of food supplementation projects at the beginning of the 1980s (Beaton and Ghassemi, 1982). Usually leakages and difficulties of targeting inputs to the most needy contrive to reduce the effectiveness of such programs. In the late 1980s large-scale government food and nutrition programs in India (Berg, 1987a), Tanzania (GOT/WHO/UNICEF, 1988), Thailand (Grant, 1987), and Indonesia (Rohde and Hendrata, 1983) were acclaimed as successful in reducing child malnutrition rates. Their success has been attributed in part to their community participation components.

The purpose of this chapter is to examine CP in government-promoted food and nutrition programs. How is CP successfully achieved through such programs? The government food and nutrition programs in India, Tanzania, Thailand, and Indonesia are used as case studies. On the basis of experience with CP in a variety of fields of development, an analytical framework for measuring CP is developed. Special attention is paid to the role of information in the design, implementation, and monitoring of the programs. Constraints to CP in government food and nutrition programs are discussed and areas requiring further research and development are identified.

Community Participation

What Is Community Participation?

Community participation is a process of a type and degree that often varies over time, even in the same project. CP has many alternative definitions, reflecting different stages of the process and suggesting that no one definition is adequate. Cohen and Uphoff (1980) considered four areas of community participation: in decision making, in implementation, by receiving benefits, and in evaluation. This ample definition probably represents the full spectrum of concepts that many people have of community participation.

Both Kadt (1982) and Muller (1983) differentiated two forms of participation: direct participation, which is participation in implementation through the mobilization of community resources, and social participation, which is participation in decision making so that community control of factors determining health is increased. A workshop on community participation in development planning and project management accepted the following definition: "In the context of development, Community Participation refers to an active process whereby beneficiaries influence the direction and execution of development projects rather than merely receiving a share of project benefits" (Paul, 1987, p. 44).

All agree, however, that community participation is not political participation but the active involvement of a community in the development process or the process of change. CP concerns the participation of the community at large, not just that of elected leaders or political representatives. The term "community" can include both the people living in a geographically defined area and a group of people with some common trait, interest, or problem (e.g., a mothers' club, a farmers' association). Two distinct modes of CP exist: one of harmonious cooperation in projects following community development lines, and the other of conflict-confrontation-negotiation on issues between people and power figures (Hollnsteiner, 1982). This chapter focuses on the project-oriented approach to CP. CP as used here is limited to the process of involving beneficiaries in the design and implementation of food and nutrition programs.

CP is essentially concerned with decision making, both at the community and the individual levels. Although CP concerns collective action, it is dependent on achieving or increasing individual decision making. The decisions to be made can cover a broad spectrum, both at the individual and community levels. These decisions are expressed simplistically in Figure 13.1. The individual decision can range from refusing services to voluntarily helping in their implementation. At the collective level, the community decision can range from not contributing to an externally conceived program through active involvement in planning and managing a community program. The linkages between individual and collective decision-making processes can be very complex, typically involving boards, committees, task forces, and other mechanisms through which the influence of individual decisions can often become greatly diluted (Brownlea, 1987). Such issues, though important, are beyond the scope of this chapter.

Information for decision making is of central importance to the CP process. Information is supplied through training, through continued

Figure 13.1. The spectrum of individual and collective dimensions of community participation in development projects

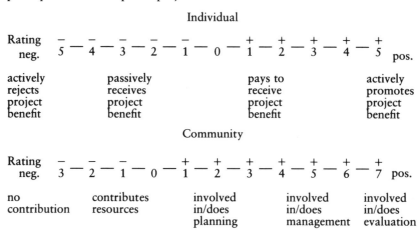

<table>
<tr><td colspan="11" align="center">Individual</td></tr>
<tr><td>Rating
neg.</td><td>−
5</td><td>−
4</td><td>−
3</td><td>−
2</td><td>−
1</td><td>0</td><td>+
1</td><td>+
2</td><td>+
3</td><td>+
4</td><td>+
5 pos.</td></tr>
</table>

| actively rejects project benefit | passively receives project benefit | | pays to receive project benefit | actively promotes project benefit |

Community

| Rating neg. | − 3 | − 2 | − 1 | 0 | + 1 | + 2 | + 3 | + 4 | + 5 | + 6 | + 7 pos. |

| no contribution | contributes resources | involved in/does planning | involved in/does management | involved in/does evaluation |

supportive supervision, and through the development of participatory research methods. Stimulation of the individual decision-making process is the essence of the conscientization approach, using participatory research methods as proposed by Freire (1974).

What Are the Objectives of Community Participation?

Although most would agree that the long-term objective of community participation is community development, the short- and medium-term objectives are subject to discussion. Five separate objectives were identified for CP in development planning and project management: sharing costs, increasing efficiency, increasing effectiveness, building beneficiary capacity, and increasing empowerment (Bamberger, 1988). The relative importance of these objectives varies depending on the promoter. Government and donor agencies emphasize efficiency. NGOs and PVOs more often emphasize empowerment and capacity building.

Similar differences of opinion exist over PHC. Some advocate selective PHC approaches (emphasizing efficiency) and others a broader approach (emphasizing empowerment) (Rifkin and Walt, 1986; Wisner, 1988; Warren, 1988; Taylor and Jolly, 1988). This debate reflects the recognized antagonism between the dual objectives of PHC, namely, improving medical impact and achieving social empowerment (Muller, 1983; Shoemaker, 1988; D. Werner, 1988b).

The efficiency-empowerment debate, unfortunately, clouds the issue and diverts proper attention from the problem—the lack of organizational capacity in communities. The establishment of PHC in poor Third World countries is most limited by the lack of local organization capacity (Chabot, 1984; Goldsmith et al., 1985). The polarization of these PHC issues has been criticized, and a middle way between the two approaches is deemed both necessary and practicable (Mosely, 1988). The less radical view of CP sees efficiency and empowerment objectives as complementary stages in a long-term evolutionary strategy. Advocates of this approach argue that empowerment is a longer-term objective that first requires the strengthening of community organization.

Differences between Government and Nongovernment Projects

Pyle (1981b) analyzed a government-community health worker program in Maharashtra State in India and compared it with the various small-scale PVO integrated nutrition and primary health care programs. The NGO projects were all successful and provided theoretical models for the government program. The government scaling-up operation of the PVO/NGO experiences was not successful. Several authors have suggested that small-scale PVO projects could not be scaled up because charismatic leadership was the most important ingredient of success (Gwatkin et al., 1980; Faruqee and Johnson, 1982). Pyle argues that the failure was associated with rational organizational and political obstacles. The principal differences that Pyle found between the government program and the original successful PVO projects are summarized below in four broad areas.

Orientation/Incentives. The PVO projects studied by Pyle were results-oriented and included task setting. Objectives were specific and time-bound, actions were targeted at the most vulnerable, and preventive nutritional and educational aspects were emphasized. Individual initiatives of workers were rewarded within a team approach. The government program lacked focus, was more curative, did not target, and was procedure-oriented, concerned with inputs. Payment was made regardless of performance. The approach was one of strict hierarchical management.

Accountability/Supervision/Training. PVO training was an on-the-job, ongoing process conducted by supportive supervisor-trainers. It emphasized problem solving based on feedback from simple information systems and flexible local administrative control. Government training was theoretical, technical, one-shot, and overloaded. Supervisors inspected (poorly). Training was undercentralized, with rigid administrative control.

Community Interaction/Self-Sufficiency. PVO projects had community diagnosis, required participation in decision making on action, provided a financial contribution for services, and used existing community groups. The government scheme had none of these characteristics.

Commitment/Time. PVO had a commitment, or political will, to implement the project that was not time-bound. The government program had political will and budgetary commitment but was extremely time-bound. Implementation was too hurried.

How to Measure Community Participation

Considering the different objectives of CP, its measurement is not simple. Several proposals to measure CP exist (UNICEF, 1981; Pyle, 1981b; Agudelo, 1983; Rifkin et al., 1988). Most include a range of process indicators that emphasize empowerment over efficiency objectives. An analytical framework is proposed in Table 13.1, which attempts to consider both efficiency and empowerment objectives of CP. The characteristics of the indicators and their ranking are given in the table and are illustrative rather than definitive. Interpretation will vary depending on the individual project. Justification for the choice of indicators is based on experience of CP in various areas of program development as discussed below.

Needs Assessment. CP in needs assessment is fundamental (Ghai, 1988). CP is most empowering when the needs assessment and action choice are done by the community with little or no external help. For many, community experience in the participatory research process is more important than whether an appropriate course of action is chosen. Mistakes are seen as part of the learning process. Experience of CP in rural development does not support this view because the choice of successful actions was seen as an important factor for establishing and maintaining CP (Gow and Vansant, 1983). CP in needs assessment should take the form of a dialogue between "experts" and the community in project development and management (Hollnsteiner, 1982), where the knowledge of both parties is maximized in deciding on appropriate actions. Rural development projects with CP in needs assessment were better sustained and had a better fit of program components (Korten, 1980; Gow and Vansant, 1983). The operationalization of such an approach is extremely labor-intensive, however (Cernea, 1983).

Participatory research methodologies are used for message development in social marketing (Griffiths, 1988a). Such CP is for making a chosen intervention (nutrition education) culturally and socioeconomically relevant. It is obviously important for achieving efficiency objectives.

Organization. The creation or strengthening of community organiza-

Table 13.1. An analytical framework for judging community participation aspects of primary health and nutrition care projects

Indicator	Ranks				
	Nothing/narrow	Restricted/small	Mean/fair	Open/good	Wide/excellent
Needs assessment/ action choice	None.	Done by outsiders with no VHC[b] involvement.	Assessment by outsiders and discussed with VHC whose interests considered.	Community does assessment and outsider helps in analysis and action choice.	Community does assessment/analyses/ action choice
Organization	Imposed with no active community/ organizational support.	Imposed but some activity, or limited community organization links.	VHC-imposed but became very active.	Uses existing community organizations.	Existing community organizations involved and controlling activities.
Leadership	One-sided organizational support dominated by elite or health staff.	CW[a] working independent of social interest groups or community support structure.	Organizational support functioning under leadership of independent CW.	VHC or organizational support active, taking initiative together with CW.	Organizational support fully represents variety of interests in community and controls community worker.
Training	Little or no training of CW or in unfamiliar language.	Lengthy preservice training of CW in remote institution with no in-service training.	Preservice CW training in local institution with little in-service training.	Short local preservice CW training followed by regular in-service training outsiders.	Short local CW preservice training, plus regular in-service training through supportive local supervisor/trainers.

Table 13.1 (continued)

Indicator	Nothing/narrow	Restricted/small	Mean/fair	Open/good	Wide/excellent
			Ranks		
Resource mobilization	No resource contribution by community. No fees for services. CW externally financed.	Fees for services, no fund-raising, VHC has no control over money collected. CW externally paid.	Community fund-raising and fees paid but no VHC control of expenditure. CW voluntary.	Occasional community fund-raising but no fees; VHC controls allocation of money. CW voluntary.	VHC raises funds, collects fees, and controls allocation of money, pays CW.
	Induced by health staff, CW supervised by health staff.	CW manages independently with some involvement of VHC. Supervision by health staff.	VHC self-managed without control of CW activities.	VHC self-managed and involved in supervision of CW.	CW responsible to and actively supervised by VHC.
Management	No clear objectives, no targeting, curative.	Process-oriented objectives, no targeting, curative more than preventive.	Impact-oriented objectives but no targeting and more curative than preventive.	Impact-oriented objective, VHC interventions targeted to at-risk groups, but more curative than preventive.	Impact-oriented objectives, CW interventions targeted at at-risk groups. Preventive and curative.
Orientation of actions	No IS,[c] or information used locally. Nobody aware of problem dimension or program progress.	Information sent to outsiders who are aware of problem dimension and program progress, but no feedback to VHC.	IS used for routine daily activities/decision making by CW, who is aware of dimension of process and program progress.	VHC receives information necessary for decision making from CW. VHC aware of problem, program progress/benefits.	Impact-oriented objectives, CW interventions targeted at at-risk groups. Preventive and curative.
Monitoring evaluation/ information exchange					VHC disseminates information so that community is aware of problems program and progress/benefits.

[a] CW = community worker
[b] VHC = village health committee
[c] IS = information system

tional capacity is important for achieving empowerment objectives but does not help in furthering short-term efficiency objectives and is very laborious and time-consuming. In Table 13.1, the lowest score is given when no community organization is used to promote activities in the community, or a committee, such as a village health committee, is imposed from outside. CP in rural development programs was most often successful when developed through existing formal or informal organizations and through more than one organization if necessary (Korten, 1980; Cohen and Uphoff, 1980; Gow and Vansant, 1983). In Panama, after political and administrative support for PHC stopped, the degree of linkage with other local organizations was a key factor for the continued existence of local health committees (Laforgia, 1986).

Leadership. The autonomy of the community organizational capacity is important for empowerment objectives. In the short term, it may be more efficient for an external agency to assume or impose leadership. Over the long term, the greater the community leadership the more likely that a program will be accepted, successful, and sustained (Gow and Vansant, 1983; Korten, 1980). A large need exists for developing (training) indigenous community leaders. In Table 13.1, the lowest rating is given when the leadership for all activities is rooted in a service system such as the health system. The highest rating is given when the community organizations control the activities of the community worker.

Training. Training has important implications for both efficiency and empowerment objectives. The building of organizational capacity through on-the-job training, following a process approach of learning by planning, was a key feature of successful community participation in rural development programs (Korten, 1980; Gow and Vansant, 1983). In successful nongovernmental PHC projects in India, in-service training was an ongoing process. It was provided by supportive supervisor-trainers and emphasized problem solving. In less successful government PHC programs, training was one-shot, theoretical, and technically overloaded. External or nonlocal institutions provided training that was divorced from subsequent nonsupportive supervision (Pyle, 1981a; Lalitha and Standley, 1988).

Resource Mobilization. This indicator is relevant to both empowerment and efficiency objectives. Voluntary local commitment of labor, time, or money can obviously lessen the cost to government of providing a service. Such commitments are also necessary for breaking paternalism, which reinforces local passivity and dependence. Resource mobilization is common in nongovernmental programs but difficult in government ones. Politicians will often resist government attempts to charge for services because they prefer to distribute free services in exchange for political compliance (Gow and Vansant, 1983; Pyle, 1981b). Communities are most willing to contribute for drugs or water and sanitation services, not nutritional ones (Laforgia, 1986; Parlato and Favin, 1982).

Management. This indicator concerns how community workers are supervised and to whom they must account. It is closely related to the organization and leadership indicators. In the short term, direct supervision by the extension agency with no link to any community organization is the most efficient scheme. Over the medium and long terms, a community worker who reports to and is paid by the community, with technical supervision provided by the extension agency, will meet both efficiency and empowerment objectives. Rural development and PHC experience favor the latter structure (Gow and Vansant, 1983; Laforgia, 1986; Pyle, 1981a). In Table 13.1, the lowest rating is given when a community worker responds exclusively to an external body such as the health service. The highest rating is given when the community worker is responsible to and supervised by the village health committee.

Orientation of Actions. This indicator is important for both efficiency and empowerment objectives. Starting small with simple activities that can soon produce visible effects was essential to successful community participation in rural development projects (Korten, 1980; Gow and Vansant, 1983). Successful nongovernmental PHC projects in India used a results-oriented approach with task setting. Objectives were specific and time-bound, and preventive and curative actions were targeted at the most vulnerable. Government programs lacked focus, were more curative, did not target, and were procedure-oriented (Pyle, 1981b). In Table 13.1, the lowest rating is given when activities are curative, there are no clear outcome objectives, and no targeting. The highest rating is given when objectives are impact-oriented, and actions are targeted at the most at-risk groups.

Monitoring, Evaluation, and Information Exchange. How information is generated and used has important implications for both empowerment and efficiency objectives. The learning by planning process, basic to empowerment, depends on a community being able to see the results of its actions. CP requires simple information systems developed for local use, capable of monitoring both activities (process) and benefits (outcomes) (Korten, 1980). Program information systems in PHC projects are often excessively complicated and seldom used for decision making at any level (Parlato and Favin, 1982). Few PHC projects have tried to disseminate results locally showing the benefits of participation (Parlato and Favin, 1982). In Table 13.1, the lowest rating is given when no information system exists. The highest rating is given when the community organization (village health committee) collects information regularly concerning the food and nutrition situation and program activities and disseminates them to the community.

Community Participation in Government Food and Nutrition Programs

The determinants of success of a program with a community participation component may be grouped into three clusters. The first is political will at the central government level (made evident, for example, by a budget commitment). The second is local administrative support (made evident by decentralized decision making). The third is the organizational capacity of the community necessary to receive inputs (Bossert and Parker, 1984). The analysis of the case studies is concentrated at the community level.

The examples chosen for analysis are the Tamil Nadu Integrated Nutrition Project, India; the Iringa Nutrition Program, Tanzania; the National Growth Monitoring Program, Thailand; and the Family Nutrition Improvement Program, Indonesia. These government programs have claimed at different times to be effective and to have community participation as an important part of their implementation strategies.[1]

To evaluate the community participation component of the projects, the analytical framework developed in Table 13.1 was applied to each one. Based on the information contained in published and unpublished sources, an analysis was performed for each indicator. The ratings of the various characteristics of the four programs are presented in Table 13.2, together with sources of information. These were confirmed on the basis of firsthand site visits in the case of Iringa and Tamil Nadu (Pelletier, 1990; Shekar, 1990). The derivation of the ratings for the four projects is explained below.

India: The Tamil Nadu Integrated Nutrition Project

The community participation characteristics of the TINP project are fair, favoring efficiency over empowerment. On the basis of the framework for analyzing community participation, TINP achieved a combined rank score on the eight indicators of 20.5/40 (55 percent). The TINP training component is good, with in-service training and supportive local supervision. Simple impact-oriented information systems, task setting,

[1] See the Appendix for brief descriptions of these programs.

Table 13.2. An analysis of the community participation characteristics of various government integrated primary health and nutrition care programs

	India[1] World Bank Tamil Nadu	Thailand[2] National programs	UPGK Balita[3]	Tanzania[4] Iringa
Needs assessment	1	1	1	2
Organization	2	1	1	4
Leadership	2	1	2	5
Training	5	1	1	4
Resource mobilization	2	1	3	5
Management	1	1	1	5
Orientation of activities	5	4	5	5
Monitoring evaluation	4	2	5	5

Sources:
[1] Murthy, 1985; Berg, 1987a.
[2] Grant, 1987; Zinn and Drake, 1988; Teller, 1986b; Zerfas, 1986; Shoemaker, 1988.
[3] Rohde and Hendrata, 1983; Priyosusilo, 1988; Zinn and Drake, 1988.
[4] GOT/WHO/UNICEF, 1988; Zinn and Drake, 1988.

and focused interventions targeted at at-risk groups all contribute to the project's efficiency.

Program objectives and results are disseminated in the community as a means for mobilizing support. The TINP has little or no community participation in needs assessment or action choice, little community articulation or link with a village health committee or local support organization, little or no mobilization of community resources (apart from some women's groups that voluntarily assist in production of the food supplement), and no community participation in project management. Although leadership is firmly planted in the service system, the community worker seems to work independently of social interest groups.

Thailand: The National Growth-Monitoring Program

Introduced in 1981 by the Ministry of Public Health, the growth-monitoring program is a component of the larger rural primary health care program and is implemented in all of Thailand's villages. In successive national development plans, emphasis has been given to community preparation for community participation through assisting the people to recognize their nutritional problems and be ready to start problem-solving interventions (Suntikitrungruang, 1984). The activities include three monthly weighings of all children under age five in the village. All children suffering second and third grade malnutrition are then weighed monthly and given food supplementation for three months. They are followed by or referred to the health service if they do not recuperate (Zinn and Drake, 1988).

An analysis of the community participation characteristics of the Thailand program in Table 13.2 reveals it to be very restricted, with a combined rank score of 11/40 (27.5 percent). There is no needs assessment, and the activities are developed vertically through the health sector, with little or no link to any community organization. Leadership rests with the health staff. Training of community workers is minimal (5-10 days) and one-shot. The community does not mobilize resources, and even the volunteers get free health care. The community "volunteers" are managed directly by health staff. The actions are fairly restricted, focused, and targeted. There is very little growth monitoring because the three monthly weighings are a screening exercise to identify malnourished children for targeting curative supplementary feeding. Preventive growth monitoring for growth promotion does not occur. The results of the weighings are used little locally for education or public dissemination. They are not discussed in any public forum or considered at meetings of the village development council.

Indonesia: The Family Nutrition Improvement Program (UPGK Balita)

The community participation aspects of the UPGK program are ranked as fair, with a combined score of 19/40 (47.5 percent). Community volunteers do not carry out a needs assessment with the community. The UPGK has no guaranteed link to a discussion forum such as a village health committee. There seems to be no mechanism to guarantee the involvement of different community associations, although there is evidence that UPGK is more effective where the weighing is developed through village women's groups (Wirawan, 1986). The original Banjarnegara model used the local women's meetings intensively as its forum of action (Rohde et al., 1975). Community workers are more linked to their Ministry of Health supervisors than to any specific community organization, but they probably work independently of specific social interest groups. Training is limited to one week with no continuous supportive supervision. Apart from the voluntary community workers, there is apparently little or no mechanism to mobilize community resources in the UPGK program, unless the community in which the project is located decides to do so. Management is done almost exclusively by extension service staff with little or no community participation.

The interventions are targeted to the most at-risk sectors of the population through growth monitoring and are impact-oriented. The actions are

focused, limited to immunization, oral rehydration, and nutrition education by the volunteer, based on the growth performance of the child.
Program objectives are results-oriented, and simple information systems
are used to track activities. Project results are displayed at the weighing
posts in the form of a chart showing the number of children in the village,
the number registered, the number weighed last month, and the number
who grew.

The UPGK was scaled up very rapidly, with the intention to correct for
any qualitative deficiencies in implementation over time. In consequence,
the program remains very vertical with limited locally predetermined actions. Its objectives are almost purely educational. Berman (1984) has
suggested that great geographical variation exists in the quality of community health worker activities in Java. Zinn and Drake (1988) found that
the ratio of children to health worker at the UPGK Balita weighing posts
ranged from 18 to 322, which also suggests great heterogeneity of
implementation.

Tanzania: The Iringa Nutrition Program

As discussed further in the Appendix, the Iringa program interventions
are a broad mix of actions, including a systems development and support
program designed to stimulate the capacity for analysis and assessment
for action (the Triple-A strategy) (Jonsson, 1988; Pelletier, 1991b). The
Triple-A strategy is fundamental to the program, as described in Chapter 11.

The community participation characteristics, presented in Table 13.2,
show that the Iringa program scores high with combined rank score of
34/40 (85 percent). Overall needs assessment was done at the regional
level by a project design team, but significant community input exists in
choosing which interventions to initiate. The village health committees
were chosen by the communities with outside assistance but have become
very active and subject to the control of existing community organizational structures. The community workers are fully under the guidance of
the existing community organizational leadership, which by design is the
same as political party leadership. Training is very decentralized and
largely based on the Triple-A cycle. Short local preservice training seems
to have been supplemented by periodic in-service training from outside
the community (regional level). No external food aid supplementation is
included in the program, and most resource problems have to be resolved
at the village level. The best example of how this has happened is the
creation of day care facilities in each community. Through applying
Triple-A at the village health council level, over time it became apparent

that children three years of age were not fed often enough because their mothers were too busy in the fields. In discussion with the village committees, day care was chosen as the most appropriate action to solve the problem. As a consequence, more than 90 percent of village councils pay for somebody to look after the village weaning-age children while the mothers work in the fields. Community health workers are also paid for by the community. Management of the community workers is the responsibility of the community health council, with technical supervision from the health system. Orientation of actions is determined by the Triple-A cycle at all levels. Through active outreach of growth monitoring, actions are concentrated in children with growth faltering. Emphasis is given to outcome objectives. Over time the capacity for Triple-A at the village level was created so that monitoring and evaluation of activities, largely carried out by the village health worker, has eventually come under the control of the village health committee.

The Iringa nutrition project has created a local administrative capacity that supports and promotes community participation in making decisions concerning nutrition. Whether this capacity can be maintained after external financing is withdrawn remains to be seen. More than 60 percent of the externally originated ongoing costs are for maintenance of the support team for the regional administrative activities in favor of the program.

Lessons Learned and Implications for Food and Nutrition Policy

This review indicates that CP, although limited, is both possible and beneficial in government food and nutrition programs. As discussed further in the Appendix, all projects claimed that the prevalence of severe malnutrition decreased by 30 to 50 percent within two to three years of project implementation. There is evidence in Tamil Nadu and Iringa that similar populations in nearby areas not covered by the projects did not experience similar improvements. In India, Thailand, and Indonesia, community participation was oriented toward achieving efficiency objectives. Only in Tanzania were both empowerment and efficiency objectives being pursued and gradually met.

Severe malnutrition is being detected and treated efficiently in these government programs, but in the absence of empowerment objectives the programs might be criticized as being palliative. It might be argued that being palliative effectively is enough and that socioeconomic development will eventually bring the remedy. Others would argue that being palliative delays socioeconomic development. All experiences of CP reviewed agree that being effective is a key requirement for achieving the degree of community organization that will permit empowerment to occur. Further program development is necessary to see whether government programs of the type analyzed are capable of evolving and becoming more empowering. The reorientation of training and management components of such programs could facilitate such a process.

Information for Decision Making in the Community

CP in needs assessment is considered essential for community participation, but of the government programs only Iringa achieved this goal. The development of methodologies for achieving CP in problem diagnosis could improve empowerment aspects of government programs. Examples of dialogue between "experts" and the community over possible actions to be taken based on the problem diagnosis are scarce (Hollnsteiner, 1982). Various documents, largely aimed at nongovernmental projects, explain how to do a community diagnosis (Brown and Brown, 1982; King et al., 1972; Galbraith, 1976; Werner, 1983; Fuerstein, 1986). An analysis of experience in NGO/PVO projects would be useful in drawing up guidelines to facilitate the future development of such activities in government programs. One difficulty preventing many government agencies from doing this is that they can provide solutions to only a limited number of the many problems the community faces.

Although the dual PHC objectives of empowerment and efficiency are apparently antagonistic, growth monitoring would seem to have the potential to help achieve both. The advantages of community-based growth monitoring for improved coverage, targeting, and screening contributes to increased program effectiveness. Experience in rural development suggests that CP is best achieved by starting small with simple activities that can soon produce visible effects before progressing to more complex problems. Growth monitoring and promotion fit this description. If adequately treated as a learning process, growth monitoring has great potential for individual and group empowerment. As shown in the Iringa nutrition program and in some instances in the Indonesian program, the feeding of information on child growth into community organizations and health and development committees can serve to promote empowerment objectives. The most advanced project in these aspects of community management of such information was the Iringa project.

The importance of social mobilization to help achieve community participation in nutrition programs is clear. Nutrition components of programs are difficult to sustain, and communities are more willing to contribute for drugs or water than for nutritional services (Laforgia, 1986; Parlato and Favin, 1982). Communities do not recognize preschool child malnutrition as a major problem when all preschool children in the community are stunted. They become the norm in the absence of an external comparison. Severely malnourished children (III grade) are most often kept in their homes and are such a small proportion that they are often unperceived by the community as a whole. CP in food and nutrition programs depends on making the problem and the benefits of preventive measures visible to the community. CP should involve the maximum number of people in a democratic review of the problem and discussion of possible solutions and goals. Community mobilization for a program depends on working initially with strategic allies in the community, such as leaders of opinion, religion, administration, and commerce, who favor gradually mobilizing the entire community on behalf of the goal. For the purpose of setting community goals and measuring their degree of attainment, some system of community-based growth monitoring or nutritional surveillance is necessary.

Despite its extensive use in food and nutrition programs, growth monitoring is still conceptually confused and surprisingly little researched (see Chapter 5 for more discussion). All of the projects reviewed here claimed to be doing growth monitoring, but all used child growth or weight information for a wide variety of purposes. A better understanding of the use of information on child growth for individual counseling, social mobilization, screening, targeting, and surveillance purposes is needed. More research is necessary to determine the appropriateness and adequacy of different indicators for these different program purposes (Taylor, 1988; Gerein, 1988).

The orientation of actions has important implications for both empowerment and efficiency objectives. All programs scored high on this indicator. Government programs typically emphasize actions over outcomes. Performances are measured on the basis of pills distributed, injections applied, lectures performed, and food packets distributed, not how many children are malnourished or grew properly last month. The adoption of impact-oriented objectives forces the need for an outcome-driven monitoring system. Monitoring systems that track impact or results facilitate achieving community participation and empowerment objectives and, through social mobilization, can help overcome bureaucratic inertia.

Implementation Issues

The organization, leadership, management, and resource mobilization indicators are interrelated and important for achieving empowerment objectives. Only in the Iringa project were these aspects well developed. Most communities need a great deal of outside support at the beginning of a project. The gradual transfer of leadership to community organizations increases sustainability and does not compromise government capacity to expand to other communities. The difficulty in government programs is getting government officials to avoid creating dependency. This problem can be resolved with well-conceived training and the correct orientation of actions.

Only the Tanzanian program scored high on the management indicator. For short-term efficiency purposes, the volunteer or community paid worker (trained in a one-shot training course) linked to a health system supervisor (inspector) is obviously the most efficient situation. In this situation, the community worker becomes the lackey of the health system (Werner, 1983). At the opposite end of the spectrum, the community worker reports to and is paid by a community organization or the health committee. In addition, these workers receive regular technical supportive supervision from the health system. This latter situation has potential efficiency benefits for the health system, but it is not easily achieved in the short term. Iringa is the best example of the mobilization of local resources in the government programs reviewed, but Tanzania is politically very favorable for doing so. The Tamil Nadu and Thailand approaches create dependency on the supply of external food resources, which inevitably blocks community development of autonomous solutions. Community resource mobilization is in the interests of program efficiency. It is in the interest of community empowerment for the community to control resources and paternalistic relationships to be broken. The achievement of this situation within government food and nutrition programs is largely dependent on political will. If that exists, the rest could be achieved with time by properly resolving the training, organization, and leadership factors.

The feasibility of participatory approaches to development obviously depends on the political and cultural climate in which a program is being implemented. For this reason, it is important to conceptualize CP as a gradual process that might start off weak in many aspects but should be designed with the intention of evolving and becoming stronger. In this light, it should be realized that to gain a rank of 2 for organization (see Table 13.1) in India may be more difficult than gaining a rank of 5 in Tanzania. In many political and cultural situations, only nongovernmental organizations are able to implement participatory approaches to development.

The adoption of impact- or results-oriented objectives can help to overcome political and cultural barriers to participatory development. Objectives such as reduction of infant mortality and child malnutrition in a community are difficult to contest on any political or cultural grounds.

Acceptance of such objectives or community goals almost inevitably leads to the need to involve the most affected in the solution of the problem. Advocacy for child survival and development goals at the international and national levels can facilitate the acceptance of such goals at the community level.

Training through supportive local supervision was key to the success of two of the programs analyzed. Tamil Nadu has developed decentralized training packages that are structured and focused on a limited number of program actions. Training is action-based learning by doing, with little theory or classroom learning. Close supportive supervision makes training a continuous process. Training in the Iringa program is less structured, emphasizes problem solving, and is a component of continuous supportive supervision. Recent analysis of PHC programs suggest that although community health workers may be capable of extending health service coverage and in many places are doing so effectively, their true potential is still not being fully realized (Scholl, 1985; Gray, 1986; Berman et al., 1987). Considerably more investment in training, supervision, and logistics is necessary than is being provided in many large-scale government PHC programs. The cost of providing such supervision is potentially onerous, however, and its practicability is open to question. In many African countries, it does not seem possible (Gray, 1986).

Training is most empowering when community members instead of government employees are trained to supervise and train the community workers. For many governments, this may prove the only affordable way of achieving high coverage. The approximation of nongovernmental and government agencies at the community level is a problem in many Third World countries, however. Inequality in the distribution of income and access to the benefits of society is great, provoking much antagonism between the state bureaucratic machinery and nongovernmental organizations at the community level. How to tap the potential of nongovernmental organizations at the community level is a key question for governments wishing to improve the nutritional status of their child populations using participatory methods. The strategy of bottom-up social mobilization in favor of adequate child growth, as is being developed in Tanzania, needs to be tested in other political environments.

14

Multisectoral Nutrition Planning: A Synthesis of Experience

F. James Levinson

During the early 1970s, a significant shift in thinking took place about the conceptualization and planning of international nutrition programs. The shift was partly a reaction to supply-oriented interventions of the past, which had not been particularly effective in reducing malnutrition and had not generated interest—or substantial funding—from development planners and decision makers. It was also consistent with a broader trend toward more systematic, indeed scientific, program planning. And it was based on a growing recognition that malnutrition is not simply a health problem but is inextricably related to food policy, agriculture, income generation, and other areas of development concern.

The new thinking manifested itself in what was often referred to as "multisectoral nutrition planning." Workshops and conferences began to organize around this theme, programs in several universities were developed to address it, and a number of international assistance agencies revamped their nutrition strategies to take this shift of direction into account. Most important, a substantial number of units, councils, and committees were established in the governments of low-income countries to carry out such planning. The idea, in short, was that systematic multidisciplinary planning would produce a combination of policy or project interventions in several development sectors, which, if well operated and well coordinated, could be effective in reducing malnutrition.

This chapter looks first at the components of nutrition planning, at least as conceptualized in the universities and some of the international agencies. Then follows a review of the multisectoral nutrition planning activity, which was undertaken for several years by units established in several low-income countries and continues to operate in a few countries.

In sharp contrast with the conceptual and technical issues, the discussion of country experiences indicates that the durability of such efforts related far more to issues of bureaucracy and politics.

Finally, the legacies of multisectoral nutrition planning and its effects on our thinking about international nutrition today and on some of our more effective programs are examined.

Nutrition Planning and Its Components

The basic components of nutrition planning articulated in the 1970s are those listed by Field (1987): (1) analysis of the nature and magnitude of the malnutrition problem; (2) assessment of the primary determinants of that malnutrition; (3) identification of promising intervention points; (4) calculation of their relative cost-effectiveness; and (5) monitoring of experience and evaluation of performance.

In fact, with or without elaborate data analysis, this sequence of systematically approaching malnutrition problem solving is generally followed today. What has changed is our thinking about the multisectoral elements of such planning (particularly components 2 and 3) and, more broadly, the evolution of a more sober, less multisectorally ambitious approach to planning and a less "nutriocentric" view of development planning.

Determinants of Malnutrition

Analysis of causality represented perhaps the most important addition to thinking about the development of nutrition programs during these years. Until the 1970s, nutrition programs had been characterized by a series of supply-oriented interventions, first employed by home economists in the 1950s conditioned primarily by First World experience, and then a series of technological interventions (protein concentrates, synthetic amino acids, and mass media education) in the 1960s. With the inception of nutrition planning came an understanding that program development needed to be preceded by a better understanding of the causal factors behind the problem. Although this conclusion was undeniably sound, the nutrition planning community, particularly universities doing research and providing advisory services, all too often made the mistakes of allowing such analysis to become overly complex, leading to untenable demands for data collection and analysis, and sometimes drawing the fallacious conclusion that specifying the importance of a cause dictates its necessary response. As Pines (1982) points out, it was assumed that because the causes of malnutrition were multisectoral, the responses also would have to be. Another problem encountered with causality analysis (usually multivariate regression analysis) was that the data used were usually procured at the national level—data that were available from nutrition or consumer expenditure surveys—while, as later learned, such analysis, to be genuinely useful, needs to be done in more geographically disaggregated fashion. Some nutrition planning has been initiated at the local level, but it never involved such sophisticated data analysis.

Although the mostly national-level analysis that was done sometimes required indiscriminate data on all conceivable determinants of malnutrition, and although the purpose of combating malnutrition sometimes seemed lost in the process, the concept of causality brought the field of international nutrition into closer touch with the realities and constraints facing low-income, malnourished populations. This proved particularly important in looking at the relative importance of real income, belief patterns, and infection in malnutrition causality.

Countless earlier nutrition education programs failed because they did not account for the income and time constraints faced by families. In contrast, recent nutrition education initiatives begin with problems as perceived by mothers themselves and work backward from these problems toward education programs.[1] This not only represents pragmatic wisdom but also, for the first time in this work, programmatic acknowledgment of a fundamental respect for both the choices and the instincts of low-income families operating in adversity and an understanding that choices usually are based on generations of trial and error where the cost of error can be fatal.

Better understanding of belief patterns and practices, in turn, revealed situations (for example, particular perceptions of diarrheal disease, which result in delayed provision of supplementary solid food in North India, Pakistan, and Afghanistan) when increases in family income per se would have relatively little effect on the nutritional status of children.

The collection of data on a wide range of possible determinants sometimes revealed situations in which addressing hygienic conditions precipitating infection and disease may have a more immediate and significant effect on malnutrition than increased food intake. (In urban Mozambique, such analysis found that the probability of a child suffering from acute

---

[1] Elmore (1982) describes this process in public policy administration as "backward mapping," which begins at the point at which administrative actions intersect private choices. (In fact, in nutrition education, the starting point would be decision making in the family.) Backward mapping determines the optimal goal based on local realities and then works backward through the structure of implementing agencies, asking at each level how and with what resources those at that level can contribute to the level below in attaining the objective. This contrasts with "forward mapping," which erroneously assumes that policy makers control the manifold processes affecting implementation.

malnutrition was roughly five times higher if it lived in a home without a latrine.)

On the basis of an analysis in Ghana, Tripp (1981) hypothesized that the primary determinant of a child's nutritional status is not family income but rather income specifically earned and controlled by the child's mother.

In some cases such analysis carried out locally, though not highly empirical in nature, led to avoiding costly mistakes. In Pakistan, some understanding of causality, coupled with information on income elasticities of demand, led to reversal of a proposal to introduce a high-status prebaked "naan" (white flour preparation) into the ration shops. In Sri Lanka, similar thinking avoided a costly milk program that in the long run would have been detrimental to the poor.

A related component of nutrition planning advocated by some practitioners was labeled "functional classification" analysis and attempted data collection in Costa Rica, Sri Lanka, and the Philippines. The idea was to collect detailed information on many different configurations of malnourished families, based on such variables as occupation, geographic area, landholding status, type of land, and family size and to gear particular interventions specifically to families with well-suited configurations of characteristics. Not unexpectedly, the data collection itself became cumbersome, and host governments quickly lost interest. Even if the data collection had been successful, it is unlikely that interventions could have been found that were refined enough to discriminate effectively among potential beneficiaries.

Nonetheless, this approach helped develop a consciousness of the importance of disaggregation in our research and targeting in our programs, concepts that characterize today's most effective planning and programmatic activities from Tamil Nadu to Iringa.

One of the most interesting undertakings of policy research to emerge from such consciousness in recent years is the three-year Food and Nutrition Policy Study initiated in Indonesia in 1987. The study attempts to disaggregate macro food consumption data by region and population groups, perform determinant analysis of malnourished population groups, and reintegrate the findings of this analysis into revised early warning and food security systems. Overall, the study seeks to integrate micro needs with macro policies in a more systematic fashion than has been the case heretofore. Significantly, the study does not precede nutrition program activity in Indonesia, which is considerable,[2] but is carried out simultane-

[2] The Indonesian National Family Nutrition Improvement Program (UPGK) and the World Bank–assisted Nutrition Intervention Pilot Project (NIPP) have been important models of integrated service delivery. They include a wide range of community nutrition interventions:

ously with an eye toward eventually using the analysis for program purposes (Soekirman, 1988).

Generally excluded in such causality analysis are what have been called the macro contextual determinants—characteristics of the society, the government, and the broader process of development that may contribute to poverty and malnutrition in the first place. (Nor for that matter has there been much marshaling of evidence on the magnitude and severity of malnutrition problems specifically to demonstrate the effects of such inequitable, nonparticipatory patterns of development.) There was little analysis of this kind in the 1970s—usually justified by our assumed inability to do much about the macro determinants—and, at least among operational entities, there is little today (Hakim and Solimano, 1976).

Identification of Intervention Points

Having some understanding of the multisectoral causality of malnutrition and correctly recognizing that multiple changes in socioeconomic conditions would be necessary to alleviate and ultimately eradicate it, we sometimes assumed that simply by identifying, with some empirical precision, the changes that were necessary, government ministries would feel compelled to respond.

This notion gave rise to national nutrition plans with long lists of multisectoral demands, which never were taken seriously except by the nutrition advocates themselves, and to the substantial problems faced by nutrition planning units described in the next section. Participants in one failed effort wrote that "contrary to logical argument the complex etiology of malnutrition does not necessarily demand a complex response. Complexity in intervention and the need for a high degree of intersectoral coordination contradict the principles of successful implementation and require a capacity beyond that of most implementing agencies" (Ross and Posanai, 1988, p. 144).

At the same time, as Berg (1987b) notes, the multisectoral thinking of that period, however unrealistic, created a sensitivity among nonnutrition professionals in many countries to the importance of nutrition concerns and led in Tamil Nadu and Indonesia to major programs that were intersectorally coordinated if not truly multisectoral. This sensitization also encouraged several relationships that have yielded significant programmatic results.

---

growth monitoring, oral rehydration, nutrition education with emphasis on breastfeeding and weaning foods, home and village gardens, and small-scale food processing and storage. The programs are well coordinated with immunization and family planning services. Rapid expansion of these integrated services during the mid- and late 1980s inevitably has strained

Nutrition with Health. Nutrition without question has added several new and important dimensions to public health activity, particularly at the community level. These include child growth monitoring, highly focused nutrition education (relating, for example, to breastfeeding, solid food supplementation, and diarrheal management) connected with the growth monitoring, and vitamin and mineral supplementation.

Nutrition with Agriculture (and Food). Although agricultural production programs often are justified by governments and international agencies as means of alleviating hunger and malnutrition, these programs, once funded, usually have been pursued in the traditional manner with premiums on productivity, yield, and higher incomes for the producers. Until recent years, the relationship between agriculture and nutrition was concerned almost solely with the nutrient content of crops, while food studies were concerned mainly with food balance sheets and with the estimation of demand projections for agricultural planning and food import purposes.

Today, in part because of sensitization to nutrition planning in many countries, the relationship is beginning to focus on other issues such as who benefits from agricultural production processes and who benefits in terms of consumption? That is, which foods are disproportionately consumed by which people and how is the food distributed?

In some countries, these issues and the analysis of consumer subsidies, at one time a concern almost solely of nutrition planning groups, have been subsumed into the now major policy area of food security analysis.

Nutrition, in a sense, has become the conscience of agriculture, arguing that increased agricultural production per se is insufficient if that production does not address hunger and malnutrition through its production or consumption effects. It is, accordingly, a notch more difficult today for governments to concentrate production disproportionately on large landholdings or to pursue policies harmful to food security at the household or local level without at least modest outcry from nutrition advocates.

National Efforts at Multisectoral Nutrition Planning and Coordination

To facilitate nutrition planning in individual countries, the United States Agency for International Development (USAID), FAO, and other assistance agencies helped several governments establish nutrition planning ca-

---

available resources, particularly trained staff. As a result, efforts are currently under way to consolidate these gains and target additional resources to the needier subdistricts.

pability. In some cases, small units were set up in national planning offices or in the office of the president or prime minister. Others were housed elsewhere or established as autonomous entities, or responsibility was given to an existing nutrition organization.

As will be indicated in the final section of this chapter, the activities initiated during these nutrition planning efforts have led to important program advances in subsequent years (though usually as sectoral programs), and the sensitization provided, particularly to groups and individuals involved in food policy and broader poverty alleviation efforts, have yielded important benefits. Yet the experience of the nutrition planning councils and coordinating bodies, beginning for the most part in the mid-1970s and lasting an average of six years, was difficult. It became clear that the technical considerations of multisectoral nutrition planning discussed heretofore in this paper were dwarfed by political and bureaucratic realities in the countries in which they operated. The history is summarized in this section, which concentrates on the experience of some of the more important initiatives and the primary issues they faced: (1) the scope of the undertakings, (2) the authority and resources provided to them and the problems of coordination they faced, and (3) the political vulnerability inherent in most of these undertakings.

Scope

Three primary examples often cited of multisectoral nutrition programs are those that were initiated in the Philippines, Colombia, and Sri Lanka in the mid-1970s. Although they all generated substantial nutrition-related interest and activity in their countries, they differed markedly in scope. The program in the Philippines, though substantial enough to require intersectoral coordination, was not a multisectoral program per se but rather a collection of direct nutrition interventions. The programs in Colombia and Sri Lanka, though not products of highly analytic planning, did seek to pursue nutritional ends through multisectoral means.

It should be clarified at the outset that broad scope as used here does not necessarily imply large-scale, nationwide, or even ultimately broad-based interventions. Rather, it suggests "nonrestrictive" in possibilities and the potential to venture beyond direct nutrition interventions into other development policies and programs with important nutritional implications, should this be warranted. In many of the countries referred to in this chapter (e.g., Costa Rica and Zambia), the scope of nutrition planning was largely limited to direct nutrition interventions, calling into question whether the planning was multisectoral in the first place (although the interventions selected may have required some interministerial coordination).

Efforts at such integrated, coordinated nutrition activity were already under way in the Philippines, although with limited resources, when President Ferdinand Marcos decided in 1974 to upgrade its status, making it, by presidential decree, a well-publicized component of his New Society program. The timing of this decree raises the distinct possibility that it was motivated, at least in part, by the then apparent failure of Marcos's land reform program, which earlier had been heralded as the president's first New Society campaign.[3] The need for a high-visibility substitute was clear, and an enlarged nutrition program was attractive because it addressed a serious, well-recognized problem particularly affecting children and their mothers throughout the Philippines (with the inherent photo opportunities this implied); provided some seemingly worthwhile programmatic responses, some of them technological in nature; and the international climate was supportive, relating in part to the then much-publicized "world food problem."

With nutrition now mandated as a national priority, a National Nutrition Council (NNC) was created to coordinate nutrition activities throughout the country. At the same time, a private organization (the Nutrition Center of the Philippines) was established by Mrs. Marcos to represent private sector involvement in nutrition.[4] Primary responsibility for implementation of the program was placed, interestingly, not with the traditional central government ministries but with local nutrition committees headed by governors or mayors.

Nutrition personnel in the country responded enthusiastically to the president's decree. A nationwide child weighing survey, Operation Timbang, was undertaken, which eventually covered most of the country, and efforts were made in some areas to make weighing an ongoing program tool. Numerous other programs were initiated, usually accompanied by T-shirts and major newspaper coverage. It soon became apparent to at least some officials in the program, however, that the political condition of the president's blessing was, in fact, high symbolic value at low cost (Florentino et al., 1982). The program consisted of numerous activities and cleverly packaged components with such names as "nutripaks," "nutrihuts," and "nutribuses," implemented in part by grass-roots workers

[3] An interesting contemporary examination of that program and its inherent limitations can be found in Kerkvliet (1976).
[4] The substantial private sector financing of the program represented one form of "under the table" taxation levied by the government in return for facilitating a favorable climate for business interests in the Philippines. This, plus funding from some municipalities, permitted minimal central government spending on the nutrition effort.

laden with the fanciful title of "Barangay nutrition scholars." Even these programs, however, reached only a small proportion of children in need. (According to one anonymous critic of a 1985 conference presentation on the Philippines, "nutripaks" reached only 7 percent of children suffering from third-degree malnutrition, while the nutrition "scholars" were found only in a quarter of the Barangays.[5])

Additionally, however, it soon became clear that the scope of the program was circumscribed. Although activities covered the whole range of nutrition service delivery—child feeding, nutrition education, nutrition-related health services, production of nutritious foods, and nutrition training—and considerable intersectoral coordination was necessary to operate these projects, the program itself was never intended to be multisectoral. In fact, license was given for a nutrition policy, not for a food policy, which in the case of the Philippines had a particularly crippling effect on nutrition. (The point is generalized by Winikoff, 1978.) Despite the rhetoric about nutrition and national development, the program had and continues to have virtually no relationship with basic production or control of assets. Significantly, despite the NNC's broad system of intersectoral coordination, it had only a marginal relationship with the National Economic Development Authority (NEDA) (Florentino et al., 1982).

While direct nutrition interventions were being undertaken, the country was facing and making a broad array of decisions with significant implications for food consumption and nutrition, but never with the direct involvement of the National Nutrition Council or any part of its apparatus. In addition, the Marcos government shied away from a proposed food price subsidy scheme—in spite of positive results of a pilot test (Garcia and Pinstrup-Andersen, 1987)—as being too expensive.[6]

There was, to be sure, no lack of trying by nutrition advocates in the country. The most significant effort was a major Food and Nutrition Plan developed under the auspices of the secretary of agriculture and consisting of "envelopes," which dealt with several of the above issues, including food price subsidies and edible oil consumption. The plan was encouraged by international assistance agencies and was even a prime agenda item

---

[5] Although some impressive results have been attributed to several of these programs over the years, these reported results usually appeared, at least to this writer, to be at odds with firsthand observation. One program statistician, when pressed for data supporting a set of such significant results, acknowledged that the numbers were dictated more by the First Lady's demands than by field observation.

[6] Pines (1982) makes the interesting point that even when major nutrition decisions are made, the nutrition community is often only peripherally involved. His examples include the Costa Rican "glass of milk a day" program, the Peruvian food stamp program, and possibly President Allende's milk import program in Chile. They reinforce the adage, common in the 1970s, that "nutrition is too important to be left to the nutritionists.

on one of the World Bank Consultative Group meetings on the Philippines. It might have provided a nutrition check on many of the decisions referred to above, but, once again, the government decided against it.

Looking broadly at nutritional levels (see, for example, UN-ACC/SCN, 1989), it appears that, as in many countries, these levels are affected primarily by national and international economic trends and the successive effects of international markets on domestic prices, employment, and, inevitably, food consumption. (Hence, for example, the expected decline in nutritional status accompanying the economic recession in 1982–84). To the extent that government policy per se, however, affected nutritional levels of malnourished population groups in the Philippines in the decade following Marcos's 1974 presidential decree, it appears that any positive effects of the NNC programs were most likely outweighed by the negative effects of overall food and agricultural policy.

If national efforts in the Philippines were limited in scope, the Food and Nutrition Program (PAN) in Colombia and the Food and Nutrition Policy Planning Division in Sri Lanka probably represented the other end of the spectrum. Ironically, although these more truly multidisciplinary initiatives may have had greater potential for positive effect on nutrition, both were dismantled while the NNC in the Philippines continues to operate.

PAN was Colombia's National Food and Nutrition Plan. It functioned during the Lopez Michelsen administration from 1974 to 1978 and then in piecemeal form until 1982. From the outset, PAN was conceptualized as a comprehensive, genuinely multisectoral undertaking to boost incomes of the small landholding *minifundistas* in the longer run, while directly addressing malnutrition problems in the short run. Though not the result of any sophisticated modeling or analysis, the multidisciplinary conceptualization appeared sound. Unlike the narrow set of actual program activities in the Philippines, PAN included interventions in agriculture (cooperatives and rural credit to boost production on smallholdings), and agroindustry (low-cost, nutritious foods to absorb some of this increased production and to substitute for imported commodities). Health *promotoras* facilitated the broad-based distribution of services. These interventions were in addition to the traditional nutrition interventions. A key component of PAN was a significant and well-targeted scheme of food coupons provided by health personnel to mothers and young children in low-income families. Importantly, the program was pegged to Colombia's well-developed "poverty map." Finally, the program grew out of a longer tradition of multisectoral efforts and received substantial financial assistance from the World Bank and USAID (Lopez, 1978).

In fact, as Uribe-Mosquera (1985) notes in his perceptive analysis, PAN avoided many traditional mistakes associated with major development programs. It was never very expensive, at its peak costing just over 1 percent of the national budget; it caused minimal distortion in resource allocation—an important attribute at least to classical economists. Food coupon prices were uncontrolled, there were few major subsidies, and PAN was never overly dependent on external assistance. Nonetheless, the program failed to survive successive changes of government and was dismantled by 1982.

In Sri Lanka, the entity responsible for nutrition planning and coordination was the Food and Nutrition Policy Planning Division (FNPPD) of the Ministry of Plan Implementation, whose minister was the president. FNPPD, headed by an agriculturalist,[7] avoided from the outset the problems of a purely public health orientation. (The major figures in the Philippines program were physicians.) The unit was responsible for a number of planning strategies, among them a Comprehensive Food and Nutrition Plan in 1986. The plan consisted of both direct nutrition interventions and well-informed specific changes in agricultural and food systems likely to have significant nutritional benefit. These included specific changes in wage rates and agricultural prices, an indexing of the value of food stamps, stabilization of open market prices, and specific developments in the subsidiary crops sector, which employs large numbers of low-income families.

In collaboration with the International Food Policy Research Institute, the unit carried out important analyses of Sri Lankan food consumption patterns and the workings of the food stamp program. Some analyses focused specifically on households designated as "ultra poor": those consuming less than 80 percent of their caloric needs and spending more than 80 percent of their incomes on food.

FNPPD carried out evaluations of the more direct nutrition interventions—among them a major review of Thriposha, the supplementary feeding program—and assumed operational responsibility for several intervention programs, including distribution of an indigenous food supplement (Kola Kenda) and a community-based program called nutrition villages.

In short, FNPPD (both conceptually and in the scope of its specific undertakings) probably most closely approximated the ideal nutrition planning entity envisaged by nutrition planning advocates and international agencies in the early and mid-1970s. As with PAN in Colombia, its eventual dismantling provides a sobering reminder of the inherent vulnerability of even the best of such entities in the precarious waters of interagency

---

[7] Although this fact normally has been considered an important plus for FNPPD, the director's nonmedical background placed him continually at odds with health officials in the country. His credibility was sometimes questioned purely on these grounds.

coordination, jealously guarded bailiwicks, and political agendas that change when a new government comes to power.

Authority, Resources, and Coordination

A hypothesis worth exploring is that in nutrition planning, as in any multisectoral endeavor, the authority given to the coordinating agency is a good reflection of a particular government's political commitment to the undertaking.[8] According to one longtime observer of such coordinating entities, they cannot simply coordinate but must have some administrative capacity and the backing of law or decree to be able to operate usefully and effectively (Thomson, 1978).

The international nutrition map is filled with cases in which such authority was not provided. The Food and Nutrition Centre (TFNC) in Tanzania was given responsibility in 1976, before the more recent regional effort in Iringa, for formulating a food and nutrition policy. Six years later the policy still had not been adopted by the government and soon thereafter was found to be "out of date" (Mutahaba, 1985). In Ghana, the National Food and Nutrition Advisory Council experienced the same lack of authority (Sai, 1978). In Jamaica, a Nutrition Advisory Council was inaugurated in 1973 but was given no executive authority. No ministry was anxious to house a purely advisory body of this nature, and only junior staff attended its meetings (Antrobus, 1978). CANAS, the nutrition planning body in Senegal, was able to get attractive nutrition language into the national plan but lacked the authority to translate such language into programs (Pines, 1982). In contrast, in the Philippines such authority was provided but only within a limited sphere of activity.

The Philippines, however, faced a trickier situation with respect to resource allocation and coordination. The decision was made to implement nutrition programs through local nutrition committees headed by governors or mayors. The rationale was twofold: first, to elicit local political support, and second, to raise the money to finance these undertakings. Neither provided an unqualified success. Marcos was reluctant to allocate substantial funds for nutrition, hoping to generate "financial self-reliance" at the local level to supplement funds raised from the private sector. In most local areas there was, on the contrary, a clear expectation of central financing for such schemes, and the idea was rejected. Local leaders, however, were generally willing to take nominal responsibility for programs

---

[8] Political commitment to a process of multisectoral nutrition planning does not necessarily imply commitment to meaningful poverty reduction, although the two have sometimes coincided. At the same time, governments that have sought to use such planning as a substitute for action have rarely been very adept or committed to the planning.

that might provide political benefit.[9] On the plus side, many of these leaders became sensitized to the problem of malnutrition and provided a political constituency for the NNC and nutrition pursuits in the country (a constituency sadly lacking in Colombia or Sri Lanka). On the minus side, such leaders were interested primarily or even exclusively in only the most visible showcase projects. At its worst, this attitude resulted in many short-lived projects and the forced entry of inappropriate technology (Florentino et al., 1982). Also, the local leaders were interested in appealing to those among their constituents with political clout but were not particularly interested in the poorest of the poor or in programs well-targeted to them. Not unexpectedly, such projects were concentrated in urban or periurban areas (such central government funds as were allocated for nutrition rarely went far from Manila). Also not unexpectedly, many dedicated persons responsible for actual operation of these programs soon became discouraged and disillusioned.

In refusing to allocate their own funds for nutrition programs, some local communities in the Philippines were expressing a reluctance to fund centrally planned projects. To help counter this argument, nutrition committees were encouraged to do their own nutrition planning at the local level. Such efforts, when they were undertaken, were at best uneven and plagued by problems of staff neither trained nor particularly interested in the endeavor. A similar effort to do multisectoral nutrition planning at the provincial level in Papua New Guinea was placed in the hands of nurses and paramedics who had completed a one-year diploma course in nutrition (Ross and Posanai, 1988).

In contrast, some efforts at decentralized planning in Africa have been relatively effective. In Zimbabwe, despite the absence of successfully coordinated efforts at the center, there has been impressive coordinating at the district level by intersectoral committees established under the leadership of the Agriculture Ministry and organized under the umbrella of a Supplementary Food Production Program. The program not only concentrates on rainfed crops, vegetable gardens, and small animal production, but also includes child feeding, nutrition education, and efforts at community mobilization that appear more successful than most such attempts. Although these district efforts and comparable efforts in the Iringa region of Tanzania do not touch larger issues of food or agricultural policy, they do suggest that intersectoral coordination of these more direct interventions at the local level is both possible and desirable.

In both Zimbabwe and Tanzania, local planning has become more nec-

---

[9] Under the martial law in force at the time, local officials had little choice in the matter. They were expected to organize programs for which they received "merit points." These points were earned solely for producing a plan, not on the basis of performance.

essary because of the increasingly decentralized decision making in these countries. Unlike capital cities with very separate ministerial domains, the planning and administration at the regional and district levels, which almost always is characterized by inadequate staff, transport, and support systems, is inherently a more intersectoral undertaking. Beginning in the late 1970s, the Tanzania Food and Nutrition Centre took advantage of this decentralization by producing situation analyses with each of the twenty regions and mobilizing support around priorities. By 1983, the Joint WHO/UNICEF Nutrition Support Program (JNSP) in Iringa was initiated, and by the late 1980s nine regions had some nutrition planning process under way.

Coordination problems in Colombia and Sri Lanka did not involve local government bodies, but rather line ministries in the central government. Almost by definition FNPPD and PAN were considered intrusive, particularly by ministries of health and agriculture that were used to having complete control of their dominions. The problem was compounded in Colombia, when PAN found more efficient ways to work outside of the well-honed channels of command (Uribe-Mosquera, 1985). Most problematic of all, perhaps, were instances in which nutrition coordinating bodies, impatient with ministerial inertia, opted to take on executive responsibility themselves for particular operational activities. One case in point was in Chile, where CONPLAN, the national planning commission, initiated a nutrition-oriented agricultural information system and a sanitation project independent of the relevant ministries (Pines, 1982). Another was FNPPD in Sri Lanka, which assumed operational control for food supplement and community nutrition activities. In both cases, antagonisms arose that may well have hastened the demise of these units.

In Indonesia, the government made no fewer than five institutional attempts at coordinating nutrition programs between 1952 and 1983. In each case and despite substantial effort, the results were disappointing (Soekirman, 1988). In Costa Rica, with its long tradition of poverty alleviation and social justice programs, the problem was not a lack of commitment to basic human needs but rather the unfortunate placement of the nutrition planning unit within the government. The Secretariat for Food and Nutrition Policy (SEPAN) was established as a semiautonomous body within the Health Ministry and staffed by officials who were not always able to hold their own within that ministry, much less coordinate the work of others. Even its legal mandate as an intersectoral planning body overlapped with responsibilities in MIDEPLAN, the Planning Ministry. Despite the creation of a National Plan for Food and Nutrition, SEPAN, like the similarly powerless Food and Nutrition Coordinating Committee in Lesotho, came to serve almost solely as a technical advisory group on nutrition. This was particularly regrettable because SEPAN might have been a logical instrument for the rational allocation of at least a portion of the funds collected through the so-called Family Allowance Law—a substantial tax on both salaries and sales to create funds for social programs.

The most extreme case of interministerial coordination problems in nutrition probably was that of Ghana in the early 1960s. When funds did become available for a nutrition coordinating council, the official in charge saw it as an opportunity for empire building. Within a few weeks he had recruited one hundred officers with little in the way of job specifications, had purchased cars, and began his own program. In time this operation was called to a halt, but by then the idea of coordinated nutrition activity no longer had the confidence of ministries and agencies in the government (Sai, 1978).

To the extent that program implementation actually emerged from multisectoral nutrition planning efforts in some of these countries, such programs often appeared piecemeal, disconnected, and without a real base of support, pointing up one of the genuine ironies of such planning. Strategies emerging from multisectoral nutrition planning and conceptually designed as a package of effective and complementary policy and program interventions undertaken by several different operational entities often ended up being diluted and disconnected precisely because no minister or ministry was able to develop substantial interest or exercise real authority.

A primary resource constraint in national-level nutrition planning is skilled personnel, a challenging problem at best and overwhelming at worst. In Colombia, the staff needed for PAN was already involved in other work in the country. Initial PAN analysis, for example, indicated the need for data that was more disagggregated or more specifically related to nutrition, but skilled, experienced persons not already fully employed in other nutrition-related work were in short supply. The problem was compounded because Colombia lacked the long history of nutrition involvement of, say, Chile or India. One stopgap measure was the use of foreign experts, but the results were mixed.

The problem was, if anything, worse in other countries. In Bolivia, a nutrition coordinating organization could be staffed only by drawing trained people away from the very programs being coordinated. The same was true of CANAS in Senegal and would have been true of a proposed coordinating agency in Sierra Leone (Pines, 1982).

A review of Papua New Guinea's experience with multisectoral nutrition planning and coordination initiated in 1978 was forthright. "The policy had set targets without adequately specifying how these targets would be achieved. The bodies given responsibility for coordinating and implementing the policy were unable to develop the necessary means. They did not have the analytical, technical, and managerial capacity to plan and implement successful projects. Simply put, the task set by the policy was too difficult. As staff turnover and failure took their toll, the enthusiasm present in 1978 was dissipated. By 1983, the nutrition planner's position had been dropped from the National Planning Office and the [other primary entities] were defunct" (Ross and Posanai, 1988, p. 142).

Politics and Vulnerability

As suggested at the outset of this examination of national nutrition planning initiatives, the effectiveness and durability of these efforts invariably had much less to do with the nature of the planning undertaken than with perceived political benefits of visible nutrition activity, administrative and bureaucratic jealousies, or well-guarded bailiwicks. Durability also related importantly to program constituencies and to the ability to survive a change in government.

An extreme case of such an effect of government change on nutrition policy and programs was that of Pakistan in the early 1970s. Until 1971, nutrition activity in the country consisted primarily of biomedical survey work. When Bangladesh was created, all such nutrition activity in Pakistan ground to a halt, not because of any a priori conceptual disagreement but simply because virtually all nutrition personnel in the country had been Bengalis. The vacuum created by the virtual exit of the entire nutrition community—and much of the public health community as well—provided an opportunity for Prime Minister Zulfikar Ali Bhutto to introduce an entirely different mode of decentralized health and nutrition services based on the people's health and work schemes he had observed in China. He also introduced the concept of consumption planning to be juxtaposed against traditional supply-oriented agricultural planning. Although an extreme example, the Pakistan case reflects the general inability of most new governments to build on the experience of their predecessors and the associated tendency to sweep clean and begin anew (Winikoff, 1978).

In Pakistan, the new beginning necessitated a fresh look at ways to provide more food and services for the poor with some positive results, whereas government change in Colombia marked the demise of PAN. The administration following the Lopez government in 1978 dropped major components of the program, and the next government in 1982 dismantled PAN altogether, transferring responsibility for many of its components to line ministries. Each of these governments was seeking a new look, which did not include the "confusing" concept of food and nutrition. It was not clear to new officials, including many at senior levels of the planning department, what the malnutrition problem was all about, because average caloric intakes were more than adequate and other data were confusing and conflicting. Additionally, multisectoral undertakings appeared too unwieldy to the new governments. Finally, after key program components were dropped in 1978, the weakened program was susceptible to legitimate criticism (Uribe-Mosquera, 1985).

Most revealing was that the dissolution of PAN did not create even a whimper of dissent. The program was wholly devoid of a political constituency to protect it, partly because it was so effectively targeted toward the rural poor and malnourished, who were politically impotent. Meanwhile, within the government, PAN already had alienated many ministerial officials by the inherently intrusive nature of its work.[10]

Although PAN was dismantled, one of its offspring, the Integrated Rural Development Program (DRI) survived intact. DRI differed from PAN in two possibly decisive ways. First, in contrast with PAN's "poverty map" beneficiaries, the recipients of DRI services were somewhat more economically and politically viable; and second, unlike PAN, DRI carefully cultivated community-level governments.

The same absence of outcry accompanied the disbanding of FNPPD in Sri Lanka in 1989. In the government reorganization following a change of presidents (but not party), the Ministry of Plan Implementation, which housed FNPPD, was merged into the Ministry of Finance and Planning. On the recommendation of the country's Administrative Reforms Commission to cut back on the number of government units, FNPPD was abolished.

To its credit, FNPPD over the years had sensitized several officials of the Ministry of Finance and Planning and generated interest among them, particularly in issues relating to food consumption. One important official actually had worked for a short time in FNPPD at the time of the unit's creation. Arguably, this sensitization and the data regularly provided by FNPPD had strengthened the hands of such persons in deliberations relating to broader policies affecting food consumption and poverty alleviation. Ironically, this very interest and analytic capacity within Finance and Planning may have argued against maintaining FNPPD intact within the same ministry.

[10] This unhappy reality was in sharp contrast with the hopeful words of one PAN program advocate, who stated in 1975, "Once you arouse the consciousness of people . . . you can never go back . . . . Continuity is bound to be there . . . . Once a program shows its benefits it would be hard to find a government in Colombia which would abandon [it]" (Lopez, 1978, p. 74). The lack of real political support calls to mind Pyle's (1981b) analysis of the similar phenomenon experienced by Project Poshak, a large experimental nutrition effort undertaken in India in the early 1970s.

More generally, for the latter years of its life FNPPD probably had been caught in a political "nether land" precisely because it followed its mandate. One of the unit's responsibilities was to recommend food and agricultural policy changes that might positively affect nutritional well-being. While most of these recommendations appeared sound, they were, by and large, not central to the decision-making process in the Ministry of Agriculture, the Ministry of Finance and Planning, or the prime minister's secretariat. The unit's exclusion from major decision making in this area became obvious when the new president announced (initially as a campaign promise) a new "Janasavia" program of income transfers to low-income families over a two-year period to replace the bulk of the food stamp and other welfare programs. The implications of the Janasavia program for nutrition and food consumption dwarfed the effects of all other programs combined and raised many critical questions, yet FNPPD was wholly excluded from the decision-making process.

At the same time, bureaucratic support for FNPPD, which might have come at least from nutrition and public health officials in the Ministry of Health, was not forthcoming—a result of many years of what the Health Ministry considered intrusion by unqualified outsiders into its domain. Finally, as in Colombia, there was no vocal political constituency within the larger population.

In sum, nutrition planning and coordinating entities during this period not only were particularly vulnerable to political change but seldom had any real choice with respect to the nature and scope of their undertakings. Some were blessed with mandates from government leaders (the Philippines and Colombia) that conferred some degree of authority although usually circumscribed by political requirements. Others represented a relatively painless (and inexpensive) means used by less interested governments to satisfy internal or international pressure. Some (the Philippines and probably Chile) were welcome to coordinate their direct nutrition projects intersectorally but were not invited to meddle in broader food or economic policy, thus inherently limiting the potential effects of their endeavors. Others (Colombia and Sri Lanka) were permitted to be genuinely multisectoral in their pursuits and recommendations, but they antagonized the bureaucracy of line ministries in the process and still did not usually have the desired effect on major government policy.

Legacies of Multisectoral Nutrition Planning

Although the proliferation of nutrition activity envisaged by nutrition advocates in the 1970s did not fully materialize in the 1980s, there has been a significant increase in nutrition program activity in recent years and, even more important, a marked improvement in the quality of such programs. Most of this activity today is sectoral and not part of multidisciplinary coordinated efforts. Yet the activity surely has been affected by and in some part the result of multisectoral nutrition planning in the 1970s.

This point deserves further elaboration. Many of the most impressive nutrition programs today—in Tamil Nadu and Indonesia, the Iringa program in Tanzania, the district-level activities in Zimbabwe, and the planned Child Nutrition and Household Food Security project in southern Lesotho, to name a few—are made up of the very components that characterized the failed United Nations-assisted Applied Nutrition Program (ANP) of the 1960s. Like the contemporary examples, the ANP included small-scale agriculture, home gardens, and small animal production. It also included nutrition education, child feeding, and environmental sanitation. In fact, the only major component of today's programs not included in the ANP was growth monitoring.

So why was the Applied Nutrition Program an acknowledged failure, while today's programs with the very same components are becoming more successful? A closer look at the Iringa JNSP program in Tanzania provides some insight—and makes clear the important legacy of nutrition planning. In Iringa very explicit attention was given and continues to be given to the causes of malnutrition. Communities as a whole and mothers and village health committees in particular were asked to think through systematically, for example, the extent to which household food inadequacy was the result of cropping problems, storage losses, or inadequate income, or the relative importance of economics, fuel scarcity, overworked mothers, and inadequate information in explaining low-nutrient intakes of children. No such thinking was ever part of the ANP. There was in Iringa, from the outset, a recognition that simply increasing food production without concentrating on those communities and families in greatest need would be futile. A process of village-level analysis was accordingly undertaken to assure that those groups most vulnerable to economic deprivation, food shortage, or child malnutrition would be specifically targeted. Targeting decisions were made at the village level, where the circumstances of each family were well-known or could easily be ascertained, thereby assuring the effectiveness of such targeting, assuming broad participation in the decisions. One important outgrowth of the targeting focus in Iringa was income-generating activities focused on women's groups. Again, this focus was absent in the ANP. For Iringa, decision making rests on a conceptual framework that is relatively simple compared with the sophisticated models of the 1970s but substantially more thoughtful than any planning or review mechanism employed in the ANP. The Iringa approach is referred to as the Triple-A cycle and seeks continually to reassess local needs through repeated cycles of assessment, analysis, and action both in the villages and through the various government levels. Finally, careful cost analysis based on malnourished children reached, systematic monitoring and evaluation, and professional management are all basic to Iringa but were largely absent in the ANP.

Each of the above elements owes some debt not simply to the techniques employed in multisectoral nutrition planning, but, perhaps more, to the systematic thinking that nutrition planning implied.

While sectoral (although usually interdepartmentally coordinated) programs are improving, those economic planners concerned at all with social or poverty issues have become more cognizant of nutrition, possibly as a result of sensitization from the nutrition planning and coordinating groups discussed earlier. Although coordination has been a weak link of multisectoral nutrition planning—and probably would argue against a dependence on such intersectoral coordination of programs in the future—benefits surely were derived from those difficult efforts by nutrition planners to bring together people with different backgrounds and disciplines to focus on malnutrition. At its best, and despite the squabbles, there was a critical mass of concerned persons who provided nutrition with more of an actual home than it has had before or since.

But this cognizance of nutrition among development planners probably emanates more from the rapidly growing importance of food policy and food security analysis—also legacies of nutrition planning—with their central focus on food consumption per se. In most countries it would be difficult to talk seriously about poverty or food insecurity without thinking of food consumption as a measure of these problems or as a measure of the success of programs designed to address them.

It was most likely this confluence of better programs on the one hand and heightened consciousness of food consumption and nutrition on the other that led to the identification of nutrition as a primary component of broader programs designed to ameliorate the (at least) short-run deleterious effects on the poor of structural adjustment. Interestingly, while nutrition programs were always second-guessed when based on developmental rationale (increased productivity, human resource potential, better learning, child survival hypothesis) or on purely humanitarian grounds, rarely a murmur of dissent is heard today when nutrition is used in the context of structural adjustment.

If most nutrition programs are likely to be sectoral in the future, pitfalls associated with such programs need to be avoided. One potential danger is that in certain cases they threaten a return to the "magic bullet," the supply-oriented intervention. This is particularly true for micronutrient programs. Consultative groups dealing with vitamin A, iron, and iodine are welcome additions to the nutrition scene, but interventions wholly focused on a single nutrient are likely to encounter some of the very problems multisectoral nutrition planning was designed to overcome.

Sectoral programs, no matter how well designed, will not help with the critically important responsibility of looking at the nutritional or consumption effects of broader policies. Experience in Sri Lanka, where this responsibility was taken seriously, indicates that, unless the work is done by individuals or groups in the actual arena of decision making, the analysis (even if sound) is likely to be only peripheral to that decision making.

One modest response may be to identify individuals already in this arena (usually in planning or finance ministries or in the offices of a president or prime minister) who already are interested in food consumption or poverty alleviation and equip them with a small professional staff and analytic capacity to review, on an ongoing basis, the major components of a country's development strategy for effects on poverty alleviation, if not specifically food consumption and nutrition. (The recently created Bureau of Health and Nutrition in Bappenas, the planning ministry in Indonesia, may have some of the characteristics necessary for this work. Another relevant model is the Food Security and Nutrition Unit [FSNU] in the Office of the President and Cabinet in Malawi. During debate over the minimum wage in Malawi, the FSNU was able to present graphically, over a period of years, the number of days required by a "minimum wage family" to purchase a 90-kg bag of maize. This clearly delineated "consumption effect" proved to be broadly persuasive in the government's decision to raise the minimum wage, with clearly positive nutritional benefit.) Such an entity, unburdened by the responsibility for coordinating or running projects and less intrusive and politically vulnerable, might be in the interest of those governments with some sincere interest in the problems of their poor (or who suddenly develop such an interest in the presence of structural adjustment programs).

The effectiveness of such an entity would be doubtful without at least one senior official willing to assume overall responsibility by providing a mandate and operational work plan to the group and then regularly feeding issues to the group as they become timely for policy decision making. Where such interested officials do not exist, nutrition advocates and sectoral personnel need to continue the work they have always done in seeking to generate such interest and commitment. But the task is unquestionably easier in 1990 than it was in 1970, and this may, in and of itself, be an important legacy.

15

Information as an Input into Food and Nutrition Policy Formation

Harold Alderman

A good field biologist knows the value of a search image, or mental map. With such an image, rare species turn up at a rate sufficient to amaze colleagues; without one, even suitable habitat may appear barren. Similarly, a word just learned seems to appear in every journal one reads in the subsequent week. It should not be surprising, then, that a modest subset of economics literature and a larger literature in political science and sociology are devoted to the role of economic ideas in the attitudes and actions of the general public. Although it may be difficult to identify cases in which a specific problem led to a focused study and from there to a policy choice, such a search severely limits the scope of possible interactions (Lindblom and Cohen, 1979). Keynes (1935, p. 383) recognized a much broader range, contending that "practical men, who believe themselves to be quite exempt from any intellectual influences, are usually the slaves of some defunct economist. Madmen in authority, who hear voices in the air, are distilling their frenzy from some academic scribbler of a few years back."[1]

Economists, of course, debate this proposition. For example, while Irwin (1989) argues that a major food policy decision of the nineteenth century, the repeal of the corn laws, was more a product of economic ideas than of shifts in power among interest groups, Stigler (1982) demurs, proposing just the contrary.

Central to the following discussion, however, is the view that this distinction need not be cast in absolute terms; interest groups consolidate their power, in part, by the generation and dissemination of information.

---

[1] Keynes himself was echoing the defunct Schiller's 1789 history lectures.

Figure 15.1. Illustration of modes of information flow for nutrition and food policy

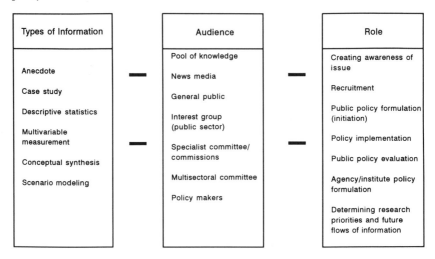

Types of Information	Audience	Role
Anecdote Case study Descriptive statistics Multivariable measurement Conceptual synthesis Scenario modeling	Pool of knowledge News media General public Interest group (public sector) Specialist committee/ commissions Multisectoral committee Policy makers	Creating awareness of issue Recruitment Public policy formulation (initiation) Policy implementation Public policy evaluation Agency/institute policy formulation Determining research priorities and future flows of information

The object of this chapter is to explore the role research plays in this path from information to food and nutrition policy. Because the final point on this pathway, food policy, is a broad aggregation of decisions regarding nutrition, health, and agriculture, the approach must be eclectic, centering on economic policy but including clinical interventions as well. The focus, however, is not on the policies per se, or on the entire political process, but on communication between researchers and individuals responsible for formulating such policies, often through a host of intermediaries.

The indirect nature of much of this communication provides the variation that makes the inquiry interesting. Figure 15.1 gives an impression of the varieties of relevant communication. There is no one-to-one correspondence between the categories of information depicted and the potential audience or between the users of the information and its role. There are, then, a great many possible combinations of elements in this simplified listing of modalities. Furthermore, paths will differ depending on the issue being researched. Research may have a long-run influence by changing the basic understanding of the issues society addresses, or it may be directed toward an immediate technical question. Moreover, policy is context. Hence the position of the analysts, the structural character of the firm or public body they are trying to influence, and the broader sociopolitical environment will all influence the form of communication.

Weiss (1977) offers three models of policy interactions: those in which problem solving responds to issues posed by decision makers; those in which research has thrown up an opportunity that can be capitalized upon; and an interactive model in which information results from a general search for knowledge. As will be discussed below, her list is perhaps too restrictive. Indeed, this framework does not explicitly recognize situations in which the research agenda is determined by the general population instead of by officials or researchers themselves.[2] Nevertheless, her key point, which is essential to the following discussion, is that research is an interactive process and is only partially defined by issue or discipline.

Clearly, the information that is most useful and the means by which it is communicated are partly determined by the nature of the problem and the audience to which the communication is directed. No individual can gather and process all information necessary for major decisions. Decision makers must consequently rely on an organizational chain through consultants, congressional aides, undersecretaries, and the like. The more links in the chain, the more communication errors, hence the importance of packaging and of review procedures. Moreover, the structure of the decision-making body itself is influenced by the nature of the information it must process (Sah and Stiglitz, 1986).

The form in which research is communicated to decision makers also influences the nature of this inquiry; the pathway from research to policy decisions seldom leaves a paper trail. This partly reflects the evolutionary nature of shifts in conventional wisdom. Moreover, effective policy interactions often require the analyst to seek anonymity to allow government officials to claim credit when they choose or to avoid appearing manipulated. A low profile may be a negotiating tool when advice is unpalatable or when analysts incorporate the voice of the relatively powerless. Timmer (1988a) discusses these issues in the context of price and marketing decisions.

Varieties of Information Processes

Beginning, admittedly somewhat arbitrarily, with the third column of Figure 15.1, one notes that information plays a key role in creating awareness of a problem. This is often an early step in a political process of recruiting interest groups or individuals into the process of seeking solutions. At this early stage the information is generally descriptive, but analysis may trace a link between a phenomenon and a previously recognized problem. The background data for the CBS documentary "Hunger

---

[2] This idea corresponds to the outside initiative model for setting agendas presented by Cobb et al. (1976).

in America," which was addressed to a nonspecialist audience and contributed to a political consensus, is an example of the former (Sims, 1983). Studies that linked malnutrition to economic consequences, including poor cognitive development, illustrate the latter. India established nutrition as a priority in the late 1960s partly on the basis of such information (Berg, 1973). In this case specialists communicated directly with policy makers, aided by their close contact during the relief effort for the Bihar famine.

In Berg's example the crisis was real and acute. The creation of a sense of crisis when a situation may be chronic and pervasive, however, may also be an important step in gaining access to the public agenda. Sims's study, which draws on a model of convergent voices for priorities for public policy developed by Cook (1981), illustrates this in the initial phase of attracting awareness to nutrition in the United States. She also implies that public attention spans are short. Hopkins (1987), however, uses a tabulation of published studies, similar to that presented by Sims, to argue that attention to hunger is somewhat cyclical, having a periodicity not unlike world food stocks and may, in fact, be causally related.

Sims also argues that general public awareness must be channeled in order to become legitimized and be placed formally on the policy agenda. She sees interest groups as having a major role in this stage, collecting and sharing information with officials as part of this process.

Generation of awareness generally pertains to situations in which policy makers have not articulated an issue, but information has a similar role in recruiting support once an issue is legitimized.[3] When there is nascent awareness of an issue or problem, then, research can become an instrument in the lobbying process. "Advocacy research" is often commissioned.[4] The available body of research is also sifted, distilled, and repackaged for presentation to a broader audience by proponents of a position. In this process nonsupportive results are often dismissed. The tendency in this process is for research results to be simplified and taken out of their qualifying context. Catchy slogans—"food first" or "small is healthy"—lend themselves both to oversimplification and to a more widespread acceptance by the greater public. Such use may not always be good science, but the quality of the research from which more popular presentations are derived is not necessarily indicated by the use to which the results are applied.

---

[3] As Cobb et al. (1976) indicate, success in setting an agenda is distinct from influencing the ultimate decision.

[4] One need not dictate the results to have advocacy research. A researcher's past work often allows a fair prediction of future work. For similar reasons, given the controversy around Operation Flood, India's large dairy development program, in the mid-1980s, the

The research environment is not, however, unaffected by the political milieu. Gould (1981) reveals how even good scientists are often very subtly influenced by their preconception. Many errors in the measurement of so-called intelligence, which Gould recounts, were eventually corrected, although often after incurring large social costs because of misguided policies. It is an open question whether the process of self-correction upon which science is based is hastened by the political nature of information. But because many agencies and organizations act as if their information has a value in recruiting allies and refuting opponents, research that has entered the policy arena receives extra scrutiny. Controversy helps define the research agenda. Governments are also willing to use research results as lobbyists do to explain or justify actions perhaps chosen on the basis of other criteria (Grosh, 1991). In such cases they are recruiting support from the general population. For example, the government of Pakistan presented descriptive statistics on the use of rationed flour at the time derationing was announced, as part of its efforts to preempt criticism of the change (Alderman, 1988).

A government's use of research for recruitment differs from the role that research may have in policy formulation. Similarly, a government's use of information on what individuals think about an issue differs from its use of information about the problem itself. Governments nevertheless regularly commission research, presumably with some intention of using it. It is probably easier to identify such cases of the direct use of research in policy implementation than in policy formulation. Often agencies or departments have institutionalized a procedure for evaluating information and using research. In such cases research likely plays a different role in the initial policy decision to establish an objective than in subsequent implementation. The Indonesian food logistics agency, Bulog, for example, regularly uses demand and supply projections to reevaluate rice and fertilizer pricing policies within the context of its stabilization objectives (Timmer, 1986). Similarly, in Jamaica, where food-related transfer programs have long been government policy, research commissioned by the government led directly to reforms of eligibility criteria (Grosh, 1991).

Where evaluation of information is not institutionalized, such as when a crisis brings a problem to the fore, governments are both in a position to commission or support research and, at the same time, may be less patient in seeing it through. For this reason, as much as because of the lack of a particular constituency for analysis, research is more likely to influence policy indirectly through redefinitions of concepts than directly through commissioned studies.

European Economic Community sought a researcher with no experience in that country to conduct an evaluation.

The slow evolution of collective or conventional wisdom, then, is likely the most pervasive influence analytical information has on policy. This pertains in particular to basic research neither designed for a specific policy nor targeted to a particular agency but which influences approaches to specific issues through synergism with other research. For example, the shift from projects designed to close the protein gap toward those aimed at meeting energy requirements, which occurred in the late 1960s and early 1970s, reflected the results of studies as well as articulate syntheses of such studies. These shifts are often overlooked as a source of policy formulation because there is often a presumption that a decision maker exists in the sense of an identifiable individual or committee that weighs evidence and reaches a conclusion (Lindblom and Cohen, 1979). Often, however, no apparent decision is made, although changes in policy follow from a general movement in ideas. Such shifts occur most rapidly among specialists and are subsequently communicated to policy makers not only through consultants but also when academics sit on government commissions or, as is often the case, in ministerial and advisory posts.

It is not only national governments that have policies. The World Bank and nongovernmental organizations have internal policies, as do agencies within governments. Because bureaucracies and civil services have different tenures from those of policy makers, their responses to outside pressures are often dampened. Internal policies, then, are often formulated in a manner distinct from the larger governmental process. Such agencies may also have different proclivities for information than legislative bodies, in part reflecting a common technocratic ideology. Bureaucracies do not, of course, respond in a uniform manner. Haas (1990), for example, presents three models of how organizations redefine problems: through incremental growth, turbulent nongrowth, and learning. Only the latter involves questioning the underlying theories of programs, although technocratic change can be part of adaptation in the first instance.[5]

A subset of internal institutional policy is research policy, such as the priorities for the Consultative Group on International Agricultural Research (CGIAR). This system, which was responsible for many of the technological improvements popularly known as the green revolution, was the object of much of the criticism directed at the seed and fertilizer revolution. As a research system, however, it may have a particular affinity for analysis, including institutionalized appraisals of its own priorities. Examples of changes in research policy could include (to continue with

---

[5] Haas (1990) presents the shift to meeting basic human needs by the World Bank as an example of learning. In a different context, the role of research in institutional policy is presented in Adams's (1985) study of the establishment of the International Monetary Fund Cereal Import Facility.

the CGIAR example) the shift away from breeding for protein as well as the system's use of feedback from early economic impact studies to include as research priorities suboptimal conditions and coarse grains (Pinstrup-Andersen et al., 1984).

Illustrations

National Nutritional Policy in Chile

Chile has an extensive history of food distribution; since 1924 all governments across the political spectrum have supported various programs to distribute supplementary food (Vial et al., 1988). This policy, along with increased provision of public health care, has contributed to a steady and rapid decline of infant mortality rates even during periods of economic decline (Castañeda, 1985; Solimano and Haignere, 1988).

One significant difference between this program and a variety of subsidy schemes is that the distribution of food to women and infants is explicitly linked to health care clinics, although other programs such as school feeding and day care centers are not. Another feature of the health care system which distinguishes the distribution program under the Pinochet junta from earlier programs is the degree to which it has been targeted. The first of two major steps in this direction was implemented in 1975, when the eligibility for supplemental foods was reduced to roughly half the previous target population by the elimination of distribution to children over six years of age and the restriction of eligibility to families that were enrolled and participating in the National Health Service, which is universally available.[6] A second major shift occurred in 1982, when quantities per recipient were reduced for general recipients, although they were increased for children in families below a socioeconomic cutoff point or for any child who indicated inadequate growth. The targeting, then, included both preventive and curative criteria.

These major changes were mainly driven by ideology and budgetary concerns. To some degree, however, this ideology is a product of the general shifts in professional opinion worldwide and therefore helps illustrate the range of interactions between researchers and policy makers, even in a country that had suspended its democratic tradition. The prevailing approach has been attributed to a particular training,[7] although proponents of targeting are not restricted to a single school or country. More

[6] Previously children up to the age of fourteen were eligible.
[7] Many of Chile's foreign advisers were trained in the University of Chicago, as was a principal Chilean proponent of targeting supplemental feeding, Miguel Cast.

likely, this orientation reflects a convergence of views also represented in professional articles and books (see, for example, Reutlinger and Selowsky, 1976). This shift may also account for roughly contemporaneous reorientations in other countries, such as Sri Lanka. Moreover, even when ideology underlies the design of programs, the experience contributes to the body of empirical evidence (see, for example, Pinstrup-Andersen, 1988b), which may then reinforce the shift in opinion.

The actual design of targeting in Chile has, however, been influenced by a variety of research efforts. Poverty maps based on census data were constructed in 1974 and 1982. The mapping was used to provide support for continuing programs and to indicate the feasibility of defining poverty on an index of readily available socioeconomic indicators. Similarly, a survey in 1985 contributed to the targeting of school feeding programs. As administrative decentralization increases (itself ideologically based), such use of data is being institutionalized. For example, each municipality administers a social stratification survey to assist in determining program eligibility, using indicators similar to those derived for the poverty maps.

Such mapping is often a stimulus for policy and may place an issue on an agenda as well as provide technical background for program design. For example, the awareness created by a nutrition risk map prepared by UNICEF in Malawi led to official recognition of the existence of malnutrition and likely contributed to a subsequent rise in the minimum wage. Similarly, the Sistema Alimentario Mexicano (SAM) was designed partly from food deficit mapping (Montanari, 1987).

In another context, a small survey in the late 1980s was employed by Chile's health minister to fend off program cuts following rising milk prices. This can be considered an example of intragovernmental lobbying. Other data have been employed in program implementation. Medical doctors have sought data to bolster their position that some supplementary foods should be provided to all children at clinics to encourage visits and weighing. This underlies both the shift to an entirely clinic-based distribution achieved in steps over a decade and provides the rationale for the two-tier distribution system in place since 1985.

Nutritionists have also contributed data to assist in choosing foods to be distributed, for example, or in monitoring criteria. The latter role, of course, is comparatively routine, but even in this case the range of communication illustrates the variety of pathways from research to implementation. In general, communication of findings is facilitated when academics enter the government. In one case, however, one of the most influential nutritionists in Chile chose to hold a public press conference presenting data on increased incidence of diarrhea, which he attributed to the distribution of a cereal substitute for milk. The budget-driven decision to remove milk distribution was subsequently reversed. Such a ploy was, of course, aided by the researcher's preexisting stature and is not an option for all researchers. It illustrates nevertheless the political use of information, even in a country which at the time had a restricted range of political activities.

Reappraisal of the Women, Infants, and Children Program (WIC) in the United States

Research has a potential role not only in policy formulation and implementation but in protecting existing programs from intergovernmental sniping as well. An example is the reauthorization of WIC under the Carter administration. An instance of internal lobbying, the example also illustrates the importance of timeliness as well as the role of a charismatic individual.

The WIC program was authorized in 1972 to provide food supplementation and nutrition education to high-risk pregnant and lactating women, infants, and children under five years of age. Although the WIC program mandates evaluation, few rigorous studies had been completed by the time the program was due for reauthorization during the Carter administration. The program was, however, supported by Robert Greenstein of the United States Department of Agriculture (USDA), the implementing agency, who based his enthusiasm largely on a gut feeling that WIC works. Using a professional network, he contacted James Austin at the Harvard School of Public Health to elicit information. By coincidence, one of Austin's students, Eileen Kennedy, was in the final phase of writing a thesis on the impact of WIC, a topic chosen years earlier on other criteria. Kennedy's research had found lower incidence of low-birth-weight babies among women participating in the program. Greenstein was thus able to locate supporting data without the usual lead time that research requires and was able to work it through the appropriate channels.

This process, largely dependent on Greenstein's experience in government, was likely also aided by the paucity of competing studies that could have been used for counterlobbying or to draw the discussion into fine points of methodology. By the time the research was published in a professional journal (Kennedy et al., 1982), other studies were also available.

This example also illustrates a point made above: policy interaction often occurs with few published trails. A similar example is the case of derationing of flour in Pakistan. Although this case differs from the reauthorization of WIC in a number of key aspects, most notably in that a body of relevant research had been assembled over a decade, a government official played a key role in disseminating research results to other cabinet members.

Greenstein's role in the evaluation of WIC stands in contrast to an incident in 1986 in which the conclusions of a study of WIC were altered by two political appointees within the USDA before its release (Marshall, 1990). Neither the principal investigator of this $6 million study, David Rush, nor the advisory committee overseeing it was allowed to comment on the revisions of the text. Although this case again illustrates that policy-orientated research is defined in an interaction between the researcher and the audience, it may also be interpreted as indicating the potential to appeal to alternative audiences. Rush et al. (1988a, 1988b) eventually published their findings that WIC reduced fetal mortality and improved infant health in a professional forum. Moreover, the role of the USDA officials was investigated by the General Accounting Office, which found no justification for the editing of the original study. A subsequent hearing before the House Select Committee on Hunger and the Senate Committee on Agriculture, at which Greenstein—no longer with the government— was a witness, provided additional publicity for Rush's results (Marshall, 1990).

The Breast versus Bottle Debate

The potential dangers of bottle-feeding of infants in developing countries were subject to more than a decade of public debate after the publication of "The Baby Food Tragedy" in the August 1973 issue of the *New Internationalist,* a magazine then recently launched with the support of Oxfam in England. The charge that promotion of bottle-feeding by multinational firms was contributing to infant mortality was based in part on field observations of Derek Jelliffe. It was then expanded upon and focused on one corporation: Nestle's. A pamphlet titled *The Baby Killer* was published by War on Want, and a subsequent German version titled *Nestle's Kills Babies* was issued. This public debate included a well-publicized libel trial, a feature on CBS's news program "60 Minutes," and a consumer boycott of all products manufactured or distributed by Nestle's and its subsidiaries (Dobbing, 1988). Other manufacturers of infant formula were attacked through shareholder resolutions. The issue, then, was largely judged by the lay public. This public debate is an example of advocacy research and of popularization of academic research.

Concurrent with this grass-roots campaign, researchers assembled a large body of data on the physiological differences between formula and human milk as well as the epidemiology of infant deaths and the correlates with the use of bottled formula.[8] Sociologists and economists also documented departures from recommended hygiene and dosage by mothers constrained by economics and education. Other researchers studied the means by which formula was advertised and distributed (Greiner, 1975). These studies, which often covered the larger issue of the decline of breastfeeding, were extracted and occasionally elaborated in the brochures and mailings by the partisans of the public debate on the promotion of infant formula (Dobbing, 1988).

A feature of this debate, which is common in public advocacy, was the appeal to authority. Often the authority is deemed such by virtue of his or her research on the topic—hence Derek Jelliffe's testimony to a subcommittee of the United States Senate. Authority is, however, also conferred by notoriety for other work, as indicated by the public role of Benjamin Spock in this issue.[9] In a related vein, an editorial in the *Lancet* criticized the WHO and UNICEF for failing to focus on the available data in their preparation for an international conference on the marketing of infant formula.

It would, however, be naive to expect that such a forum would be conducted like an academic seminar. Although research contributed to a climate that made an international code a political imperative, it was only one of many actors on the main stage. This main stage was the 1981 Geneva conference, at which the United States was the lone dissenter (for ideological reasons) against a draft of an international code for marketing alternatives to breastmilk.

The sponsoring United Nations bodies have, of course, no means of enforcing compliance with this or any other guidelines. Although sponsors of the boycott against Nestle's continued their campaign and negotiations with Nestle's, the Geneva guidelines were intended as foundations for regulations to be enacted by national governments. In Kenya, a group of researchers and government officials met to discuss the WHO/UNICEF guidelines in the context of a country-specific data base (Elliot et al., 1985). The combination of survey data and international guidelines likely contributed to the subsequent passage of legislation on marketing of infant formula.

Nuances, such as the fact that a child may be bottle-fed because it is sick rather than vice versa, influence professional opinion but generally

[8] Much of the research available in the 1970s is summarized in Jelliffe and Jelliffe (1978). This work had been published in the *American Journal of Clinical Nutrition* the previous year.

[9] When a professional takes a partisan role it often comes at a cost in terms of academic reputation. In this politicized atmosphere, few statements on the biochemistry of human milk were divorced from charges that the researcher had traded his integrity for a grant or, conversely, had intentions to undermine the capitalist system.

are obscured in public debates. They may, however, have a role in policy implementation, particularly when the debate has shifted from the public to the professional arena. In this particular instance, improved methodology may change the magnitude of estimated benefits to breastfeeding but not the overall advantage (see, for example, Habicht et al., 1985). Although such studies are directed at a specialized audience, refinements of methodology are themselves likely prompted by the degree of controversy.

Crop Breeding Priorities for International Research Centers

Most nutritionists and national planners recognized a need to deal with what was termed the "protein gap" in the two decades following World War II. They were encouraged in these endeavors by the United Nations Protein Advisory Group. Some of the strategies advocated, such as promotion of fish protein concentrates or leaf protein powders, at the time seemed like technological magic bullets but in retrospect seem like solutions seeking problems. Indeed, the absence of a social and economic context for these attempted solutions was a major contributor to the enthusiasm for the new multidisciplinary approaches to nutritional planning that were endorsed in the early 1970s.[10] This was a general trend, but specific research findings contributed to the shift away from seeking means for protein fortification. This example, as well as the following, then, are examples of research influencing policy mainly through the redefinition of issues as viewed by professionals.

It is noteworthy that the shift of emphasis was promoted by research in various disciplines. For example, Sukhatme as well as Gopalan used survey data to indicate that protein deficiencies seldom were observed in food consumption data except where calories were also lacking (Joy, 1973). Other researchers calculated the costs of formulated foods and found them prohibitively expensive compared to traditional diets (Orr, 1972), and clinical nutritionists questioned whether kwashiorkor and marasmus were clinically distinct deficiency diseases. This body of information, coming from a variety of sources, provided signals to plant breeders in several research centers.

This debate was mediated in part by economic analysis. For example, Ryan et al. (1974) calculated the nutritional constraints in diets in South India and the potential gains from research on sorghum varieties and recommended against a protein breeding objective for the International Center for Research in the Semi-Arid Tropics. Similar calculations by

[10] This approach is itself going through reappraisal (see Berg, 1987a, and Field, 1987, as well as Chapter 14 of this book).

Pinstrup-Andersen (1971) influenced research at the Colombian Institute of Agriculture and the Centro Internacional de Agricultura Tropical, where a high-lysine variety of maize had been developed. It was pointed out that this variety yielded fewer calories per acre than other high-yielding varieties with lower lysine contents. Moreover, consumer preferences, which would translate into prices received by farmers, did not favor the cultivars of the high-lysine variety because the gene that increased the lysine was also linked to those that controlled milling properties. The audience for this research was the research community itself, albeit across disciplines; it was directed neither to a general public nor to a legislative body.

Harriss (1987) argues that agricultural research was late in using such information, but this judgment hinges on the definition of the relative term "late." To be sure, the reevaluation of the protein gap had begun while breeding for protein was still in the ascendancy, but nutritionists themselves debated the perspective for several years. Indeed, because of fads and false starts in any scientific discipline, a rapid adoption of a new priority carries risks as well as potential gains. In another context, Timmer (1988a) argues that experienced policy makers are skeptical of new approaches, precisely because they have seen other fads billed as new professional insights. Timmer is surely correct in warning economists who deal with government officials. In the case of protein strategies, however, many officials proved too slow to respond to a reorientation with staying power; in the early 1980s, for example, Egypt justified its regressive subsidy on frozen chicken and meat on the basis of the requirement for animal protein, and until recently the Chinese government has promoted consumption of animal protein on nutritional grounds.

Food Security as a Concept and a Strategy

Harriss (1987) gives particular attention to the role of agricultural research in increasing food availability. Another approach to the economics of nutrition, however, emphasizes the importance of purchasing power rather than aggregate food supply. This perspective underlies a number of general policy shifts. To a degree, the increased receptiveness to the inclusion of compensatory programs in structural adjustment packages voiced by the World Bank and the IMF (WB-IMF, 1987, 1989) provides an example, as does the implementation of a number of targeted transfer programs. Any attempt to trace a precise pathway from a specific research effort to such policy statements would be misleading. Nevertheless, some discussion is useful, inasmuch as this essay maintains that it is in the creation of such schools of thought that research has some of its most pervasive influence.

Key papers that express the perspective of improving nutrition by focusing more on purchasing power than on aggregate food availability include Reutlinger and Selowsky (1976), Reutlinger and van Holst Pellekan (1986), and Sen (1981). The logic of these arguments is not new either as a concept or as a guideline for policy; Dreze (1988) indicates the role such a perspective played in famine policy in India in the nineteenth century. Nevertheless, the more recent studies have contributed to a school of thought that has quantified such notions and applied them to issues currently being considered by various policy makers.[11] An example with which the author is familiar is the approach to Afghan refugee repatriation proposed by the World Food Program and the United Nations high commissioner for refugees in 1989. This strategy for the repatriation of an estimated 3 million refugees is based on cash grants to returning families as well as open market sales of commodities, which private retailers would be free to market within Afghanistan. Various advisers who participated in drafting this approach made references to the research papers on food security cited above; yet none of those papers were presented to the policy makers, who bear ultimate responsibility for the program. It is, moreover, quite likely that the policy makers who supported the proposal are not aware of the link between such papers and the plan of action.

Similarly, the incorporation of social concerns into structural adjustment programs, either in the design of the adjustment strategy or, more often, in fashioning compensatory programs,[12] partially reflects this body of research on the feasibility of targeting of transfer programs. Because many schools of thought coexist, however, advocacy research also plays a significant role in convincing planners that such programs are desirable. For example, UNICEF has played a highly visible role regarding the particular issue of the social costs of macroeconomic policies, obtaining a fair amount of media coverage with the publication of its annual report on the state of the world's children as well as with Cornia et al. (1988).

Such shifts of professional opinion or ascendancy of schools of thought are not linear progressions. They differ markedly from what leading philosopher of science T. S. Kuhn (1970) has termed "paradigm shifts." Although the phrase is currently in circulation, the examples Kuhn originally discussed, the Copernican and quantum mechanics revolutions, surely indicate that such shifts pertain to major, pervasive changes in how scientists structure the information they process. There may be candidates

---

[11] See, for example, the case studies in Pinstrup-Andersen (1988b).

[12] An example is the Program of Actions to Mitigate the Social Costs of Adjustment (PAMSCAD) drawn up by Ghana in 1987 with foreign donor and World Bank support.

for paradigm shifts in the social sciences as well, but they are at best rare. Shifts in policy perspectives or prevailing wisdom, however, occur continuously, perhaps with a movement that is more like a pendulum than a linear progression.

Institutions might indeed be torn asunder by paradigm shifts, yet new directions may evolve in the light of changing consensual knowledge. The incremental shifts in the World Bank discussed by Haas (1990) or referred to above may lead to new policies but stay within the context of neoclassical economics.

Kuhn's (1970) perspective is, nevertheless, relevant to these movements in professional perspective. Kuhn argues that a paradigm shift occurs with the accumulation of anomalies—phenomena that are not in concordance with theory. New theories do not necessarily explain all evidence better than their predecessors, at least at first, but they allow the resolution of anomalies. Similarly, social sciences, as well as public policy, regularly must confront the accumulated evidence that systems are at variance with predictions. The discordant facts collected contribute, then, to movements in worldviews, although rarely can the pressure for reformulation be traced to a single finding.

Expansion of Vitamin A Research

Large-scale efforts have been made to fortify foods with vitamin A or to administer the vitamin to large numbers of children. For example, a series of research efforts in India took research from animal models through clinical trials and pilot projects to a program covering a portion of the majority of Indian states (Swaminathan et al., 1970; Vijayaraghavan et al., 1975). Similar efforts occurred in other countries. Although the body of clinical and field research that has contributed to the design of such programs differs in many respects from the social science research that is the main focus of this essay, recent attempts to broaden vitamin A supplementation programs illustrate how individuals and nonprofit groups use research results to lobby for further research. Thus it introduces a perspective on the supply of research.

Vitamin A prophylaxis programs are primarily motivated to prevent severe avitaminosis, which leads to blindness and death. Blindness is comparatively common in a number of settings, but clinical symptoms are seldom observed in more than a small percent of the at-risk population. Consequently, such programs are at a comparative disadvantage in competing for a share of a health care budget.[13] Recent research, however, provides evidence that mild vitamin A deficiency is associated with increased morbidity and mortality and may be reversed with supplementation (Sommer et al., 1983; Barclay et al., 1987; Beaton et al., 1993). This finding has a direct bearing on the value of prophylaxis and has galvanized principal researchers in the field to press for new programs.

In this effort they had an influential ally, Martin Forman of USAID, who had also played a key role in funding earlier research. Forman combined the original evidence on the efficacy of supplementation with new evidence on the extent of vitamin A deficiency in Africa, a region that had not been considered a priority in initial prevalence studies, to press for more research funding. In alliance with Helen Keller International, a nonprofit organization, he took preliminary results from field trials to the House Select Committee on Hunger. The appeal of a magic bullet, the potential applicability for Africa while the Ethiopian famine was in the news, and the interest of Representative Mickey Leland, among others, combined to result in a three-year $30 million allocation for vitamin A research as an element of a special Child Survival Fund.

This example can be taken to illustrate the political nature of research allocations. It also indicates the role of individuals who are not researchers themselves in taking research findings into the lobbying process. It is noteworthy, also, that the lobbying was aimed at Congress; USAID does not usually favor earmarks because funds are rarely additional and earmarks reduce the flexibility for within-agency budget allocations.

This example also illustrates another point that is relevant beyond the specific issue. It was argued above that policy research is context-specific, even if generalizations may be derived from a variety of experiences. It might appear, then, that clinical results are more transferable than economic research. In particular, priorities for nutrition policy may be based on findings in other countries, although implementation may require local research. This does not, however, seem to be the case with the recent findings on vitamin A, nor was it apparently so with oral rehydration therapy.

How much research is enough is a broad question and surely depends on the relative risks of errors of commission and omission. Current programs to supplement diets with vitamin A in Tanzania and Indonesia were likely influenced by the specific research conducted there. Elsewhere policy makers have been less enthusiastic, requiring evidence from their own

---

[13] Dr. Alfred Sommer (personal communication) contends that in India the efforts of a private citizen, Dr. Venkaswami (an ophthalmologist), played a crucial role in promoting the transition from early research to a public program.

countries.[14] In at least one country (Bangladesh), however, such research has been resisted because the available evidence is sufficiently convincing that some people feel it would be unethical to give a placebo to control groups. This irony reflects the fact that, in general, the information necessary to initiate a policy differs from that necessary to prevent an action.[15]

Discussion

In certain contexts information has political value in the sense that it can be used to recruit supporters. It also has a value in the sense that it is presented in introductory courses in the theory of industrial organization, namely, to reduce uncertainty and shift prior expectations of gains and losses following from different decisions. In both cases one acquires and disseminates information according to this value and depending on the cost of its acquisition.

Some efforts to quantify the returns to research have been made, for example, in regard to agricultural research (Evenson and Kislev, 1976). It is more difficult, however, to quantify returns to food and nutrition policy research. Some policy measures are justified on the basis of income distribution and merit goods, and therefore, the benefits of research that influences these measures are hard to quantify.

To illustrate, the Pakistan subsidy example provides a comparatively transparent link from research to policy change; a research effort that cost in the neighborhood of $200,000 led to a policy change that, fairly conservatively, can be shown to save 20 percent of the subsidy budget in the first year alone (Alderman, 1988). The savings, then, were approximately $40 million in 1987. Similar calculations could be made for reforms in Chile, Jamaica, Sri Lanka, and elsewhere. The scale of such policies virtually guarantees that fiscal savings from improved delivery would dwarf the costs of research. The economic gains, however, are far more complicated. In the Pakistan example the alternative subsidy program may have actually increased distortion of the price of flour at the margin. Moreover, though a reduction in the budget deficit may have salutary macroeconomic implications, conventional cost-benefit analysis

---

[14] The author found an extreme case of this viewpoint in a 1986 editorial in the *Muslim*, a leading newspaper in Pakistan. It was argued that there was no relevant evidence for the increased probability of genetic disorders with first cousin marriages because no study had been conducted in Pakistan.

[15] It is easier to dispose than to propose. This general statement can draw upon statistics and rhetoric for elaboration. As is well known, one can reject a null hypothesis, but one does not accept it. Moreover, one rarely reports failure to reject as a core of a journal article (Begg and Berlin, 1988).

evaluates changes in transfers only in terms of generally hard-to-elucidate distributional weights.

From a cost-effectiveness perspective, however, the potential saving from research that improves targeting or delivery of services is virtually certain to be higher than the cost of the research. This observation by itself does not indicate an underinvestment in policy research; one also needs to know how much of this potential is realized. This implies, of course, that the effectiveness of research is determined not only by the information generated but by the manner of communication. Manner implies something different than quality, for the concern here is the political context of policy research; much information is generated to counter the information promoted by other interest groups.

Different interest groups, however, have different abilities to generate information. Discussion of the impact of information on policy must, then, return to the endogeneity of the research agenda. Under the induced innovation hypothesis the generation of information responds to impersonal price signals (Binswanger and Ruttan, 1978). De Janvry (1978), however, indicates that agricultural research priorities often are dictated not by price signals alone but by the interests of a subset of the population (see also Alderman, 1984). This idea probably can be generalized beyond agriculture; funding of policy-oriented research is determined simultaneously with current policy.

Shocks, however, contribute to new directions in policy. They are not ruled out even by an extreme form of this hypothesis of simultaneity. Even if the range of probable findings is restricted by the statement of the question, research results are not perfectly determined by the agenda. Unanticipated results can be captured by other interest groups and exploited. Moreover, often there are several funding sources, reflecting, in part, diversity of current policy perspectives and the varying social roles played by the different forms of information from investigative journalism to elaborate data collection and analysis.

Information as a political tool is a special case of the issue of competing information. A particular concern for the topic under discussion is whether quality of information matters. I have tacitly assumed that any influence of information on policy, particularly that derived from economic and social science research, would lead to higher social welfare. But the possibility of misinterpretations, facts taken out of context, and other errors becomes a near certainty when the complexity and volume of information needed for major policy choices is taken into consideration. This is often taken as an argument for less policy intervention. The appropriateness of this recommendation, however, depends in part on whether the process of information generation is self-correcting.

The idealized version of the scientific method depicts a linear process in which new and better research replaces outmoded information and failed theories.[16] The noted historian of science Stephen J. Gould has devoted twenty years of essays to illustrating that human failings of the practitioners and the collective social context divert this process into cul-de-sacs and side paths, yet the basic abstraction remains apt. This may, however, be more likely for the physical sciences, in which replicability is both possible and practiced, than for the social sciences, which are never divorced from historic—and nonreplicable—contexts.

McCloskey (1985) studies how economists have dealt with this aspect of their discipline. He argues that the profession has elevated positivism over other methods of persuasion, which are, in fact, powerful means of communication. A similar trend is toward increased reliance on mathematical proofs that are self-contained in the sense that their validity does not depend on social context. These tendencies may be appropriate when the communication is directed toward other economists. It is a theme of this chapter that such professional communication, distilled and often trivialized, is a major pathway, however indirect, from economic research to policy formation.

This long-run tendency for self-correction and dissemination of ideas is, of course, philosophically comforting and perhaps solace to an adviser waiting in the under secretary's anteroom. But one needs only to type a few letters on the qwerty keyboard or seek a Stirling motor to recall that short-term technological decisions have long-term consequences. Similarly, policy choices, regardless of their quality, change the trajectory of an economy in a manner that restricts subsequent options. Later choices, including corrections of previous errors, then, come at a path-dependent cost (David, 1985). Therefore, even if science is self-correcting, short-term dominance of bad ideas incurs major costs. This is often recognized in the case of the continuing tension between economic populism and principles of macroeconomic management and international trade. It is also the case for food policy.

How, then, can researchers and funders of research increase the probability that research has salutary effects on policy design? Ironically, this may occur if the political nature of information is explicitly acknowledged.[17] This is not an argument for abandoning scientific objectivity, but

---

[16] Similarly, Polyani (1962) argues that an "invisible hand" regulates the scientific community without outside direction. He sees conservative community values of reasonableness and replicability being balanced by the esteem of originality.

[17] The discussion at this point pertains to the communication of research to policy makers. But the political nature of advocacy research can reinforce intellectual rigor (Cherias, 1990). Results that are most discomforting to political interests or accepted wisdom require impeccable methodology to fend off challenges.

it does recognize that usable knowledge is often normative and more rapidly assimilated when communicated accordingly. Moreover, usable knowledge implies a user; communication that bears in mind both the type of user and the objective should be more effective (Gailbraith, 1988).

The examples presented above depict this spectrum. It should be clear that, although political expediency usually holds sway in policy decisions, research often guides the implementation of policies chosen on other grounds. Moreover, research gives momentum to cautious bureaucrats and to interest groups. As illustrated, this may happen when research quantifies what supporters of a policy believe to be the case. Similarly, the examples discussed illustrate a portion of the range of possible interactions where research effort can generate findings that are then employed to recruit uncommitted individuals—laymen, professionals, administrators, or politicians according to the issue—or to recruit funding to increase the volume of supportive evidence. Knowledge of the types of evidence needed to influence decisions can guide the nature of the research. For example, in certain situations evidence is required to confirm that results in other communities are applicable to local conditions. This suggests a different scale and design of research than that which might be indicated when the prior expectations of the scientific community—or policy makers—are more diffuse. Similarly, research aimed at guiding the implementation of existing policy can be designed to meet a different set of objectives and addressed to a more specialized audience than research aimed at defining policy priorities.

The examples presented also indicate that individuals do matter; Forman, Greenstein, Jelliffe, and Venkaswami were noted in the illustrations less for their own research than for their roles in shepherding research toward actions. Conversely, the two adversaries of Rush were shown to delay, if not negate, the impact of a $6 million research project. A scientist does not necessarily dilute the quality of his or her efforts or compromise professional integrity if key actors are identified and included in discussions as a research effort matures. At least, such interactions will highlight findings. Moreover, if begun early in the process, they may contribute to the project's design and the generation of usable knowledge.[18]

Most good researchers recognize that technical research skills are by no means perfectly correlated with the ability to write a grant or raise funds and often design their research efforts to acquire or include these skills. Because these proposals generally attempt to predict the importance

---

[18] Flexibility is also needed. Not only do key individuals shift responsibilities and interests, but new issues enter the policy research during the long gestation of many research efforts.

of the research and, therefore, implicitly assume a user and a communication channel, it is actually not a major shift from current research practices to acknowledge these users and interest groups explicitly. Once these are acknowledged, research efforts that gain the skills to communicate to these groups as well as (not in lieu of) to the general scientific community would maximize the value of the knowledge acquired.

16

The Role of Information in
Enhancing Child Growth and
Improved Nutrition: A Synthesis

David Pelletier

The earlier chapters in this volume reveal various ways information can be used to improve nutrition. Information at the individual level can improve screening or education, as in the case of growth monitoring, and national data sources, focused research studies, and conventional wisdom can influence policy analysis. The range of required information further includes operations research to assist in the design of programs and evaluation studies to determine effectiveness and cost-effectiveness of various intervention strategies and for other purposes. Thus it appears that information can and should play an important role in efforts to improve nutrition. Because of the generally weak state of national capabilities for gathering, analyzing, and using information in these diverse ways, however, the identification of information needs is only the beginning of the process of determining how those needs can best be met. This chapter will attempt to synthesize the roles of information in formulating and implementing food and nutrition policies and programs and examine the implications for efforts to strengthen the use of information in developing countries.

Categories of Information

As a first step in the synthesis, the information needs identified in the earlier drafts of each chapter were listed and then grouped into categories

Table 16.1. Categories of information required in support of actions to improve nutrition, as suggested by contributors to this volume.

Category of information or knowledge	Chapters reflecting this need
1. Information to initiate and sustain political support at various administrative levels	8, 15
2. Knowledge of factors affecting food, nutrition, and health at household and individual levels	2, 3, 4, 10, 11, 12
3. Knowledge of effective intervention strategies and important design features	2, 3, 4, 5, 6, 8, 9, 10, 11, 12
4. Prior experience with interventions in the national setting	10, 11
5. Community perceptions, priorities, and probable reaction to proposed changes	4, 7, 11, 12
6. Implementation bottlenecks: ex ante assessment and ongoing feedback	5, 10
7. Social and political reactions to the introduced changes by local populations and interest groups	5, 7, 10, 11, 12
8. Behavioral changes in the population: positive or negative, anticipated or unanticipated	4, 6, 7, 8, 10, 11, 12
9. Changes in the food, nutritional, or health status of the population	3, 7, 8, 11, 12
10. Cost and cost-effectiveness of strategies	5, 10
11. Improved methodologies for information gathering, analysis, and use	3, 4, 5, 6, 14

Note: In commissioning the chapters for this volume, the editors asked authors to identify the role(s) of information and/or key information needs as they relate to the subject of each chapter. Most authors were asked to consider the role of information at the levels of households, communities, and national governments. In the interest of brevity, these sections of the chapters have been largely deleted, but their overall implications are described in this chapter.

as shown in Table 16.1. The first nine categories can be viewed as quasi-sequential (although they are in fact interactive) in that political support must be developed (category 1), often in tandem with or closely followed by some form of causal analysis (category 2), which proceeds to a selection of interventions (3,4), a complex implementation process with successive refinements (5–8), and, it is to be hoped, positive impact on the food, nutrition, or health situation (9). Information on cost and cost-effectiveness (10) is an important component of categories 1, 3, and 4; however, because of its particular data requirements, it is listed separately. Finally, a number of methodological questions remain concerning the generation of information itself (11). When conceptualized at the national level, the first nine categories of information have the potential to form an

Figure 16.1. Categories and sources of information required for evolving successful nutrition action

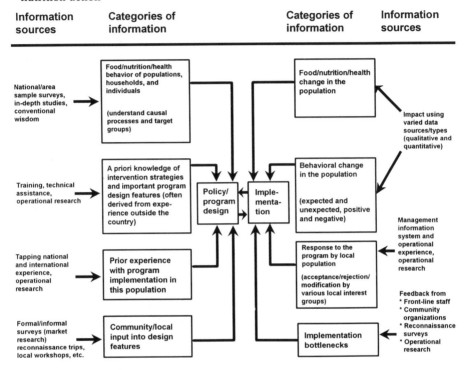

Information sources	Categories of information		Categories of information	Information sources

iterative loop (Figure 16.1) ideally held together by a dynamic relationship between policy/program design decisions and experience gained during implementation. In fact, as described by Field (1985), such a relationship is usually weak or nonexistent at the national level, and intellectually rational master plans quickly fall apart in the face of a variety of administrative, logistic, and sociopolitical obstacles at various administrative levels. Experience has clearly demonstrated the impossibility of planning for all contingencies and bottlenecks at the outset and, thus, the need for a built-in system for detecting problems and responding with necessary adjustments. Flexible guidelines, therefore, are preferable to rigid master plans.

Although the need for flexibility has been given much attention in the literature, and ongoing monitoring and evaluation systems are common, the general conclusion from large-scale rural development projects (Johnston and Clark, 1982; McFarland, 1989; Murphy and Marchant, 1988; Roberts, 1989; World Bank, 1988; Ahmed and Bamberger, 1988) and nutrition programs (Musgrove, 1989; Subbarao, 1989) is that the monitoring and evaluation systems and the programs they are intended to inform are still too insensitive to the variety of problems that occur at the interface of the program and the community (categories 4–8 in Table 16.1). Instead, most previous attempts to improve nutrition policies and programs through information strategies have emphasized problem identification, causal analysis, and targeting on the one hand (categories 1–2) and crude measures of behavioral change and nutritional impact on the other (categories 8–9). Thus the contextual details have been left inside the "black box of implementation" largely hidden from program planners and managers.

Even when managers are well aware of some of these problems, programs often lack the flexibility to make the necessary changes. An important reason for this lack is the institutional separation of planners from program managers, each having access to a different set of information and their own set of bureaucratic objectives and incentive systems. Although not depicted in Figure 16.1, this is a major obstacle to achieving the learning-by-doing approach described above. The solution would require not only more effective information transfer across institutional boundaries but also strong policy support for reorganizing bureaucratic objectives and reward systems to create a receptive climate for incorporating lessons from the field into evolving implementation plans. The importance of this is illustrated by the relatively limited success with farming systems research at the national level, which was not able to induce such changes (Farrington, 1989).

The above discussion focuses on the role of information for policy and program development and implementation from a national (i.e., capital city) perspective. An important question is the extent to which, or in what form, such a loop can be operationalized at lower levels. When applied at these lower levels, it is clear that some of the categories of information in Figure 16.1 either do not apply or are dealt with in the normal course of implementation without the need for interinstitutional communication. For instance, in community programs bottlenecks to implementation arising from local politics or social reaction to proposed actions (the downfall of many centrally designed and implemented programs) can be identified and corrected immediately, without reconnaissance surveys, operational research, or other formal systems required by higher administrative levels. Some form of vertical communication is required, however, when these bottlenecks involve material or technical inputs from government or other external agencies.

The experience from the Iringa program (Pelletier, 1991b) is particularly enlightening in this regard. In that program, the Triple-A cycle (assessment, analysis, action) was developed and implemented in a sufficiently generalized way to permit its application to information-to-action loops at every entry level, from mother to household, community, district and so on up to the national level. It was also intended to be applied to problems ranging from growth faltering in an individual child or community bottlenecks to implementation at household, community, or regional levels. In effect, the concept implies nothing more than an institutionalized practice of identifying and solving problems, but its generalizability across institutional levels and problem types makes it particularly powerful. Although a unifying concept like the Triple-A cycle does not obviate the need for formal information transfer in some cases and changes in bureaucratic objectives and reward systems, it does assist with these insofar as the cycle is applied from the bottom up so that assistance is sought only from higher levels when it cannot be found at lower levels. This places primary responsibility for solving problems on households and communities, and places government agencies in a supportive role to communities.

Despite the apparent success of the Triple-A cycle in the Iringa program, it is recognized that the receptivity toward and capacity for adopting community-based programs differ across national settings. Moreover, although a community-based approach does lend itself to program applications, it cannot assist with the diverse set of nutrition-related policy decisions, which must be made at the national level. Thus information strategies must account for these differences, as reflected in the remainder of this chapter, although some version of the information-to-action loop depicted in Figure 16.1 underlies the discussion in each case.

Use of Information at the Household or Child Level

The fundamental objective of the loop involving the use of information at the household or child level is to influence maternal or household behavior in favor of improved nutrition. As revealed by the review of experiences in nutrition education (Chapter 4), it is now widely accepted that this objective can be most effectively met when the clients for this information (mothers and households) are involved in the process of problem identification, causal analysis, and search for solutions—a radical departure for the prescriptive approach still found in most developing countries. Implicit in the search for solutions is a process of assessing the feasibility with which various options might be implemented in individual cases in light of prevailing constraints (availability of income and food, environmental sanitation, time, intrahousehold social support, and so on), which may take some experimentation before sustainable solutions are found.

This "ideal" model of effective nutrition education is best exemplified by Iringa's Triple-A cycle as applied at the household level.

The application of an information-to-action loop at the household, as opposed to national, level has the great advantages that specific, concrete information on contributing factors and implementation constraints can be rapidly exchanged between mother and health worker; a solution can be found in a single session; and the interval between sessions (when the action plan can be modified) can be measured in weeks rather than years. Its great disadvantage is the need for well-trained, well-supervised, well-staffed cadres of health workers to facilitate these changes, the sustainability of which is obviously uncertain in most developing countries under current levels of support for nutrition, particularly nutrition education.

As illustrated in Chapter 5, growth monitoring has potential not only for education but for targeting that education to those most in need, thereby reducing the health workers' monthly caseload and focusing scarce resources on the malnourished. This screening step need not be done monthly (though the growth monitoring for education should be), but quarterly (as in some Iringa villages) or biannually (as in ANEP). Although these programs still required unusually high levels of staffing, training, and supervision, such design features are useful to contain costs and increase efficiency. Such features would be especially important where the prevalence of malnutrition is relatively low and less important where it is widespread.

If this were the only benefit of growth monitoring, however, a health worker in high-prevalence areas might dispense with screening altogether and simply stagger visits to each household, analogous to the common practice of dispensing iron and folate supplements to all pregnant women without invoking expensive screening procedures. In fact, growth monitoring has at least two other potential advantages. One is based on the hypothesis that it makes malnutrition visible to mothers and involves them in the diagnosis, a precondition for effective nutrition education. A study by Ruel (1990) supports this hypothesis in that Basotho mothers receiving high-quality nutrition education in combination with growth charts improved their nutrition knowledge to a far greater extent that those receiving nutrition education alone. Indeed, this effect was even greater in the higher-risk segment of the sample (lower-educated, primiparous mothers with malnourished children). The second potential advantage occurs when growth monitoring is used to encourage community participation in activities to improve nutrition. As noted by Shrimpton (Chapter 13), growth monitoring can feasibly be managed by communities—an important consideration when trying to encourage participation—and provides some outcome information, which is important for sustaining motivation to improve nutrition. Both of these potential advantages, however, also require a well-organized program to support the education and community development activities, apart from the support and supervision of the weighing- and plotting-related tasks.

Despite these theoretical advantages of growth monitoring as a source of information for education and motivation at individual and household levels, few programs appear to have the other ingredients necessary for success. The existence of successful growth-monitoring programs demonstrates that it can be done under certain conditions, but too often the process of weighing and plotting becomes an end in itself (Chapter 5). Given what appear to be the rather special conditions required for successful growth monitoring, more feasible, creative alternatives for nutrition education that involve mothers or households in the problem-solving process are needed. These might involve, for instance, direct attention to a variety of proximate contributors to growth faltering (feeding practices before, during, and after illness, disease prevention and management), which are the ultimate targets for behavioral change in any case. These might be added to the very popular community-based day care programs like those in Iringa and Colombia. The opportunities for developing participatory approaches to nutrition education should generally be much greater in community-based programs than in clinic-based ones because of proximity to the local causes of malnutrition and greater opportunity for individual attention and follow-up.

Use of Information at the Community Level

Any change within a community—in economic activities, environmental sanitation, child care practices, or other aspects of life—must harmonize with preexisting household and individual behavior, sociopolitical institutions, and ecological characteristics (categories 5–8 in Table 16.1). This requires information on these preexisting characteristics and some degree of prediction concerning the ripples of change which the innovations may induce, not only in the domains targeted for change but also in those with functional links to the target domains. The complexity of this undertaking is well illustrated in several chapters in this volume, notably those concerning changes in women's roles (Chapter 7), water and sanitation (Chapter 9), household and individual food consumption (Chapter 11), and agriculture (Chapter 12). From the perspective of a national government, the difficulty of this task is magnified further by cultural diversity and local historical experiences in development, economic patterns, and natural ecology, factors that greatly condition the nature and magnitude of effects of policy changes and project activities.

It is useful in this regard to distinguish three approaches for community development, defined broadly as planned change in some aspect of individual, household, or community behavior. One approach is based on a centrally designed set of policies or programs applied uniformly across all subpopulations, without regard to local circumstances. Examples include agricultural price or marketing policy, a fixed package of seed, fertilizer, credit, and extension advice in a national agricultural program, or a standard set of nutrition education messages. The second approach involves decentralized design or implementation of programs and projects to improve the fit with local needs, as in regional- or district-level planning. Examples may include developing the capability to manage local buffer stocks in areas expected to be negatively affected by national food price and marketing policy; modifying eligibility criteria, the size of credit packages, or the timing of repayment of agricultural loans to suit local conditions; or tailoring nutrition education messages to prevailing practices based on cultural norms. The third approach to community development emphasizes the strengthening and support of the local community to diagnose its own problems, define its own intervention strategies (within limits), and implement the necessary changes with selective support from outside the community as appropriate. An example might be the training and support of community-based primary health care catalysts to initiate multisectoral changes as required based on local conditions.

As discussed in Chapter 13 and elsewhere (Pelletier and Shrimpton, 1994), successful community-based nutrition programs contained elements of all three approaches. The Tamil Nadu and Dominican Republic programs both achieved good fit with the needs of the population, derived from extensive experience or ex ante operational research. Both, however, had a heavy element of central design and neither approached national coverage. It appears that the quality of information that went into the design of the programs and the experience of the planners were at least as important as the locus of decision making, bearing in mind that all the programs were decentralized to some level below the central government. Of course, when evaluated in terms of empowerment—considered by some to be necessary for sustainability—the four programs differ widely, and the programs from Iringa and Colombia placed greater emphasis on this aspect.

Thus the three approaches described above (centralized planning, decentralized planning, and community-based planning) not only differ markedly in the extent to which local circumstances are addressed in the development process but also in the nature of the information used in

Figure 16.2. Relationships among knowledge, information, resources, and change agents for community development

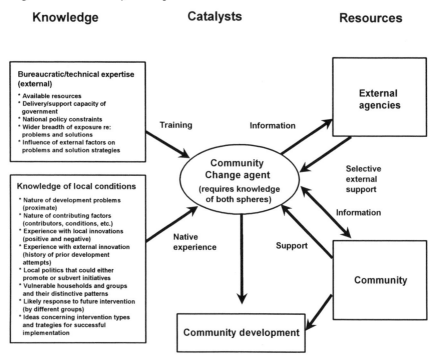

Knowledge **Catalysts** **Resources**

decision making. Figure 16.2 illustrates the two distinct spheres of information which would ideally be used in attempting to harmonize community needs and potential with the constraints and opportunities for external support (from government or nongovernmental organizations). The first of the three approaches described above uses only bureaucratic/technical information in reaching policy and program design decisions, the second supplements this with knowledge of local conditions, and the third takes a more insular approach to change in that knowledge of external factors may be fragmentary.

As indicated in the figure, the presence of a change agent within or in proximity to the community would be one way to unite the technical and local spheres of knowledge during the design or implementation of community changes. Such a change agent is typified by the ideal of a well-trained and well-supported multisectoral PHC worker (a government employee or, more typically, a member of the community). The prevailing model of change agents, however, is a government extension worker with knowledge in only one sector (e.g., agriculture or health) who acts more as an implementer of vertical programs than a source of creative energy for development. This approach reflects the vertical orientation, the lack of flexibility for decentralized planning and implementation, and the training received by extension staff in most development programs. A promising area for research and organizational experimentation would be to reconceptualize the role and training of such extension staff, as well as the programs of which they are a part, so that they become the vital link between the community (including the community change agents) and support required from outside the community in any sector of activity. Although NGOs would have the comparative advantage to foster such an approach (because they operate locally and are generally not as bureaucratically constrained), it would be especially desirable to experiment with government extension services as well, precisely because of the scope of their activities and the volume of resources they control.

Another dimension in which the three approaches differ is in their ability to respond to feedback in making midcourse adjustments in program design. The complexities inherent in predicting the variety of ripple effects brought on by planned innovations, some of them potentially undesirable, suggest that more emphasis is needed in evolving successive refinements in program design over time rather than designing an inflexible program from the outset. Lack of flexibility for decentralized decision making is likely to mean a much longer lag between the identification of implementation problems and appropriate adjustments. Although various mechanisms could be found for shortening the time required for information to reach the decision makers (through an efficient and sensitive management information system or strong capacity for operations research), the diversity in the types of problems may argue against the adoption of uniform remedies. Thus even if the ex ante design is performed centrally, there are strong arguments in favor of providing the flexibility for decentralized implementation and adjustments to shorten the time lag implicit in the learning-by-doing approach.

Finally, a trained community-based change agent should be able to assist the community in identifying and addressing any number of community problems, from sanitation disposal and water handling and storage to child day care or disease management. An important role for the change agent would be to educate the community on the need for change in any of these areas and, with the community, decide on a plan of action. An information system in this case might have a close correspondence between the indicators for problem diagnosis and those for monitoring and evaluation (e.g., number of households using latrines, number depleting food stocks). Because of the conceptually unifying properties of child growth, which is theoretically sensitive to all such changes at community level, growth monitoring is often recommended as a useful tool for diagnosing community problems and subsequent evaluation of outcomes (Chapter 13). Although many programs express interest in using growth monitoring to stimulate community development, only the Iringa program can be said to have achieved this purpose. By contrast, most were using growth monitoring successfully for individual-level applications (screening or education). Presumably, this reflects underlying weaknesses in community organization and the larger number of external factors that may interfere with community development efforts as opposed to screening or education (e.g., the need for frequent material or technical assistance from government). Growth monitoring is supposed to help strengthen community organizations, and indeed all of the programs created organizational structures to manage growth-monitoring activities. These structures, however, appear to be insufficient because only in the Iringa program were they functioning for community development.[1]

Thus, although growth monitoring can be a catalyst for community development and is useful for nutrition eduction, the strategy apparently also has some demanding preconditions for success that are often not met in practice. An important consideration in designing community-level information systems is whether to invest in the training and supervision of the growth-monitoring related activities (including, as in the Iringa case, education of the public concerning the links between child weight and community and household characteristics) or to concentrate instead on an expanded list of basic community needs, which might be more readily understood and more directly valued by the community. Another consideration is whether growth monitoring, a new activity within reach of the community's capabilities and with spin-offs in strengthening community structures, is a worthwhile, superior strategy for social mobilization. Finally, if growth monitoring is already an integral part of a planned or an existing community program because of its application at the individual level (i.e., education and screening), then the marginal cost of also using it to stimulate community development may not be great, provided it does not interfere with its original functions.

Use of Information at the National Level

The preceding sections illustrate that some version of the loop of activities depicted in Figure 16.1 can be applied to decisions and actions taken

---

[1] Even in the Iringa program, it was apparent that the community's ability to request material or technical assistance from government sometimes exceeded government's ability

at the level of households and communities as well as nationally. A particular challenge to meeting information needs at the national level, however, is that the types, quantity, and organization of information differ in important respects from those at lower levels. This is illustrated by two approaches to the problem, multisectoral nutritional planning and nutritional surveillance, both of which have met with variable success at best, depending upon how the activities themselves and their objectives are defined. This problem is discussed below, followed by consideration of the role of national sample surveys as a source of information for various categories of decisions.

Nutritional Surveillance versus Monitoring

Although it differs in significant ways from the original WHO and Cornell conceptualizations (WHO, 1976; Mason et al., 1984), the most commonly recognized form of nutritional surveillance[2] in developing countries is actually nutrition monitoring. The latter refers to a system for monitoring the nutritional status of a population over time and space, on the assumption that such information is useful for a variety of purposes (Habicht et al., 1978; Habicht, 1990). This monitoring usually takes the form of weights or heights of children attending health centers or schools, aggregated to various administrative levels. In the absence of ancillary information linked to these indicators of nutritional status, the most common applications are for general problem identification (useful for political sensitization and advocacy), for geographic targeting, and (usually overlooked) for stimulating the collection of additional information on the causes of the problem through other means (Valverde et al., 1982; Gross et al., 1987; Bondad et al., 1984). Unfortunately, experiences from Central America and Panama, where such systems have received a great deal of attention, reveal few if any instances when the information was used for the intended purpose (Arnauld et al., 1990). This greatly simplified form of nutritional surveillance is similar to experiences from other countries, as revealed in a review of nutritional surveillance in ten countries (UNICEF, 1992a).

This poor performance of nutrition monitoring at the national level is partly a result of the complexity of the decision-making process at that

---

to provide it, causing long delays and frustration in completing some community projects (Pelletier, 1991b).

[2] Defined as watching over nutrition in order to make decisions that will improve the nutritional status of populations. Under this concept, nutritional surveillance includes a wide range of activities related to policy and planning, program management and evaluation, and timely warning.

level (Chapter 15), as well as to deficiencies in the information itself even if clear political will did exist. The latter stems from the inappropriate assumption that information useful at one level is also useful at higher levels. For instance, a single data point on the weight-for-age of a child can, in principle, be immediately followed up with a diagnosis of causes and a search for feasible solutions by mother and health worker. It requires more time and ancillary information to do this at the community level (using a community prevalence estimate as a catalyst for change), but because the natural, behavioral, and political ecology of malnutrition is already known at that level (or can be easily determined) nutrition monitoring can still be effective.

Except in the case of political sensitization and advocacy, a vastly different approach is required at the national level, however, when presented with only a prevalence estimate. In Table 16.1, information at the national level on the levels and time trends of underweight children has potential utility only for categories 1 and 8. If the other categories in Table 16.1 are important for success in designing and implementing nutrition actions at the national level, then it is clear that an information system which devotes most of its resources to processing nutritional status data would be quite incomplete. Despite attempts to clarify this point and to suggest ways to collect some required ancillary data (WHO, 1976; Mason et al., 1984), many attempts to create nutritional surveillance systems in developing countries have been based exclusively on such data and with disappointing results. At the opposite end of the spectrum have been countries that embarked on multisectoral nutritional planning as a strategy to meet a far greater range of information needs in an integrated manner, with equally disappointing results with respect to the originally stated objectives (see Chapter 14).

In a sense, then, nutritional surveillance (narrowly conceived as nutrition monitoring) and multisectoral nutrition planning are extreme efforts to meet the information needs for nutrition policies and programs, with the former often being implemented in an overly simplistic fashion and the latter in an overly ambitious fashion. Both approaches tended to overlook the importance of implementation issues, represented by categories 3–7 of Table 16.1. As discussed by Field (1985), this oversight is characteristic of the "intellectual establishment" approach in which centralized planning of policies and programs takes precedence over administrative and logistic constraints. Related to this is the greater emphasis placed on ex ante design of policies and programs than on a learning-by-doing approach (Korten, 1980).

*The Role of National Sample Surveys in Food and
Nutrition Policy Analysis*

Household sample surveys, which have now been conducted in many developing countries,[3] are an important source of data for nutritional surveillance (in its broader sense) and food policy analysis. The strength of these surveys is their greater representativeness and the greater range of ancillary information against which indicators of nutritional status and food consumption can be compared. When analyzed cross sectionally, these surveys are instrumental in identifying the groups most vulnerable to malnutrition and deficits in food consumption at household or individual levels. They are also indispensable for estimating a variety of parameters for use in food policy analysis such as income and price elasticities of demand. When analyzed over time, they can reveal trends in malnutrition and food consumption in the population as a whole or among important subgroups, and price elasticities of demand and supply can be estimated with greater confidence.

In analyzing the usefulness of national sample surveys in national policy and planning decisions, the technical characteristics of the data are an important consideration. As reflected in Table 16.2, it is important to distinguish between analyses and policy decisions based on indicators of child nutritional status versus those based on estimates of household food consumption. In addition, it is necessary to distinguish among a number of analytical purposes and policy/planning applications ranging from simple prevalence estimation for initial political sensitization, to functional classification for policy/program targeting, and to causal analysis at varying levels of detail for policy and program design decisions.

From a technical perspective, indicators of child nutrition have the advantages for sensitization purposes that they can be measured in a relatively simple manner, interpreted in relation to current or chronic conditions, and shown to be related to functional outcomes with clear policy significance (e.g., risk of mortality, morbidity, reduced adult work capacity). Quantitative estimates of household food (energy) consumption, by contrast, are considerably more difficult to collect; they are also less easily interpreted because of uncertainties in setting a socially and economically acceptable level of energy requirements, including physical activity, against which the adequacy of consumption can be evaluated (FAO/WHO/UNU, 1985). Thus both the cutoff level for defining inadequate

---

[3] Empirical examples with nutritional status as the outcome include Valverde et al. (1978); Harrell et al. (1989); Haaga et al. (1986); Pelletier and Msukwa (1991); Teller et al. (1990); Sahn (1990); and Alderman (1990). Examples with food access as the outcome include the LSMS surveys (e.g., Glewwe, 1986; Greer and Thorbecke, 1986).

Table 16.2. Utility of national sample surveys for different purposes

		Type of outcome variable	
Analytical purpose	Application	Nutritional status of young children	Household food consumption
Identifying size and magnitude of the problem	Political sensitization	Good	Fair
Functional classification	Sensitization, targeting	Good	Good/Fair
Causal analysis macrolevel	National sectoral priorities	Fair	Good/Fair
Causal analysis microlevel	Designing specific program features	Poor	Good for some, poor for others
All of the above	Planning at subnational levels	Limited[a]	Limited[a]

Note: All ratings are subject to qualifications (see text) and based on characteristics intrinsic to measurement of each outcome variable and the independent variables. Measurement of independent variables is assumed to be at a fairly general level (except for household income and expenditure data) because of constraints in large, general-purpose surveys.

[a] Depends upon the level of disaggregation desired in relation to the design and sample size of the survey and the degree of heterogeneity in relevant characteristics within the country. All of the limitations described in the text apply at subnational levels as well, although smaller sample sizes are more likely to add to the difficulty.

consumption in a given population group and the extent of misclassification bias are unclear. The latter can inflate estimates of prevalence to a far greater extent than do anthropometric indicators because of random measurement error in estimates of household consumption. These technical characteristics also diminish the utility of these indicators in functional classifications because the interpretation of consumption differences across functional groups is confounded by probable variation in energy requirements across these groups as a function of the physical requirements of occupations, farm types, and the like—a factor that generally cannot be adequately taken into account in the analysis.[4]

Although variant forms of the above system represent perhaps the most common applications of national sample surveys (especially those using child nutritional status as the outcome), such data can be used for other policy and planning purposes. For convenience, these are referred to as

[4] The seriousness of this factor depends on how detailed the functional classification is. Because poor households are generally involved in more manual labor, on average, than the nonpoor, adjusting for this factor would only increase the difference in consumption (relative to requirements) between the poor and nonpoor, but the direction of such an effect cannot always be predicted when the functional classification is disaggregated further.

"causal analysis" in Table 16.2, although these data alone do not demonstrate causality with a high degree of plausibility by scientific standards. Moreover, two levels of causality analysis (and the decisions that can be supported by such analysis) must be distinguished (micro and macro) depending upon the detail with which variables were collected.

The distinction between macrolevel and microlevel causal analysis is particularly clear where child nutritional status is the outcome. This is because of the multifactorial etiology of protein-energy malnutrition (much less so in the case of household food consumption shortfalls) and in large part because of the rather subtle, contextual nature of the causes, which are difficult or impossible to capture in a national survey. For instances, household water and sanitation conditions are often used either as a proxy for chronic morbidity (because of increased risk of exposure to pathogens in households with poor water and sanitation conditions) or to estimate the relative contribution of water versus sanitation or other factors to PEM. A common method of assessing water and sanitation conditions is to inquire into the source of drinking water (e.g., piped, bore hole, river, pond) and method of human waste disposal (e.g., latrine, bush, or as source of manure).

One hoped-for policy implication of analysis based on such variables might be to help decide priorities within the health sector (viz., the importance of water versus sanitation to PEM) or between the health and other sectors (viz., the importance of water and sanitation to PEM relative to that of household income or food consumption, for instance). In Table 16.2, this is referred to as macrolevel causal analysis because the water and sanitation variables represent fairly crude indicators of the influence of health-related factors on PEM. They fail to capture some related microbehavioral and microenvironmental processes that influence PEM in concert with or independent of the measured variables. Examples of microprocesses might be the seasonal nature of water sources, the possibilities for contamination before collection or en route to its use (e.g., in storage), the influence of personal hygiene on exposure to pathogens (e.g., handwashing before feeding young children), alternative possibilities for environmental contamination such as proximity of animals to dwellings, and so on. Statistically, the result is that data on water and sanitation, as usually collected in national surveys, capture only a proportion of the variance in the morbidity-related influence on PEM.[5] The result is under-

---

[5] Similarly, a more direct assessment of morbidity, such as the occurrence of various symptoms or illnesses in the week or two before the survey, captures information on morbidity only during that period. Thus it captures only a proportion of the variance in the long-term morbidity-related influence on PEM (DeKlerk et al., 1989). The size of that proportion depends upon the ratio of intrachild to interchild variance in morbidity over the long term,

estimation (to an unknown extent) of the total effect of morbidity on PEM and, to a lesser extent, of the potential for improved water and sanitation to improve PEM. Moreover, when these effects are estimated simultaneously with those from other factors (e.g., income or food consumption) conclusions concerning the relative importance of each are influenced not only by the true relative importance (unobservable) but also by the relative magnitude of slippage in the measurement of each variable.

The above considerations are not generally discussed to any great extent in the literature on food and nutrition policy analysis, although they do receive more attention in the epidemiological literature (Rosner et al., 1990; DeKlerk et al., 1989; Alam et al., 1989a). For all practical purposes, they represent limitations that analysts (and policy makers) must tolerate until more information is available on the relative size of measurement errors in variables of this type, which could then be used to adjust the estimates of statistical effects. Apart from this, however, it is clear from the above example that information from this type of analysis is, at best, useful only for making broad intersectoral and intrasectoral policy decisions concerning the effects of several factors on PEM. Information from this source cannot assist with more detailed program design decisions, such as the education messages to accompany water and sanitation programs to overcome the hidden sources of contamination or infection, the other types of environmental improvement required, or the cultural factors that limit the use of facilities such as latrines and improved water sources. As revealed by the earlier chapters in this volume, these factors can be of major importance in determining the effectiveness of programs and the impact of policies. The major implication for designing information strategies to support policy and program design decisions, therefore, is that additional mechanisms must be established for collecting information on these contextual, microbehavioral, and microenvironmental processes. These mechanisms might range from localized in-depth quantitative studies in some cases to qualitative investigations of varying scope and duration in others.

These technical difficulties apply more to analysis of child nutritional status than to household food consumption as the outcome variable. This partly reflects greater multifactorial etiology in child nutritional status than in household food consumption, and it also reflects the potential for national income and expenditure surveys to collect such data in great detail (i.e., highly disaggregated by income source and expenditure cate-

---

by analogy with the proofs developed in the literature on dietary epidemiology (Beaton et al., 1979; Liu et al., 1978). There are currently no estimates available from the literature for the value of this ratio in the case of morbidity.

gories). In addition, there are inherently tighter linkages (behaviorally and statistically) among categories of income and expenditures, with expenditure on food (often used as the measure of food consumption) being but one. Thus such data are generally adequate for estimating demand elasticities for the whole population and subgroups of interest for policy purposes, including demand for calories from all sources or from specific commodities. Such results are of central importance to food policy analysis and may be considered a form of macrolevel or microlevel causal analysis, depending on whether and to what extent disaggregation is employed (viz., functional groups, income sources, and commodity consumed).

Even in the case of analysis of household food economics, however, these data are inadequate for shedding light on important microlevel processes. For instance, it is impossible to determine the intrahousehold consumption of food (e.g., to assess the potential for improving the food intake of specific categories of household members); nor is it possible to find alternative (nonprice, nonincome) mechanisms for increasing the total or commodity-specific consumption by population groups (e.g., by intervening on factors related to processing or preparation time, fuel requirements and availability, and the like, as discussed in Chapter 11). Thus it is still relevant to distinguish between the use of such data for broad policy decisions (e.g., which commodity to subsidize to increase the household food consumption of selected functional groups) and the use for more detailed design decisions. As in the case of nutritional status outcomes, these latter questions must generally be addressed through more in-depth quantitative or qualitative investigations.

Apart from these technical considerations, the more positive experience observed in incorporating food economics data into government decision making may be attributable to at least two other factors. First, the relevant consumer economics theory and methodologies are better developed and more widely understood by government economists in developing countries than are analogous applications in nutrition. Second, the institutional basis for food and economic policy analysis and decisions is more clearly defined in government bureaucracies, despite the variation across countries in the degree to which food policy analysis is concerned with demand versus supply analysis and the degree of disaggregated analysis by target groups. The improvements in theory, analytical methods and case studies of applying food policy analysis to nutritional status outcomes (e.g., von Braun et al., 1989a,b; Sahn, 1990; Alderman, 1990), and increased sensitization of economic planners and policy makers to the relevance of such applications, may make it possible to improve the use of national survey data in relation to nutritional status outcomes.

Strategies for Providing Information

To satisfy information needs at household, community, and national levels, the focus must be on the different uses of information and the development of effective strategies for its collection and use, as opposed to a more narrow focus on types of information (e.g., specific indicators) or sources of information (e.g, surveys versus monitoring systems). Identifying the most appropriate processes depends upon the level at which information will be used (household to national) and the specific applications at that level (e.g., policy formulation versus program design, management, or evaluation). One lesson from nutritional surveillance, national program monitoring, and evaluation or other attempts to meet information needs through large, integrated information systems is that they are inadequate for meeting the diverse information needs across countries and over time. Although certain information elements may well be common to many or most applications (e.g., indicators of nutritional status or its proximate determinants), the frequency, timeliness, accuracy, and level at which these are required should receive careful review and should not obscure the range of other information needed to complete the loop between information and effective action (Figure 16.1).

National-Level Information Strategies

The major issue regarding information strategies at the national level is the institutional context for gathering, analyzing, interpreting, disseminating, and using information. For the first three of these steps, the range of possible institutions includes national statistical offices (NSO), sectoral planning, monitoring, and evaluation units (PM&E) at national and subnational levels (these three functions are sometimes separated institutionally), cross-sectoral institutions such as food and nutrition policy/planning units (FNPU), university researchers and research centers, professional (private) research firms, and NGOs. Donor missions, consultants, and external researchers also play significant roles in collecting new information and synthesizing existing information. As indicated in Chapter 15, the audiences for information produced by these institutions include policy makers, multisectoral committees, specialist commissions, public and private interest groups, professional organizations, donors, NGOs, the news media, and the general public.

Despite these long lists of potential information providers and audiences, the actual situation in many countries is that relatively few institutions play a significant role in generating data, fewer still are involved in meaningful analysis and interpretation of it, and it is disseminated to only a fraction of the possible audiences—often in inappropriate forms. The result is much wasted effort in data collection and many missed opportunities for analysis, interpretation, and dissemination to important interest groups.

As illustrated in Chapter 15, the timing of demand for specific pieces of information is often so unpredictable that answers must be provided based on existing knowledge and information rather than information collected to meet that specific need. This situation increases the importance of conventional wisdom (as perceived by decision makers), the pool of existing knowledge among technicians, recognized authoritative sources of information, and professional networks as a means for providing answers as and when required. An enlightening case study in this regard comes from Chile, where improvements in health services, nutritional status, and infant mortality were sustained for more than two decades through effective use of program-generated information, impact evaluations, and ad hoc surveys by scientists, health professionals and professional organizations to maintain government support for programs (Vio et al., 1992). In contrast, an effort to formalize this information into a centralized nutritional surveillance system in 1983 was discontinued after only three years because its separation from decision makers rendered it ineffective.

Given this situation, one set of strategies for improving the quality of decisions is to ensure that professional networks are created and maintained; that information is regularly shared among professionals, bureaucrats and technicians; and that every opportunity is taken to influence conventional wisdom as held by policy makers and others. This can be achieved through creation or strengthening of relevant professional associations; encouraging networking among them; developing or capitalizing upon existing working groups, seminars, workshops, or symposia aimed at different audiences (technicians, bureaucrats, policy makers, and donors); and looking for windows of opportunity to reach policy makers through direct or indirect means and formal or informal channels. These are all in addition to the more formalized multisectoral committees that are supposed to fulfill these functions.

Apart from these and other strategies, it is necessary to determine the content of the messages to the various audiences, which should be done on the basis of the most pressing policy issues at the time or emerging policy issues. Regular meetings between planners, academics, and researchers would assist in identifying the policy issues, probing the state of knowledge and areas of agreement and disagreement concerning each, and outlining the implications for further analysis or research or policy options. It would be naive to expect that such a process would result in a consensus on many or most issues, but it would serve the useful purpose of achieving greater clarity on the various dimensions of a given problem and the beginnings of a decision-making algorithm.

A prior assumption underlying the above strategies is that a pool of experienced and well-trained professionals exists to take part in such activities and that they have the time and motivation to do so. The development of such a pool of professionals should clearly be a medium- to long-term priority of all countries, complemented by external expertise in the interim.

Apart from improving the sharing and use of existing information through the above strategies, several of the stages in the loop depicted in Figure 16.1 require collection, analysis, interpretation, and use of new information. As shown in the figure, these information needs must be met through a combination of data sources and methodologies, depending upon the requirements for timeliness, representativeness, form of analysis, and various user requirements. Table 16.3 arranges the possible sources of data in relation to the possible institutions that may participate in its collection, analysis, interpretation, and dissemination to illustrate the range of possibilities that may exist. Some institutions have a clear comparative advantage to undertake certain activities (e.g., NSO for national surveys), but it is not possible to specify fully those relationships in the table because of variations in local circumstances. Moreover, in many or most cases, there are clear advantages to separating responsibility for data collection, analysis, interpretation, and dissemination among different institutions. For instance, experience has shown that a NSO should not normally be expected to undertake detailed investigative analysis of national survey data because of other demands on its time, whereas that may be an appropriate role for a FNPU, PM&E, university researchers, or others, depending upon the local context. Similarly, the task of synthesizing information from many sources may be appropriate for a FNPU, researchers, and donor missions.

One of the primary factors constraining the potential of information in many developing countries is that data and information in various stages of preparation are not shared across institutional lines. The experience in the United States is enlightening in this regard in that much of the investigative analysis of national survey (and census) data is performed by uni-

Table 16.3. Institutional basis for information collection, analysis, interpretation, and dissemination (varies by country)

Information type	NSO	PM&E[a]	FNPU	University	Professional research firms	NGOs	Donor missions and consultants	External researchers
National surveys	X							
Area baseline surveys		X		X	X	X		
Investigative surveys								
Rapid		X		X	X	X		X
Long-term				X	X			X
Operations research								
Rapid		X		X	X	X	X	X
Long-term		X			X			
Program monitoring								
Ad hoc		X		X	X	X		X
In-built		X						
Program evaluation								
Demonstration projects		X		X		X		X
Pilot projects		X		X		X		X
Full-scale programs		X		X		X		X
National monitoring systems	X	X						
Timely warning systems		X					X	
Information synthesis (for policy and planning)		X	X	X			X	X

[a]This includes PM&E units at national, regional, and district levels and, for certain program-related information types, program managers and functionaries at lower levels.

versities and research centers rather than by the data-collection agencies themselves (e.g., National Center for Health Statistics or U.S. Census Bureau). Because those data sources are intended to address a wide variety of possible research questions, many of which are unspecified when the data are collected, the ability to exploit them to their fullest depends crucially upon making the data available to a large number of researchers. This is largely a question of efficiency, but it also relates to the need for verifiability in a scientific sense. The ability to increase the data-sharing and information yield from public data sets in developing countries would require policy changes in many countries concerning the classified nature of some data sets and improvements in the pool of trained researchers, computer facilities, and support. Outside agencies could play an important role in this area by encouraging or requiring that any data collected through their efforts be made available to local analysts (not just research institutions), along with the required training and computing facilities.

The most readily available pool of highly trained professionals capable of making a larger contribution is located in national universities. Here also a number of constraints appear to exist. One is that the professional link between university researchers and planners and policy makers is often weaker than desired. Another constraint is that the quantity and quality of research output from university researchers is limited in some cases by teaching and administrative duties and the absence of graduate training programs. University-based research centers are a valuable resource for meeting a variety of information needs, especially if they can draw on the expertise of the teaching faculty, but they often lack a secure base of core support to improve the volume and quality of staff and research output. Finally, one of the most basic factors limiting the contribution of university expertise to national planning and policy making is that academics are often viewed as a potential political liability, in which case policies regarding access to government data and representation on government committees may be designed to limit their involvement.

Another aspect of Table 16.3 requiring special comment concerns the role of professional (i.e., private sector) research and consulting firms. Compared to developed countries, this is a particularly weak dimension of the information-generating systems of developing countries and one that would have many advantages if strengthened. First, it would offer governments and donors a mechanism for meeting ad hoc information needs in a flexible manner and without incurring the cost burden implied by developing a government unit to meet those needs. Second, the salaries of professionals in these firms would likely be higher than those available in the public sector and comparable to other private sector work (e.g., banks and insurance companies), thereby attracting better talent. Third, the development of such firms would lessen the dependency on foreign researchers and consultants and contribute to development of national capacities (and a pool of professionals who could, at some later time, enter public service). This is an especially pressing need for African countries, which might benefit from the experience of several Latin American and Asian countries that are already developing such capacities in the private sector.

In keeping with the suggestion that some institutional separation be maintained between data collection/analysis and interpretation/synthesis, it is important that at least one institution be responsible for keeping abreast of all food- and nutrition-related activities in the country for synthesizing results as required for specific policy and program decisions and for acting as an information clearinghouse for others. Ideally, this would be the function of the FNPU, at least some of whose staff should be reserved for this purpose while others may be more involved in project-specific data analysis and interpretation. This FNPU should have good knowledge of available food- and nutrition-related information and perhaps be the central node of the network of professionals discussed above, but not that it should presume to control all government action bearing on food and nutrition issues as attempted by multisectoral nutrition planning.

Finally, as reflected in Table 16.3, the suggestion is not being advanced here that all the information needs of government could or should be met through time-consuming, detailed, quantitative surveys. To the contrary, an equally large effort is needed to strengthen the capacity for and practice of conducting short-term, qualitative investigations to develop hypotheses and follow up on leads from analysis of data from surveys, ongoing monitoring systems, and timely warning systems to troubleshoot for problems in policy or program implementation and in program evaluation (Filstead, 1979; Longhurst, 1981; Pacey, 1982; Pelletier and Msukwa, 1990; Rhoades, 1985; Scrimshaw and Hurtado, 1987). Although a great deal of useful information can be gleaned from short-term follow-up investigations, the rationale for strengthening capacities in these areas has been virtually ignored in favor of the quantitative model. Efforts to strengthen skills in these areas are likely to yield high returns whenever rapid investigations substitute for longer-term surveys; whenever they provide information for decision making where surveys would have been impossible; and whenever they improve the design, analysis, and interpretation of data from quantitative surveys based on a more sound appreciation of the local context of human behavior.

Community-Level Information Strategies

As illustrated in Figure 16.2, the basic objective of information strategies at the community level is to bring together two spheres of knowledge in some manner during the design and implementation of actions. Depending upon the prevailing politico-administrative arrangements, this might be accomplished by the delegation of responsibility for program planning and implementation to the district level or by empowering the communities themselves to plan and implement actions. In the former case, the information strategy should be geared toward generating information for district officials concerning the relevant community-level opportunities and constraints for development, but the design decisions ultimately rest with government officials. District planners would undertake investigations into local conditions using a variety of methods as outlined at the national level, but emphasizing rapid, qualitative ones. In the latter case (as illustrated by Iringa), the information strategy consists of the training of change agent(s) within the community, possible sensitization and mobilization of the wider community itself, and ongoing supportive supervision of community initiative by district-level government.

In practice, the distinction is not as clear as it may seem because programs planned at the district level can often undergo substantial modifications and refinements at the community level during implementation; likewise, so-called community initiatives are often, in fact, suggested by government representatives in the course of "supportive supervision." The important point from an efficiency perspective is that sufficient community consultation and dialogue take place to ensure good fit between actions and needs in a technical sense and good understanding of and support for project objectives on the part of community leaders and the public. Although community participation in the full empowerment sense is desirable for other reasons, it is expensive to initiate because of the training required and it may not fit with existing political and administrative realities. The review of community-based projects (Pelletier and Shrimpton, 1994) suggests that successful programs can be developed using a pragmatic mix of strategies as appropriate for local conditions and, by inference, that the quality of information may be more important than the locus of control in the program.

The distinction between district-level planning and community-based planning is important for understanding whether and how communities may play a role in generating and using information. This is illustrated below in the case of the most common type of information—that obtained from growth monitoring. When communities have been trained (or empowered) to plan their own actions, regular community growth monitoring provides information on categories 1 and 9 in Table 16.1, and the community is supposed to take responsibility for the intervening steps through the use of existing knowledge at the community level. In this case, growth monitoring serves to impart community ownership and responsibility for the process itself and any resulting actions. Also, when the results from growth monitoring or progress reports on implementation are reported to higher levels, they provide an indication of community performance for administrative supervisors. These performance indicators (as seen in Iringa) may include whether reports are received regularly, the numbers weighed, and so on, rather than the prevalence of underweight children per se. In this case, community-based growth monitoring is a strategy to achieve community participation and is a management tool.

In the case of planning at the district level, a single growth-monitoring campaign at the community level provides an estimate of the prevalence of underweight children but none of the contextual details required for steps 2–8 (Table 16.1). The latter must be obtained either by detailed interviews and formal surveys in a sample of communities or through dialogue with such communities (e.g., through focus group discussions) in much the same fashion that the community might interact with a local change agent. Of the two information-gathering strategies, the qualitative dialogue is likely to be more practical and more likely to promote support for subsequent activities. In this way, the district planners might obtain sufficient insight into local conditions to go back to their offices and design actions that meet existing needs and are socially and politically acceptable to the population of the district even though only a sample of communities may have been consulted. There is, thus, none of the interest in growth monitoring as an ongoing mobilization and management tool, and it may not be necessary unless the resulting program requires it as a continuous process (e.g., nutrition education targeted to the malnourished). In fact, unless the estimate of prevalence at baseline is important for subsequent impact evaluation or for enlisting community participation during the diagnostic phase, growth monitoring may not be needed at all in this type of program planning.[6] Instead, attention might focus on understanding in a qualitative sense the dynamics of the local economy and food system, child care and feeding practices, environmental sanitation, use of health care, and so on. This approach eliminates what may be a bit of mystique concerning growth monitoring from the community's perspective and permit a discussion of facets of community life which are familiar and of immediate importance to the people.

[6] This assumes that the results of growth monitoring are not going to be systematically analyzed in relation to other individual or household characteristics as in a functional classification, a step that is usually well beyond the capacity of communities and often of districts.

Implicit in this approach is the notion that communities should not be enlisted regularly to collect and transmit data to higher levels unless it can be used by the communities themselves. When the locus of decision making is at district or higher levels, the communities would be incapable of collecting and transmitting the required range of information (much of it contextual, which cannot be reduced to simple indicators), and the incentives for doing so would exist only if the community (or its leaders) felt there was a reasonable chance that some of its perceived needs were going to be met as a result. Moreover, when the effort is structured such that primary control over resources and actions is external to the community and the available resources may be insufficient for covering all communities at the outset, the entire incentive system is predisposed to exaggerating the problems. The proposed alternatives are either to grant sufficient control to the community, in which case information gathering and use are seen as furthering the interests of the community itself, or for the district agencies to undertake the investigations required for planning, monitoring, or evaluation as described above.

Whether the community-level strategy is based on district planning or community empowerment, it is clear that one of the great needs is for training of staff at the appropriate levels. With the district approach, training is needed for the program planners and extension workers on the broad perspective concerning the causes and potential solutions to nutrition problems; on the rationale and methods to enlist community support (if not participation) for projects; on methods for performing community diagnostics; and on experience from other settings in the range of intervention strategies and design features that may prove successful. With the community empowerment approach, training is required for the change agents (be they extension workers or community members) on some of the same issues but also on the menu of possibilities for material or technical support that exist outside the community. Although this approach should not strive to create a dependency on such support, there is often a need for some support, about which the change agent must have realistic expectations and communicate them to the community.

Finally, it must be acknowledged that considerable administrative obstacles to decentralized planning often exist within governments and donors, which often limit the effectiveness of the above approaches. Even if some budgetary decisions and ultimate project approval authority are delegated to the district level (which is usually not the case), there is a need for support from the central level for requisitions of materials and technical assistance, training, transportation, personnel matters, and others, any one of which can seriously impede the process. The fact that budgetary and approval authority is usually not completely delegated further complicates the picture. Among other things, this means that district planners must be capable of preparing well-justified proposals for consideration at the central level, which adds to the training, administrative effort, delays, and uncertainties. In addition, administrative procedures of donors may preclude funding small projects,[7] may earmark only certain activities, may impose specific procurement procedures, and create other obstacles. Thus though there is widespread agreement that decentralized project planning and implementation is ultimately required, a number of policy and procedural questions remain to be addressed before this can operate effectively.

Household-Level Information Strategies

The earlier chapters in this volume provide abundant evidence that the primary consideration in attempting to change household or individual behavior through nutrition eduction is whether the available government resources are sufficient to implement the strategy. Whether or not nutrition education includes growth monitoring, a well-trained, well-supervised, well-staffed cadre of change agents seems to be a prerequisite for success. Unfortunately, such a cadre does not usually exist, and thus much of what passes for nutrition education or growth monitoring is a poorly implemented form of those activities. Growth monitoring has too often been perceived as an inexpensive way around this constraint, with the result that poor nutrition education is now accompanied by scales and growth charts in many settings. This situation is unfortunate because growth monitoring does appear to hold potential advantages over nutrition education alone and has potential applications beyond nutrition education (e.g., screening, social mobilization, program management), as borne out in several successful community-based programs.

Because of the reality of inadequate human resources to cover the entire at-risk population, one of the biggest advantages of growth monitoring is its ability to identify the individuals at highest risk for severe malnutrition or its consequences, who should then receive intensive education and attention from a health worker. This screening function, which is conceptually distinct from the educative one, should be emphasized in all growth-monitoring programs and steps taken to enable follow-up with the high-risk children. This procedure is simpler in community-based programs that allow health workers to make home visits at some later time. In clinic-based programs, however, follow-up education must occur dur-

---

[7] Proposals from several districts, however, might be aggregated into a package suitable for funding by large donors.

ing the same session (i.e., same day) as growth monitoring to minimize the burden on mothers. If this cannot be accomplished by rearranging clinic schedules, staff responsibilities, and other constraints, serious consideration should be given to discontinuing growth monitoring in favor of other uses of staff time. Creative solutions may be found, however, as in the use of clinic-based volunteers (peers of the mothers drawn from the communities around the clinics) who could be trained by clinic staff to conduct the education or, conversely, to do the weighing (screening) and leave the high-quality education to the clinic staff. The first step, however, is for program managers and administrators to recognize the problems with growth monitoring and resolve either to correct them or to drop growth monitoring altogether.

The problem with using growth monitoring for screening purposes is, of course, that nutrition education is directed solely or primarily to mothers of malnourished children, in contrast to a preventive approach that would seek to intervene before malnutrition occurs. Nonetheless, until the means can be found to overcome the human resource constraint, it would be preferable to concentrate resources on the most needy rather than pretending that the preventive strategy is working. This is, in fact, what several of the successful community-based programs have done (Chapters 4 and 5). There may well be creative ways to overcome the human resource constraint in clinic- and community-based programs, but there may not be sufficient recognition of the problem and commitment to address it. Now that the mechanics of weighing and plotting have been implemented in many settings, it may be time to launch a growth-monitoring improvement program with all of the advocacy and promise that accompanied the original implementation of growth monitoring, but this time with more attention to solving some of the fundamental operational constraints. This would also encourage emerging community-based programs to pay attention to these operational details and avoid some of the failures of the past.

Although most of the discussion concerning nutrition education focuses on the mother and child as the objects of that education, it is clear from the chapters in this volume that the perspective should be broadened to include other caretakers (siblings, grandmothers, community caretakers), other influential household members (fathers, uncles), and more than simply the proximate determinants of child malnutrition. The importance of such issues as alcoholism, male control of income, and impacts of technological change is becoming increasingly apparent, and these are areas in which programming lags well behind knowledge. One of the many challenges ahead is to find ways to reach these other audiences and address the broader issues through strategies at the national, community, and household levels.

Concluding Remarks

The preceding sections present, in the aggregate, an extremely ambitious set of activities to strengthen the use of information to improve nutrition, so much so that it is beyond the realm of possibility of any country to implement them all. But it is not the intent of this chapter to suggest that they should all be implemented. Instead, the purpose has been to provide a more complete model of the types of information and information processes required for effective actions to improve the household food and nutrition situation in developing countries (Figure 16.1), whether those actions are at the national, community, or household levels. The administrative levels, institutions and information requiring most urgent attention must be decided at the country level based on preexisting conditions, the nature of nutrition-related actions at present, and a host of other considerations. The present chapter is only an attempt to assist the process of rationalizing which areas might require strengthening.

One of the important conclusions is that the types of data, data collection, and data analysis required at household, community, and national levels are different. If nothing else, this may help to dispel the notion that a food and nutrition information system can be based solely or largely on the regular collection and processing of simple indicators of food or nutritional status. This may be the starting point or a component of many systems, but the perspective presented here emphasizes the inadequacy of this information alone. To complete the link between problem identification and nutritional improvement, attention must be given to a variety of implementation issues, many of which imply a role for information.

Another conclusion is that, given the diversity of information types and institutions required for their collection, analysis, and interpretation at the national level, it would be unwise or impossible to try to integrate these too tightly in a bureaucratic sense. The case of Chile cited earlier provides an object lesson in the futility and counterproductive nature of such an effort. This is a major departure from the lessons from developing timely warning systems, in which a premium is placed on tight bureaucratic linkages (Brooks et al., 1985; Muhloff, 1990). Instead, attention should be given to ensure that the information from varied sources is integrated by one or more focal institutions but that the collection, analysis, and access to data and information be designed to discourage its monopolization by a few individuals or institutions.

Although the focus of this chapter is on the generation of information and the development of multiple channels for its dissemination and use, it bears emphasizing that the information should include or be closely followed by recommendations for action whenever feasible. The practice of producing reports that lack an action orientation is far too common, especially at the national level, and assumes that someone else will see the relevance of the information and follow through in an appropriate fashion. When there are strong disincentives to taking initiative, as in most bureaucracies, such reports simply encourage inaction. Thus the goal should be to provide not only the empirical and analytical basis for conclusions but also a set of action-oriented recommendations (expressed as options when possible) with a demonstrable link to the analysis.

Finally, it is apparent that the biggest single need is for training and institution building. This includes graduate training at the national level in areas related to food and nutrition policy and programs, at the subnational levels in community planning-related fields, and at the community level to strengthen cadres of health workers and supervisors in light of recent experience with community-based nutrition programs. This is clearly a massive and long-term undertaking, but it has the highest long-term benefits for nutrition and national development in general.

17

Enhancing Child Growth and Nutrition: Lessons for Action

Per Pinstrup-Andersen, David Pelletier, and Harold Alderman

Despite any progress that has been made in ensuring adequate growth and nutrition for preschool children, no intervention can claim to have had sufficient success to have relegated malnutrition to a historical footnote. Therefore, the search for innovations that will improve programs continues. At times, the frustration with the rate of progress also encourages the setting up of dichotomies in which an innovation is defined as much by how it differs from others as it is as an underlying model of effective intervention. In organizing this volume, we have indirectly encouraged this process, not only by including a diverse set of specialists but by placing a particular emphasis on the flow of information and on process as opposed to technology and materials. This theme is developed by several authors in discussing community participation.

This chapter develops some variations on that theme, with an emphasis on identifying how external agencies, including government agencies, can most effectively assist in reaching nutritional goals. In an effort to avoid defining this approach mainly in terms of what it is not, we seek to establish the role of community participation as a common element in an array of interventions. In so doing, we build upon the experience of programs reviewed here which are conceptualized in frameworks distinct from—but not necessarily antithetical to—participatory approaches.

For example, although there is a temptation to define community participation by distinguishing it from top-down projects, we endeavor to indicate how resources external to the community are essential ingredients in such programs. Similarly, the distinction between participatory and

335

technological solutions—the latter often derided as magic bullets by advocates of community approaches—may be unnecessary because improvements in delivery systems often are key features of technological innovations. This, in turn, implies that an understanding of individual and household as well as community behavior is an element of both broad categories of nutrition interventions.

Individual and Household Behavior

Available evidence strongly supports our belief that household members behave rationally, given their goals and preferences, relative power, and the constraints (particularly resource, time, information, and cultural constraints) within which they make decisions. On this premise, there are three entry points for nutrition intervention in households with malnourished members: (1) changing the goals and preferences of the malnourished individual or his or her guardian, (2) altering the relative power of malnourished individuals within the households, and (3) alleviating existing constraints.

Nutrition education has traditionally aimed at changing goals and preferences. The evidence presented in Chapters 3, 4, and 5, however, indicates that the alleviation of existing information constraints is more likely to result in nutritional improvements. The difference between attempting to change preferences and attempting to enhance household access to relevant information is not subtle. It is based on different assumptions regarding household rationality and has important implications for the design and implementation of nutrition education programs.

Traditionally, nutrition education has been prescriptive rather than participatory. The prescriptive approach, which is based on the medical model of compliance by the patient, has not been successful in nutrition education. The participatory approaches implemented in recent years, particularly the social marketing approach, have been more successful. Their success is based on an understanding of past and current behavior and emphasis on the transfer of information relevant to the circumstances of the target households, rather than general prescriptions.

Even the participatory approaches, however, have been limited by resource and time constraints in the target households and lack of power by high-risk household members.

Changes in household behavior are contingent on household resources. Similarly, attempts to improve nutrition through transfer of resources, such as food or monetary income, to the household are usually more successful if accompanied by nutrition education and information. Although there is now strong empirical evidence supporting the presence of these complementarities, they often remain ignored or overlooked in the design and implementation of interventions.

As discussed in Chapter 9, complementarity between and among individual interventions is not limited to nutrition education and household resources. Substitution between individual interventions is also common. While complementarity implies that the presence of one intervention or factor enhances the effect of another, substitution refers to a situation in which one intervention or factor may fully or partially substitute for another. The presence or absence of complementarities and substitution is critical for the design and implementation of interventions. Lack of measurable effect of single interventions, such as food supplementation, access to improved drinking water, nutrition education, and improved sanitary conditions, is largely a result of failure to deal explicitly with complementarities and substitution in design and implementation. For example, as pointed out in Chapter 9, if several effective pathways for pathogen exposure exist, interventions to block one may have scant effect on infectious diseases and thus nutrition. Efforts to provide clean drinking water in a situation of very poor sanitary conditions illustrate the point. Other illustrations can be seen in the effectiveness of formal versus nutrition education, household versus community constraints, and quantity versus quality of water available.

Two important lessons for the design and implementation of nutrition interventions result from the above. First, sufficient knowledge about the intended beneficiaries to identify factors likely to interact with and affect interventions is essential; and second, in most cases, single interventions are unlikely to be effective.

Having dealt with the first entry point for influencing nutrition through changes in household behavior, let us move to the second: altering the relative power of the malnourished individual within the household. The most serious nutrition risks are generally found in children younger than three years and in pregnant and lactating women. In low-income households of most developing countries, these individuals possess little power or control over household resources and their allocation among household members. Thus, though the assumption of rationality implies that each household member pursues his or her goals in the most efficient manner, the relative power of the individual together with the extent to which the welfare of others coincides with his or her goals will influence the allocation of household resources.

Child care, including child nutrition, has traditionally been the responsibility of the mother. Thus, relative to fathers, mothers may place a higher priority on the well-being of the child and allocate resources accordingly.

Although existing evidence is not consistent, several studies have confirmed that women allocate a larger share of household resources on goods and services important to child health and nutrition. As further discussed in Chapters 3, 6, and 7, efforts to enhance women's status, education, income, and access to technology and productive resources are likely to strengthen their relative power over household resources. This, in turn, would be expected to result in a higher household priority on the nutritional status of women and children. Another obvious, though less-studied, strategy is to better understand which information, education, and participatory methods may help redirect some of the resources they control toward improved nutrition for women and children.

The third entry point to nutrition improvement is through changes in household resource constraints, that is, by changing the availability of income and other material resources, time, and knowledge. Knowledge constraints were discussed above. Time constraints, particularly those of women, are critical for the design and implementation of interventions. The time women need to spend to participate in and derive benefits from intervention programs is not a free good. The more time needed for participation in a program, the less time is available for child care, food preparation, agricultural work, and other income-generating activities. Reduced time spent on these activities may result in negative nutrition effects that partially or totally outweigh potential positive effects from the intervention. In spite of a large body of evidence showing that women in low-income households generally are faced with serious time constraints, the design of interventions in primary health care, food, and nutrition often fails to address this shortcoming. The opportunity cost of such time—in income or nutrition forgone—is a user fee just the same as monetary user fees. If these fees are high, the service becomes prohibitively expensive.

The importance of material resource constraints—or poverty—in efforts to improve nutrition is widely recognized and needs no justification here. Malnutrition is strongly correlated with poverty, but increased household incomes alone, although usually necessary, may be insufficient to alleviate malnutrition in the short run. Household food consumption is likely to increase, but knowledge about nutrition and the prevalence and severity of infectious diseases may not be affected. Thus complementarities may prohibit nutrition effects. A large body of empirical evidence from recent research supports this notion. Increased income, whether from expanded commercialization of small-scale agriculture, wage employment, or food-related transfers, generally shows little or no significant effect on nutritional status in the short run unless accompanied by interventions to reduce infectious diseases or increase knowledge about nutrition. In the short run, the principal nutrition effect of increased income operates through enhanced food consumption and, if accessible, increased use of health care. In the longer run, households earning higher incomes will demand improvements in health care, sanitary conditions, access to water, and education. Meeting these demands may require community action, such as provision of water and sanitation, and enhanced supply of primary health care by the public or private sector. Thus, although the short-run nutrition effects are often disappointing, alleviating poverty will eventually alleviate malnutrition. Integrating efforts to alleviate household-level resource constraints with efforts to reduce infectious diseases and increase nutrition knowledge will usually result in strong positive nutrition effects both in the short and long run.

Policy-Level Interventions

National policies play a major role in a community-based approach to the alleviation of malnutrition. They influence nutritional status irrespective of community action. Policies affecting food or nonfood prices, wage rates, employment, transfers, and health care affect nutrition (positively or negatively) without the need for community action. Such effects may be strong. Therefore, although the focus of efforts to alleviate nutrition may be on the community, it is critical to consider explicit expected nutrition effects in the design and implementation of these broader policies and to seek to improve nutrition through these policies to the extent feasible.

The nutrition effects of national policies vary across countries and among population groups within a given country. Some policies, however, have shown a strong, consistently positive effect. Although the policy choice for a particular country and time period should be based on appropriate economic analyses of costs and benefits, policies that have shown a consistently positive effect across communities and countries deserve particular attention.

Breastfeeding is a basic component of a strategy to reduce infant mortality and malnutrition, particularly in environments of poor sanitation. Thus national or regional breastfeeding promotion programs, proven successful in some countries, should have high priority where recommended breastfeeding practices are not extensively followed. The protection and support of breastfeeding are important in all settings. Three sources of nutritional risks associated with breastfeeding—nonexclusive breastfeeding for the first six months, inappropriate feeding during weaning, and conflicts with the mother's employment and income-earning opportunities—should be explicitly addressed in such programs. Inappropriate breastfeeding and weaning practices are critically important in most cases of malnutrition among children younger than two years of age. Thus national support to facilitate improved weaning practices is likely to be needed generally. As further discussed in Chapter 11, nutrition education to promote improved child feeding through appropriate weaning foods has been successful in enhancing child growth. To be successful, however, the nature of national support may need to vary across communities. A prepackaged national program is not likely to be effective across communities.

Short birth intervals, high parity, young maternal age, and large family sizes all contribute significantly to existing malnutrition in preschool children and women in most developing countries (Chapter 10). Thus effective family planning programs are likely to contribute to improved health and nutrition. Because of their demonstrated effect on health and nutrition, such programs should be promoted even where reduced population growth is not a goal.

As discussed in several chapters, formal education of women has been demonstrated to have a positive effect on nutrition in many countries, although the causal relationships between improved formal education and the nutritional status of children are not fully understood (Chapter 3). The magnitude of the effect will vary across households and communities, but the probability of a significant and positive effect is high in most cases. Furthermore, nutrition improvements brought about by enhanced formal education of women are more likely to be self-sustaining than most other interventions. Thus positive nutrition effects are one of many reasons for the promotion of formal education of low-income women.

Access to primary health care services is of paramount importance in efforts to alleviate malnutrition. Their effect on the prevalence and severity of infectious diseases is particularly important. As discussed in Chapter 8, however, health interventions, such as oral rehydration services and immunizations, can reduce child mortality although morbidity and malnutrition remain high. Indeed, the worldwide downward trend in child mortality even in countries with economic stagnation and rudimentary nutrition programs provides a major impetus for technology-oriented approaches to nutritional interventions (van der Gaag et al., 1991). Health services are usually necessary but not sufficient to alleviate malnutrition. Their effect on nutrition may be negligible in the absence of other interventions. Furthermore, the nature of appropriate services may vary across communities and should be tailored to the needs and opportunities of the target community.

In view of the strong causal relationship between poverty and malnutrition, policies and programs to enhance low-income households' access to resources are likely to reduce nutritional risks. Transfer programs such as food supplementation, food price subsidies, food stamp programs, poverty relief programs, and unemployment compensation may be effective in the short run, but they usually do not result in self-sustaining improvements in households' access to resources. Therefore, though these interventions may be needed for short-term relief, policies and programs to strengthen the income-generating capabilities of the poor, including employment generation, education and skill development, enhanced access to productive resources, and technological change to increase labor productivity, are needed to ensure long-term, self-sustaining alleviation of poverty and malnutrition.

The nutrition effects of policies to maintain low prices for food and other basic necessities such as housing and transportation are equivocal. While the immediate effects on the purchasing power of low-income households who are net buyers is positive, the effect on those who derive their income from production and distribution of these goods will be negative. Furthermore, in the longer run, artificially low prices to producers will reduce production and create shortages of the particular commodities. The negative effects on the poor in production and distribution as well as the adverse effect on production may be alleviated by explicit government subsidies that allow decreases in consumer prices without corresponding decreases in producer prices. Maintaining such subsidies, however, may result in unsustainable fiscal costs unless the subsidies are effectively targeted to the poor and malnourished.

Policies and programs to reduce costs of production and distribution per unit of food, such as technological change in agriculture, improved rural infrastructure, and related investments, offer great potential for enhancing real incomes of low-income food consumers without adversely affecting low-income producers.

Agricultural policies are of particular interest in efforts to alleviate malnutrition for two principal reasons. First, in most low-income countries, the majority of the malnourished reside in rural areas and many depend directly or indirectly on agriculture for their income and food security. Therefore, policies that affect costs and revenues in the agricultural sector are likely to affect the incomes of the poor. Second, food occupies a large share of the total household budget among poor and malnourished consumers. Thus agricultural policies that affect food prices will affect the ability of poor consumers to meet their energy and nutrient requirements. As further discussed in Chapter 12, agricultural policies and programs may also affect nutrition through changes in the demand for time of members of low-income rural households; energy expenditures; and, in the case of irrigation and water management, infectious diseases.

Community Action

National policies and programs influence the socioeconomic environment within which households act. Even the most favorable policies, however, cannot hope to eliminate malnutrition completely. The need for further action, the nature of such action, and the resulting effect on nutrition depend on the existing socioeconomic environment. Moreover, the success of policies depends on implementation at local levels. Thus the interaction between national policies and more localized programs is an important consideration in the planning of both.

Communities can play an important role in diagnosing and finding solutions to their nutrition-related problems. They can provide location-specific information to be considered in the design and implementation of feasible and cost-effective interventions. Community participation in primary health care and nutrition has been promoted since the Alma Ata Declaration but with limited success. Most nutrition interventions continue to be based on the traditional top-down model. Interventions are designed outside the community, and only by chance does an intervention offered to a community match the existing problems, constraints, and opportunities for their alleviation. Community participation, where it exists, is usually limited to assisting outside project officers in the implementation of the predesigned interventions to ensure compliance.

Several recent nutrition programs are an important exception to this generally sad state of affairs. These programs, some of which are briefly described in the Appendix, provide a more enlightened approach. Most of them benefit from community participation in the design and implementation of the interventions. Rather than a prepackaged intervention, the content of the programs is tailored to the intended beneficiaries. As a consequence, the content varies among programs. The process also varies but less than the content. Community meetings, focus group meetings, household surveys, and other media generate the information and enthusiasm for community action. Community-based growth monitoring offers great promise as a lead activity to identify children with poor growth and to stimulate mothers and communities into action. Growth monitoring is a source of information which, in addition to providing an indication to the mother of a health and nutrition problem, may be successfully used as a rallying point for community action. In itself, however, growth monitoring is unlikely to influence nutrition. To have an effect, it must result in corrective measures suited for the causes of the problem. Some such measures can be taken by the household with or without external support, while others can be taken only by the community.

As further discussed in Chapters 4 and 5, attempts to link growth monitoring exclusively to prescriptive nutrition education have generally not been successful and should be discontinued. Growth monitoring should instead be linked closely with a household and community-level assessment of the causes of growth failure and opportunities for their alleviation (UNICEF, 1992a; Anonymous 1, 1989; Anonymous 2, 1989). Such opportunities may include nutrition education, but it is equally likely that a transfer of resources, such as food or health care services, or community-level improvements in water and sanitation may be needed.

Although the volume offers evidence on successful nutrition projects that employ community participation, a reader who recalls the enthusiasm generated by past community-based development approaches such as Comilla and Sarvodaya may be justified in having some reservations when Iringa and Grameen are proposed as models. What obstacles, then, can be anticipated in realizing the potential of participatory approaches?

One reason real community action in health and nutrition interventions has been so limited is the general lack of community organization within which nutrition interventions can operate. Lack of homogeneity makes organization more difficult. Resource ownership, income levels, nutritional status, and general standards of living may vary significantly among households, and local power structures may not favor nutrition improvements over other action. Furthermore, if community empowerment and organization serve to strengthen the existing power structure, nutrition may not benefit. But if they threaten the existing power structure, they will be resisted. Thus, as in the case of the design and implementation of nutrition interventions, efforts to strengthen community mobilization and action should pay attention to the existing community structure.

Thus national and regional (e.g., district-level) programs are needed to support community action. Such support should assist communities in developing and implementing appropriate intervention strategies, including the articulation of demand for external support. In addition, national and regional support should be able to respond effectively and efficiently to the expressed needs and demands of the communities in an effective and timely manner. Where national support has traditionally been based on the transfer of prepackaged interventions, innovative institutional and attitudinal changes are likely to be needed to accommodate the new approach.

A long time frame is often required to nurture participation by the beneficiaries of projects. It is often quicker to build structures and to staff them from outside than to nurture the trust and communication required for community-based projects. Guidelines for vertical program design are easier to formulate than guidelines for a process that by its very nature is experimental and has changing goals. Institutional incentives, then, have often encouraged approaches that could be more rapidly implemented from above, even at the cost of sustainability.

Recently, however, a number of agencies have begun to see the long-run advantages of fostering community participation. It is described, for example, as a major component of the World Bank's strategy for poverty alleviation (World Bank, 1992, chap. 6) and is a central theme in UNICEF's nutrition strategy (UNICEF, 1989b). This, of course, points to a major irony. Must community participation be confined to local organizations and perhaps some NGOs, or can national or international agencies and outside researchers complement the process? The growing body of experience, some of which is reviewed in this volume, provides some guidelines for this interaction.

Lessons for the Design and Implementation of Government Action

The previous chapters present clear evidence of the importance of location-specificity in nutrition problems and their solutions. The nature and determinants of child nutrition, as well as the constraints to adequate nutrition and the opportunities for their removal, vary among households, communities, and countries, and so must approaches for sustainable nutrition improvement. Most successful nutrition interventions are tailored to the specific circumstances of the target households and individuals. These interventions frequently include supply-oriented, technology-based components. But these components are carefully chosen and integrated in the intervention strategy for a particular community or group of households. Efforts to alleviate child malnutrition across countries or across all high-risk household groups within a given country by means of a prepackaged general solution have failed in the past and will fail if tried again. Because of the high degree of location-specificity, the content of the interventions is seldom generalizable across communities. The process, however, appears to be more generalizable.

In the successful interventions reviewed for this book, the process began with a solid understanding of the nutrition problem at the community level, the causes of the problem, and the opportunities and feasibility of potential solutions. In most cases, the intended beneficiaries played a major role in the generation of the necessary information. Where they did not, agencies external to the target community placed high priority from the outset on obtaining such information. Past experience has shown that a high degree of participation by intended beneficiaries in problem diagnosis, and the design and implementation of interventions greatly enhances the probability of access.

Ideally, at-risk households—as a group or community—should identify the problems, the potential and acceptable solutions, and the nature of external assistance needed. The latter is particularly important; solutions to nutrition problems usually require outside resources. The argument that the community can solve its own nutrition problems without additional resources is usually false.

On the other hand, traditional nutrition interventions based on the assumption that specialized agencies external to the community are better equipped than the community of intended beneficiaries to design the content of the interventions run the risk of promoting inappropriate technologies or addressing secondary problems. Instead of prepackaged interventions for widespread application, external agencies, such as government agencies, should offer an array or menu of intervention components from which each community could choose. The most important of these components were discussed in the previous section of this chapter. A change from prepackaged interventions for widespread application to a menu of options will require stronger institutional, administrative, and logistical frameworks, particularly those related to the delivery of goods and services, including health care, food or food entitlements, and information. It will also require attitudinal changes at all levels.

Government agencies also should make available information about the technical and economic feasibility of various options, and they should provide technical assistance to communities to initiate and strengthen their capabilities to undertake the above process. In other words, government participation in community action might be more appropriate than community participation in action designed and implemented by external agencies.

Because action will be problem-oriented and at least partly designed by the intended beneficiaries, a participatory approach is likely to result in more sustainable improvements, a characteristic that is critical yet often missing in solution-focused approaches. Precisely because the latter approaches are focused on specific solutions and technologies in search of fitting problems, questions of replicability and scaling up tend to take priority over long-term sustainability of impact. Based on the experience to date, we believe that sustainability should take priority over many other considerations, including scaling up and replicability. For most countries, this would translate to many small-scale projects tailored to the population to be served, in contrast to scaling up and replication of a given package of interventions that are successful in other communities and countries.

Past research, evaluation, and experience from nutrition intervention and related action provide much information useful to facilitate the above approach. In particular, several recent successful community nutrition programs in various developing countries have enhanced our understanding of how to tackle nutrition problems effectively at the community and household levels. Although more such programs may be needed, the time has come to create a strong multiplier effect, not by replicating programs that were successful in one setting to new settings where they will fail but by sharing the lessons learned with communities everywhere, to design and implement their own solutions with external assistance tailored to the needs and opportunities.

Intervention implementation procedures established by government agencies outside the community have traditionally been rigid and difficult to change, accrued experience and information notwithstanding. Flexibility should be built into project design and implementation to permit adjustments suggested by location-specific information and experience gained during project implementation.

Through this process, care must be taken to ensure that projects designed to benefit the poorest—and often the least organized—communities are not captured by local nonpoor power blocs. Thus government does need to maintain a monitoring role. This may be done in conjunction with NGO groups, which, although often external to the community, have long-term and localized relationships with the intended program beneficiaries. The assumption that NGOs can be a catalyst and can assist the poor in voicing their needs may be tacit in many cases and requires case-by-case assessment.

Although a technology-based generalized approach is unlikely to be successful in alleviating malnutrition, modern technology can be an important component of a broader, tailored intervention. Identifying the appropriate components of an intervention program for a particular community, including the technology-based components, is critical for success.

Similarly, the policy environment is critical for the success of community-level efforts. The often ignored nutrition effects of government policies not explicitly aimed at nutrition may be very important indeed. Food price policies; employment, wage, and income policies; subsidy, tax, and other transfer policies; and agricultural policies are obvious examples. Many other macroeconomic and sectoral policies may affect nutrition through their effects on income, food security, time allocation, sanitary conditions, and behavior among low-income households. Individual communities usually have little or no influence on the design of such policies. But the effects will differ among communities and households and should be considered when designing community action. Furthermore, at the national level, expected nutrition effects of these broader policies should be explicitly considered. Attempts should be made to enhance positive and reduce negative nutrition effects at the time of policy design and implementation. Due consideration should be given to other policy goals and the cost of alternative solutions to the nutrition problems.

A change of intervention approach from government programs, with or without community participation, to community action with government participation can be successful only if based on the accumulated knowledge about the critical issues, much of which is synthesized in previous chapters. Some of the research and training we believe to be most critical for success are discussed below.

Needs for Action-Oriented Research and Training

Research needs identified for each of the topics treated in this book are presented in the appropriate chapters and will not be repeated here. This section will present only the most urgent needs for research and training in support of immediate action.

Applied research on the implementation of nutrition projects is urgently needed. Past and current project implementation efforts suffer from a lack of operationally useful and scientifically sound information about virtually all aspects of implementation. Household responses to various interventions and implementation approaches, and how compatibility between household desires and intervention approaches can be enhanced, must be determined through research. We still need to find ways to ensure sustainability in nutrition improvements. Research on nutrition-related community action, including community mobilization, empowerment, and organization; nutrition intervention; and articulation of needs for external support are urgently needed. The functioning of local power structures and how to deal with them in community-based nutrition action is poorly understood and requires applied research.

Similarly, political economy and institutional issues with direct bearing on the effectiveness of national and regional support of nutrition interventions are poorly understood. Research on these topics and on the nutritional effects of broader government policies of the types mentioned above are needed to guide institutional changes.

Much of the above research is expected to result in generalizable findings. In addition, there is a need to undertake monitoring and related operations-oriented research aimed at the improvement of specific projects.

This book discusses several successful nutrition intervention projects.

There are others that we know of, and there are probably still many other successful projects that we do not know of. These are probably small-scale, highly individualized projects sharply focused on solving well-defined problems in the target communities. Many are probably assisted by nongovernmental organizations, and many probably practice the approach we advocate. They are successful because they are tailored to the target community. Because they are small and are administered by highly dedicated individuals from within and outside the community who have little time, interest, or money for public relations, they are poorly known outside the community. These projects could provide important lessons for the design and implementation of small-scale projects elsewhere. Therefore, efforts should be made to identify some of these projects for monitoring and process and impact evaluation. It is important to stress that the purpose of such evaluation is to learn from these projects rather than to duplicate them in other locations.

Evaluation of the impact of nutrition interventions is necessary not only to assess the impact of a particular intervention and make the necessary modifications but also to learn how to design better interventions in the future. Yet, while process evaluations are common, impact evaluations are scarce, poorly done, and often inconclusive. Empirically tested, scientifically sound, and operationally feasible evaluation methods must be developed.

Training must be given priority in efforts to strengthen national and community capacity to solve nutrition problems. Proper training can assist intended beneficiaries and others in the target communities in diagnosing their nutrition problems, identifying the cases and feasible solutions, mobilizing community resources, articulating and seeking external support, and implementing feasible and sustainable solutions. Such training should be aimed at people living in the target community, including selected intended beneficiaries who may function as change agents, as well as relevant public sector employees such as community health and nutrition workers and agricultural extensionists. Training is also needed for public sector employees at the national and regional levels to facilitate community efforts and to design and implement external support programs that are responsive to the expressed demands of the communities. Such training should combine technical and sociological aspects with emphasis on changing attitudes among government officials from a top-down to a bottom-up approach. Finally, there is a need for training in the area of economic analysis of policies and programs with emphasis on their nutrition effects.

APPENDIX

Description of Community-Based
Health and Nutrition Projects

This appendix provides a brief overview of eight community-based health and nutrition projects discussed in this volume. These projects have been highlighted in most cases because of their successful implementation or positive impact on child nutritional status. Because so few successful experiences are available for analysis, several of the authors have examined these programs in an attempt to extract lessons for the future. Although a variety of details concerning these projects are described and analyzed in the relevant chapters, their more general characteristics have been included here to minimize repetition.

Integrated Child Development Scheme (ICDS), India

The ICDS is a national public health care program, started in 1975, implemented by Indian state governments, and assisted financially by the central government through the collaborative efforts of the ministries of Social Welfare, Human Resources, Child Development, Rural Development and Health. In addition, a portion of food supplements in the project are provided by CARE and WFP. The goal of ICDS is to improve nutrition and health services to children under six years (known as undersixes) and to pregnant and lactating women (PLW). Its overall stated objectives are

The material in this appendix is drawn from earlier drafts of the chapters written by Maria Teresa Cerqueira and Christine Olson, Marie Ruel, David Pelletier, and Roger Shrimpton and from the sources cited by those authors. Their implicit contributions to this appendix are gratefully acknowledged, as is the assistance of Karen Isakson in compiling this information.

Table A-1. India/Integrated Child Development Scheme (ICDS) (initiated in 1975)

Program size and target groups

Program size (Target population)		Targeting methodology	
1975	1.5 mil. <6y & PLW	*Geographic*	Entire blocks according to socioeconomic and anthropometric criteria
1986	32 mil.	*Group*	<6y & PLW
1989	36 mil. (28 mil. <6y, 6.6 mil. PLW)	*Individual*	Malnourished <6y & PLW

Information and evaluation features

Management information system		Evaluation methodology	
Info reported	Service delivered—Yes GM data—Yes Morbidity/mortality—Yes	*Data Sources*	GM, annual health/nutrition surveys
Freq. of reports	Monthly	*Design*	Pre-post comparison— Yes
Levels reported to	Central		Comparison groups— Yes
Downward feedback	Quarterly program reports printed for feedback to states, districts, and blocks		Control for confounders—Yes (drought) Statistical tests—Yes
Local Use	Screening, NED, referrals	*Nutritional Indicators*	W/A, AC of preschoolers

Program effectiveness and cost

Physical growth	Total budget cost	Annual cost per capita	Funding sources
1976 low W/A (<70%) 42%	1988–89 US $100 mil	Not available	*National* 93.5%
1980 37%			*External* 6.5% total
1982 17%			UNICEF 3.5%
1984–88 Severe malnutrition down by 37% in drought-free vs. 5% in drought-affected areas			Bilateral aid (mostly USAID) 3%
			Suppl. food costs 45% covered by states, 40% by CARE, 15% by WFP

Source: Subbarao (1989).

to enhance mothers' capabilities to provide good physical and psycho-social child development and to reduce the prevalence of malnutrition, morbidity, and mortality. Interventions for undersixes include growth monitoring two to four times annually, medical checkups and referrals, oral rehydration therapy, immunizations, nutrition education (NED), and informal preschool education. PLW receive prenatal and postnatal care, iron and folate supplementation, and food supplements if malnourished. Services are targeted according to socioeconomic and anthropometric criteria. The program has grown from a targeted coverage of 1.5 million children under six in 1975 to 36 million in 1989 (28 million undersixes and 6.6 million PLW). In 1976, 42 percent of children were less than 70 percent of normal weight for age (W/A); by 1982, this number had decreased to 17 percent. Between 42 and 63 percent of undersixes have growth charts in program areas.

Program staffing corresponds to the pyramidal structure of the Indian government. The central ICDS management team consists of twenty officers, each state has an ICDS director and two to four officers, and districts have program officer training teams. At the block level, there is one health supervisor for six multipurpose health workers (MPHWs). These supervisors receive three months' training in management and supervisory skills at state training centers. At the community level, there is one MPHW per 5,000 population, two community health workers (CHWs) per community, and one ICDS field supervisor per 17 to 20 CHWs. CHWs receive three months' preservice training at district training centers and one week continuing education every two years. The project cost $100 million in 1988–89. The Indian national government covered 93.5 percent, and UNICEF and bilateral aid sources covered the remaining 6.5 percent. State governments covered 45 percent of food supplement costs, and CARE and WFP covered the remaining 55 percent.

Tamil Nadu Integrated Nutrition Program (TINP), India

TINP was initiated in 1980 as a joint venture by the Tamil Nadu state government and the World Bank as an attempt to create a replicable model of an integrated nutrition intervention program. It was implemented by the state government in coordination with existing national PHC programs like ICDS. The program strives to achieve universal coverage of basic health and nutrition services for children and pregnant and lactating women in a low-income rural region in south India, as well as intensive short-term supplementary feeding for strictly targeted subgroups. It is conceived and organized largely as a vertical program, al-

Table A-2. India/Tamil Nadu Integrated Nutrition Program (TINP) (initiated in 1980)

Program size and target groups

Program size (Target population)		Targeting methodology	
1989	1.1 mil 6-36m, 280,000 PLWs	*Geographic*	Low-income, rural communities
		Group	GM of 6-36m
		Individual	Underweights

Information and evaluation features

Management information system		Evaluation methodology	
Info reported	Service deliv/GM/morbid/mortal data from 30 village registers converted to 27 indicators in 15 monthly reports	*Data sources*	GM, morbidity/mortality info/registers in program areas, nutritional surveillance info in nonprogram areas, several cross-sectoral surveys 1980–86
Freq. of reports	Monthly, quarterly, half-yearly	*Design*	Pre-post comparison—Yes
Levels reported to	Multiple levels		Comparison groups—Yes (staggered design)
Downward feedback	Corrective action initiated by central office via several feedback loops to villages. Project newsletter.		Control for confounders—No
Local use	Village results displayed in office; individual screening, NED, referrals	*Nutritional indicators*	Statistical tests—No W/A of <5y

Table A-2 (continued)

	Program effectiveness and cost			
Physical growth	Total budget cost	Annual cost per capita		Funding sources
WA <70%	1980/89 $100 mil	*Per capita* $0.81	*National*	$55.7 mil (incl
1980 19% (control area 17%)	1984 $8,475,000 (29% food)	*Per beneficiary* $9.41		$16.6 for food suppl)
1984 13% (control area 17%)		*With suppl feeding* $20.00	*External*	$44.3 mil
1986 10% (control area 20%)				
Results from staggered implementation				
Phase I 55% less severe maln of 6-36m over 72 mos.				
Phase II 24% less over 48 mos.				
Phase III 35% less over 38 mos.				
1982–83 Severe maln declined from 19.3% to 12.6%, compared with increases (25.3% to 30%) in non-program communities. Signs of clinical maln reduced from 21.4 to 3.4%. Biologically signif impact occurred from 1st to 5th year.				

Sources: Berg (1987b) and Shekar (1989).

though a substantial effort was made to include information from earlier research in Tamil Nadu, local insights into nutrition problems, and experience from outside India in the detailed planning of the program. Maternal and child health (MCH) services are provided by community nutrition workers, ayahs, and MPHWs operating out of one community nutrition center per 1,500 people. For 6- to 36-month-olds, services include medical referrals, immunizations, ORT, health and NED, vitamin A injections, and deworming. Underweight children receive home visits and 90-day supplementary feeding. Pregnant and lactating women receive iron and folate supplements, tetanus toxoid, food supplements if malnourished, health referrals, and assistance in organizing women's working groups (WWG) for income-generating activities (IGA) and health and NED. In 1989, the program's coverage was a population base of 17 million in nine districts, which reached 1.1 million 6- to 36-month-olds and 280,000 PLW. From 1980 to 1986, severe malnutrition (defined as less than 70 percent of normal W/A) in program areas was seen to decrease from 19 percent to 7 to 10 percent compared with control areas, where the rate remained at 17 percent or higher.

The staffing at local level consists of one community nutrition worker (CNW) per 1,500 population (four to five villages, estimate one per 100 children), one MPHW per 5,000 population, and one ayah per community. Local-level staff are supervised by program staff, one per ten CNWs, in twice-monthly visits. CNW training consists of two months at block headquarters with the last ten days on site together with MPHWs. Training emphasizes management, administration, communication skills, growth monitoring and promotion (GMP), nutrition education, and record-keeping. Continuing education is provided by community nutrition instructors (themselves trained for two months at the College of Home Science), operating out of block-level offices. District teams also provided bimonthly in-service continuing education. Designed on a large scale, the program attempts to include cost-saving measures to demonstrate sustainability options for other regions. Total program costs came to $100 million over the period from 1980 to 1989. The World Bank provided $44.3 million of the total costs, while $55.7 million (including $16.6 million for food supplements) was provided by the Indian state government. Per capita annual costs were $0.81, or $9.42 per beneficiary.

National Family Nutrition Program (UPGK), Indonesia

The UPGK national program in Indonesia, reoriented since 1978 to an integrated approach, is implemented by the Ministry of Health–Nutrition

Table A-3. Indonesia/National Nutrition Program (UPKG) (initiated in 1980)

Program size and target groups

Program size (target population)	Targeting methodology	
1985 6 mil <5y	Geographic	27 provinces with highest IMR, rural poor areas and urban slums with functioning health centers
1988 25.5 mil <5y	Group	<5y, PLW, children 6–14y
	Individual	Moderate/severe maln children and failure to grow

Information and evaluation features

Management information system	Evaluation methodology	
Info reported	Service deliv—Yes	Data sources	GM, surveys
	GM data—Yes from CNW reports	Design	Pre-post comparison— Yes (in some provinces only)
	Morbid/Mortal—Unclear		Comparison groups—Yes
Freq. of reports	Monthly/CNWs, analyzed quarterly		Control for confounders—Unclear
Levels reported to	Health care and multiple levels		Statistical tests— Unclear
Downward feedback	Yes in a quarterly evaluation, also lateral via MOH nutr. info network	Nutritional indicators	W/A
Local use	In some cases, monthly weighing info displayed at village weighing posts; screening, NED, referrals		

Program effectiveness and cost

Physical growth	Total budget cost	Annual cost per capita	Funding sources	
1978 maln/<5y nationally 14.1% 1986 maln/<5y 12.8%; 25% <5y (6.2 mil) showed consistent weight gain. Avg. weight for comparison children fell <WNL at 13 mos (for program children never dropped). By end of weaning, 40% of program children better nourished than nonprogram children. Growth curve of NED children flattened after 7 mos (control at 5 mos.)	1989 $35.2 mil, excl research and development funds (USAID)	$2 per capita	*National* *World Bank*	30% ($11 mil) 70% ($24.2 mil)

Sources: Priyosusilo (1988), Rohde and Hendrata (1983), Zinn and Drake (1988).

Directorate, with technical assistance from Manoff International Incorporation and the World Bank. The primary focus of the program is education. Services for children under five include monthly growth monitoring, immunizations, vitamin A supplementation, food coupons if moderately or severely malnourished, ORT, medical referrals, and NED. PLW receive iron, NED, food supplementation demonstrations, medical referrals for illness, and education regarding home vegetable gardens. Provinces with the highest infant mortality rates—and with functioning health centers—were targeted, whether rural poor or urban slums. In 1987, the targeted population was 6 million children under five. By 1988, that number had risen to 25.5 million children, with an estimated 47 percent of all children being weighed monthly. Nationally in 1978, 14.1 percent of children under five were considered malnourished. In 1986, the number of malnourished children had dropped to 12.8 percent, and 40 percent of program children were noted to be better nourished than nonprogram children. While the average weight for comparison children consistently fell below normal at 13 months, it almost never dropped in program children.

In the operation of UPGK, communities select one volunteer community health worker per 100 children to carry out the project activities. They are given preservice GMP training for three to five days. Technical supervision and ongoing continuing education are provided monthly by government health center staff, ideally one per 10 CHWs, but ranging from 18 to 320 CHWs. Total project costs in 1989 came to $35.2 million, of which 30 percent was covered by the national government and 70 percent by external sources. Annual costs per capita were estimated at $2, or $11 to $12 per child.

National Nutrition and Primary Health Care Program (NPHC), Thailand

The NPHC program in Thailand began in 1982 as an integrated program implemented and financially supported by the government ministries of Health, Agriculture and Cooperatives, Education and Interior, with 6 percent external funds. Its objectives are to assist both the rural and urban poor to recognize their nutritional problems and begin problem-solving interventions. Interventions to reach these goals include establishment of child care centers with ORT, medical referrals, immunizations, parasite control, health/NED, and community and school training in nutrition and food production. Children under five receive growth monitoring four times annually and vitamin A supplementation. Moderate and severely

Table A-4. Thailand/National Nutrition and Primary Health Care Program (NPHC) (initiated in 1982)

Program size and target groups

Program size (Target population)		Targeting methodology	
		Geographic	Rural areas and urban slums
1985	1.5 mil <5y	*Group*	<5y, PLW and 6-14y
1989	2.5 mil <5y		

Information and evaluation features

Management information system		Evaluation methodology	
		Data sources	GM
Info reported	Service deliv—Unclear	*Design*	Pre-post comparison—Yes
	GM data—Yes		countrywide
	Morbid/mortal— Unclear		Comparison groups— Yes
Freq. of reports	quarterly		Control for confounders—No
Levels reported to	Health center and multiple upper levels,		Statistical tests— No
	incl MOH Nutr Surveillance Unit	*Nutritional indicators*	W/A of preschoolers
Downward feedback	Village reps sent to decision makers for action,		
	prog adjust and feedback; minimal use		
Local use	Screening, NED, referrals		

Table A-4. (continued)

Program effectiveness and cost

Physical growth	Total budget cost	Annual cost per capita	Funding sources
1983 Severe maln <5y 2%, mod 13%, mild 36%	1972–76 National Nutrition and PHC budget: $350,000	No data available	*National* 1982–86—76% ($10 mil) 1987–91—94% ($14 mil)
1988 Severe maln 0.04%, mod 2%, mild 20% (down 80% since 1980). In this time period, Thailand experienced considerable socioeconomic development including advances in education and health; therefore unsure which activities are responsible for improved nutritional status.	1982–86 $13.1 mil 1987–91 $14.93 mil		*External* 1982–86 24% total UNICEF 15% USAID 9% 1987–91 6% total UNICEF 5.5% USAID 0.5%

Sources: Teller (1986a, 1986b) and Zerfas (1986).

malnourished children receive monthly GM and food supplementation for 90 days, with referral to a health center if recuperation fails in that time. PLW receive prenatal and postnatal care, including food, iron, and iodine supplementation. The program targeted a population of 1.5 million children under five in 1985 and grew to 2.5 million in 1989. Severe malnutrition of these children stood at 2 percent in 1983 and moderate malnutrition at 13 percent. In 1988, severe malnutrition was 0.04 percent and moderate was 2 percent, representing an 80 percent drop. Because Thailand experienced considerable overall socioeconomic development at this time, these drops cannot exclusively be attributed to effects of NPHC, although 98.4 percent of villages are covered in the program, and 84.8 percent of children under three years were receiving quarterly GM.

At the community level, village leaders and volunteers receive two to five days of preservice training in program planning, implementation, monitoring, and evaluation, with periodic follow-up continuing education and retraining. CNWs, community nutrition leaders, and fund managers are supervised by regional health center staff and village committees. Total project costs from 1982 to 1986 were $13.1 million, of which 76 percent was covered by the national government and 24 percent by UNICEF and USAID. From 1987 to 1991, the total budget projection was $14.93 million, of which 94 percent would come from the national budget and 6 percent from UNICEF and USAID. No data are available on annual costs per capita.

Iringa Nutrition Project (INP), Tanzania

The INP began in 1983 as a pilot project of the Tanzanian government in a region of high IMR. It involves the collaborative efforts of the ministries of Planning, Health, Education, and Agriculture and the Tanzanian Food and Nutrition Center. Funding was provided by the Joint Nutrition Support Program (JNSP) of WHO, UNICEF, and the Italian government. The objectives of the INP are to decrease infant and child mortality rates, to decrease morbidity and malnutrition, and to raise maternal nutritional status. It places heavy emphasis on increasing the capabilities of all levels of society to use the Triple-A cycle—to assess, analyze, and act—against immediate and root causes of ill health and malnutrition. Strategies for accomplishing these goals include regular village health days (monthly or quarterly), including GMP, child care/feeding centers, immunization, promotion of weaning food preparations, control of common childhood illnesses, ORT, and home visits for the severely malnourished. There are no external food supplements. In addition to physical rehabilitation of

Table A-5. Tanzania/Iringa Nutrition Project (INP) (initiated in 1983)

Program size and target groups

Program size (target population)		Targeting methodology
1984–88	46,000 <5y	
	Geographic Groups	Pilot areas in region of high IMR <5y & PLW. Families, schoolchildren and community members at-large for nutrition, food security, and community mobilization activities.
	Individual	Severely underweights addressed most intensively

Information and evaluation features

Management information system		Evaluation methodology
Info reported	Service deliv—Yes GM data—Yes Morbid/mortal—Yes Village reports of community actions discussed at VHC meetings	*Data sources* GM, HH survey 1988 *Design* Pre-post comparison—Yes Comparison groups—Yes Control for confounders—No Statistical tests—No
Freq. of reports	Quarterly	*Nutritional indicators* W/A <5y
Levels reported to	Local village councils for management and motivation, health center and multiple upper levels/ computerized reg'l analysis	
Downward feedback	Yes, via management meetings at several levels. Triple-A cycle activated at multiple levels to intervene and supervise.	
Local use	Screening, NED, referrals, community mobilization	

Table A-5. (continued)

	Program effectiveness and cost		
Physical growth	Total budget cost	Annual cost per capita	Funding sources
1984 Moderate underweight (W/A <80%) 56%, severe maln 6.3%	1983–87 $3.48 mil total -Personnel 39.4% -Vehicles 13.2% -Local transport 12.8% -Supplies 17.3% -Infrst rehab 46.0%	$3.60 startup $5.30 expansion $8.05 ongoing $16.95 total	National 15% ($470,000) -villages 66% -regions 21% -districts 12% -central 2% External 85%
1988 Moderate underwt 38% (32% drop), severe maln 1.8% (70% drop)			

Sources: GOT/WHO/UNICEF (1988); Pelletier (1991b).

infrastructure, such as health centers and water and sanitation systems, village-based activities include community mobilization training at all levels in the Triple-A cycle to mobilize actors to address context-specific problems. It also includes technical training of staff to analyze PEM problems, NED, water and environment sanitation, household food security, CHW, child care training, and income-generating activities for women's working groups. From 1984 to 1988, INP's total population coverage area was 230,000, including 46,000 children under five years. From 1984 to 1988 the prevalence of total underweight (less than 80 percent W/A) children decreased from 55.9 to 38 percent, and the prevalence of severely malnourished children (less than 60 percent W/A) decreased from 6.3 percent to 1.8 percent.

Integrated into the existing administrative structure, the project makes use of village councils and village health committees (VHC) in implementation and supervision. Specific INP implementation committees coordinate with government ministries for the involvement of extension workers regarding local needs. GMP and teaching activities are carried out by two CHWs per community, in addition to traditional birth attendants and healers and 3.5 child day care attendants per village. They are directly supervised by VHCs with technical support from government health center staff. Training and monthly management supervision are provided as well by regional supervisors, one per twelve CHWs. CHWs receive six months of preservice training by regional trainers, three months in the classroom and the remainder in the field, in addition to on-site in-service continuing education conducted twice monthly by district staff. Total project costs from 1983 to 1987 were $3.58 million, 15 percent of which was covered by the Tanzanian national government and 85 percent by JNSP. Annual costs per child are estimated at $16.95. Broken down according to various costs in different project phases, they are $3.60 per child in the start-up phase, $5.30 per child in expansion areas, and $8.05 per child ongoing.

Embu Growth Monitoring Program (Embu GMP), Kenya

The Embu GMP is a community-operated growth-monitoring project that began in 1987 in Embu District, Kenya, with a target population of 13,500 children under five in two administrative locations. It is implemented by the Ministry of Health with a modest amount of funding from UNICEF, including weighing equipment. Its primary focus is to extend the national facility-based growth-monitoring program's activities into the villages. Its objectives are to decrease mothers' traveling time to clinics,

Table A-6. Kenya/Growth Monitoring Program (GMP) (initiated in 1985)

Program size and target groups		
Program size (target population)	**Targeting methodology**	
Embu	5,000 <5y	*Geographic*	Pilot area with rural cash cropping, high population density, no other community development activities
		Group	5m to 5y
		Individual	Underweights

Information and evaluation features	
Management information system	**Evaluation methodology**
	Data sources	GM data, qualitative review of process; no impact analysis performed
Info reported	Service deliv—No
	GM—Yes
	Morbid/mortal— No
Freq. of reports	Monthly
Levels reported to	Health centers and multiple upper levels
Downward feedback	None
Local use	NED, referral

Program effectiveness and cost		
Physical growth	**Total budget cost**	**Annual cost per capita**	**Funding sources**
No information available	$12,500 over 2 years + equipment/supplies	Est. $1.25 although no conclusive info available	*National* Existing district-level and supervisory staff *External* $12,500 plus weighing equipment, (UNICEF) training, supplies

Source: Oniang'o (1989).

to increase GMP coverage, to provide health/NED to mothers to help them improve health conditions for their children, and to motivate mothers to action by actively involving them in local program operation. Project activities at village level include GM by community volunteers for children under five, NED counseling, and medical referrals for food supplementation for the severely malnourished. In 1987, an estimated 5,000 children (37 percent) in the area were being monitored for growth, and most mothers were able to explain trends in the child growth curve.

The program is introduced to communities by a government GM implementation team of medical staff from district level. At the community level, activities are implemented by five community-selected volunteers who form a GM committee. They attend a three-day preservice training seminar and receive ongoing supervision by one nutritionist per nine villages. The marginal cost of implementing the project was $12,500 (from UNICEF), corresponding to approximately $1.60 per child per year, but this figure does not include the personnel-related costs for the three-member district implementation team.

Applied Nutrition Education Program (ANEP), Dominican Republic

The Applied Nutrition Education Program (ANEP) is a joint initiative by Caritas Dominicana/CRS and USAID to replace a food distribution program in the Dominican Republic that for fifteen years had not appeared to improve the nutritional situation. In 1983, under a USAID operational program grant and with technical assistance from Logical Technical Services Corporation, ANEP was implemented as a community-based, grass-roots strategy to improve the nutritional status of children in 90 poor, rural communities. At the core of the strategy is the integration of child GMP with health and nutrition education. Educational messages and techniques have been carefully developed as the primary focus of the program. Mothers' and families' awareness of child growth, health, and nutrition is raised, and they become more self-reliant and better able to improve health conditions. All children in the community are weighed every six months, and high-risk children (under two years or under 75 percent W/A) are weighed monthly and receive home visits for additional assessment and education contact. Coverage has grown from an estimated 1,236 children under five in 1983 to 8,798 in 1987. The project boasts 70 percent coverage and 85 percent of high-risk cases. In 1983, moderate to severe malnutrition (under 75 percent W/A) stood at 14.6 percent; in 1986, it had dropped to 6.9 percent. Overall, malnutrition was reduced by 31 to 43 percent in a period of national economic stagnation. An

Table A-7. Dominican Republic/Applied Nutrition Education Program (ANEP) (initiated in 1983)

Program size and target groups		
Program size (target population)	Targeting methodology	
1983 1,236<5y	Geographic	Low-income, rural communities with high malnutrition incidence or risk factors and existing community organizations <5y
1986 6,035<5y		
1987 8,700<5y	Group	
	Individual	Children <75% WA or <2y

Information and evaluation features		
Management information system	Evaluation methodology	
Info reported	Service deliv/GM/Morbid/Mortal data converted from registers to 20 coverage indicators	Data sources	GM, pre/post KAP study survey of nonprogram communities. MOH nutritional surveillance data over entire period.
Freq. of reports	Monthly	Design	Pre-post comparison—Yes
Levels reported to	Multiple upper levels		Comparison groups—Yes
Downward feedback	Yes, from center to regions to communities		Control for confounders—Yes
Local use	Screening, NED, referrals; community results displayed		Statistical tests—Yes
		Nutritional indicators	W/A

Table A-7. (*continued*)

| | Program effectiveness and cost | | |
Physical growth	Total budget cost	Annual cost per capita	Funding sources
1983 Mod/severe maln (<75% W/A) 14.6% 1986 6.9% (50% drop, 2–3 years participation) Overall maln reduced by 31%–43% in period of national economic stagnation	$305,809 over 3 yrs. (incl. local costs and in-kind contributions, without technical assistance)	$23.17 (Total cost/8,798 number ever enrolled) $25.91 with technical assistance	*National* 0 *External* 100% (USAID) CRS/Caritas in-kind contributions 11.5%

Sources: Shrimpton (1989) and USAID (1988).

evaluation disclosed significant behavioral change in key health and nutrition practices as well.

A total of seventy-two community promoters implement the program at the community level, in a ratio of one per 100 children. They are supervised by seven program supervisors (one per ten promoters) in bimonthly visits. Central program management is accomplished by four specialized staff members who provide monthly supervision and conduct collective quarterly meetings for training and evaluation. Upper-level supervisors, using participatory methods, provide promoters with twelve-day preservice training on site with emphasis on administration, GM, NED, communication, and data processing. Thereafter, they meet quarterly with promoters for 1.5-day sessions of training and evaluation. Total cost of the project from 1983 to 1987 was $305,809, including local costs and in-kind contributions. Annual cost per beneficiary was $23.17, based on 8,798 children. Funding was heavily dependent on external sources (90 percent from USAID) with the balance provided through in-kind contributions from CRS.

Hogares de Bienestar Infantil (HBI), Colombia

HBI is an important component of the Colombian government plan to eradicate urban poverty. Begun in 1987 through the Institute for Family Welfare (ICBF), an autonomous branch of the Ministry of Health, it co-opts community organizations to help in program implementation. HBI seeks to improve development, health, and nutritional status of children under seven years by strengthening the family unit, increasing income, and improving living conditions, particularly in families of poor single working mothers. There is no individual targeting in the program. It facilitates creation of community-operated day care centers in the homes of community-selected mothers, which provide children with 70 percent of their daily nutritional requirements in an environment promoting positive psychosocial development. Mothers are provided loans to improve their kitchen and toilet facilities to meet the standards for participating in the program. The homes are managed by parent associations that are allocated both enriched flour and money from ICBF to buy food to feed the children. GM is provided three times annually. By the end of 1988, the program included 350,000 preschool children.

ICBF animators introduce the program to leaders in urban communities known to have inadequate water, sanitation, and housing facilities. Community leaders, including the heads of existing community organizations, organize a parents' association and select suitable volunteer day care pro-

Table A-8. Colombia/Community Day Care Homes Program (HBI) (initiated in 1987)

Program size and target groups

Program size (target population)		Targeting methodology	
1988 350,000 <7y	*Geographic*	High-poverty urban areas based on census indicators, i.e. water, poor sanitation, crowding
1989 400,000 <7y; 25,000 daycare homes	*Group*	<7y of poor single working mothers at risk for maln or abandonment. Program biased for older children (median age 3y), thereby missing highest maln-risk group—6 to 18m).
1990 1 mil <7y (projected)	*Individual*	None.

Information and evaluation features

Management information system		Evaluation methodology	
Info reported	Service deliv—Yes GM data—Yes Morbid/mortal—No	*Data sources* *Design*	GM data; 1987 survey of main prevalence Pre-post comparison—Yes (via GM only) Comparison group—No Control for confounders—No Statistical tests—No
Freq. of reports	Monthly/Quarterly	*Nutritional indicators*	W/A
Levels reported to	Parent association and multiple upper levels		
Downward feedback	Minimal. Board presents activity and accounts reviews to both ICBF and parent associations		
Local use	None		

Program effectiveness and cost

Physical growth	Total budget cost		Annual cost per capita	Funding sources
Moderate/severe PEM (WA<80%) reduced from 30% at entry to 20% at end of first four months	1988 50.0% 25.0% 20.0% 7.0% 0.5%	$4.5 mil food child day care fees initial setup costs teaching materials supervision	$127	Government— Institute for Family Welfare

Source: Shrimpton (1989).

viders, one per fifteen children. Local assembly boards, composed of parent representatives from the day care centers, manage ICBF funds. ICBF's 139 zonal offices provide direct implementation support, supervision, and technical resources in nutrition, social work, psychology, and education. Community organizations receive training on fiscal and operational aspects. Day care providers are trained one week on day care activities to promote child psychosocial development and sound nutrition, in addition to supervisory training. Because of the community's major role in implementation, the expansion of HBI has not raised ICBF's staffing needs significantly. In 1988, the project cost the Colombian government $4.5 million, roughly 30 percent of ICBF's budget. Annual cost per capita was $118, excluding parental contributions of up to $10 per month.

References

Aaby, P., J. Bukh, I. Lisse, and A. Smits. 1983. "Measles Mortality, State of Nutrition, and Family Structure: A Community Study from Guinea-Bissau." *Journal of Infectious Diseases* 147: 693–701.

Aarons, A., H. Hawes, and J. Gayton. 1979. *Child to Child*. London: Macmillan.

Abdullah, M. 1989. "The Effect of Seasonality on Intrahousehold Food Distribution and Nutrition in Bangladesh." In *Seasonal Variability in Third World Agriculture: The Consequences for Food Security,* ed. D. E. Sahn. Baltimore: Johns Hopkins University Press.

Abdullah, M., and E. F. Wheeler. 1985. "Seasonal Variations and the Intra-Household Distribution of Food in a Bangladeshi Village." *American Journal of Clinical Nutrition* 41 (6): 1305–1313.

Abrams, B., and C. Berman. 1993. "Women, Nutrition, and Health." *Current Problems in Obstetrics, Gynecology, and Fertility* 16 (1): 3–61.

ACC/SCN (Administrative Committee on Coordination/Subcommittee on Nutrition). 1992. *Second Report on the World Nutrition Situation*. Vol. 1: *Global and Regional Results*. Geneva, Switzerland: World Health Organization.

Achterberg, C. 1991. "Effective Nutrition Communication for Behavior Change." Report of the Sixth International Conference of the International Nutrition Planners Forum. Washington, D.C.: USAID and the Nutrition Foundation.

Adadevoh, S. W., C. Hobbs, and T. E. Elkins. 1989. "The Relation of the True Conjugate to Maternal Height and Obstetric Performance in Ghanaians." *International Journal of Gynecology and Obstetrics* (IRELAND) 28 (3): 243–251.

Adair, L. S. 1987. "Nutrition in the Reproductive Years." In *Nutritional Anthropology,* ed. F. E. Johnston. New York: Alan R. Liss.

Adair, L. S., B. M. Popkin, E. Bisgrove, and C. Barba. 1990. *A Longitudinal Analysis of the Patterns and Determinants of Women's Nutrition in the Philip-*

pines. Maternal Nutrition and Health Care Program, Report No. 1. Washington, D.C.: International Center for Research on Women.

Adams, R. 1985. "The Creation of the IMF Cereal Import Facility." *World Development* 11 (7): 549–563.

AED (Academy for Educational Development). 1988. "Growth Monitoring and Promotion: Issues and Actions." A Report of an Advisory Meeting Sponsored by the Nutrition Communication Project of the Academy for Educational Development in Coordination with the Office of Nutrition of AID. Washington, D.C.: AED.

Agudelo, C. A. 1983. *Community Participation in Health Activities, Some Concepts and Appraisal Criteria*. Bulletin of the Pan American Health Organization No. 17: 375–385.

Ahmed, V., and M. Bamberger. 1988. *Monitoring and Evaluating Development Projects: The South Asian Experience*. Washington, D.C.: World Bank.

Ainsworth, M. 1991. "Economic Aspects of Child Fostering in Côte d'Ivoire." World Bank, Washington, D.C. Mimeographed.

Akin, J. S., C. C. Griffin, D. K. Guilkey, and B. M. Popkin. 1985. *The Demand for Primary Health Services in the Third World*. Totowa, N.J.: Rowman and Allanheld.

Akintola, F. O., O. Areola, and A. Faniran. 1980. "The Elements of Quality and Social Costs of Rural Water Supply and Utilization." *Water Supply and Management* 4 (4): 275–282.

Alam, N., F. J. Henry, and M. M. Rahaman. 1989a. "Reporting Errors in One-Week Diarrhea Recall Surveys: Experience from a Prospective Study in Rural Bangladesh." *International Journal of Epidemiology* 18 (3): 697–700.

Alam, N., B. Wojtyniak, F. J. Henry, and M. M. Rahaman. 1989b. "Mothers' Personal and Domestic Hygiene and Diarrhoea Incidence in Young Children in Rural Bangladesh." *International Journal of Epidemiology* 18 (1): 242–247.

Alam, N., B. Wojtyniak, and M. M. Rahaman. 1989c. "Anthropometric Indicators and Risk of Death." *American Journal of Clinical Nutrition* 49 (5): 884–888.

Alderman, H. 1991. "Food Subsidies and the Poor." In *Essays on Poverty, Equity and Growth*, ed. G. Psacharopoulos. Elmsford, N.Y.: Pergamon Press.

Alderman, H. 1990. *Nutritional Status in Ghana and Its Determinants*. Social Dimensions of Adjustments in Sub-Saharan Africa, Working Paper No. 3. Washington, D.C.: World Bank.

Alderman, H. 1988. "The Twilight of Flour Rationing in Pakistan." *Food Policy* 13 (4): 245–257.

Alderman, H. 1987a. *Cooperative Dairy Development in Karnataka, India: An Assessment*. Research Report 64. Washington, D.C.: International Food Policy Research Institute.

Alderman, H. 1987b. "Allocation of Goods through Non-Price Mechanisms: Evidence of Distribution by Willingness to Wait." *Journal of Development Economics* 25 (1): 105–124.

Alderman, H. 1986. *The Effect of Food Price and Income Changes on the Acquisition of Food by Low-Income Households*. Washington, D.C.: International Food Policy Research Institute.

Alderman, H. 1984. "Attributing Technological Bias to Public Goods." *Journal of Development Economics* 14 (3): 375–393.

Alderman, H., and J. von Braun. 1986. *Egypt's Food Subsidy Policy: Evaluation of Effects and Policy Options for the 1980s.* Final Report to United States Agency for International Development. Washington, D.C.: International Food Policy Research Institute.

Alderman, H., and J. von Braun. 1984. *The Effects of the Egyptian Food Ration and Subsidy System on Income Distribution and Consumption.* IFPRI Research Report no. 45. Washington, D.C.: IFPRI.

Allen, L. H., J. R. Backstrand, A. Chávez, and G. H. Pelto. 1992. *People Cannot Live by Tortillas Alone: The Results of the Mexico Nutrition CRSP.* Human Nutrition Collaborative Research Support Program. Washington, D.C.: USAID, Office of Nutrition.

Almroth, S., and M. Latham. 1982. "Breastfeeding Practices in Rural Jamaica." *Journal of Tropical Pediatrics* (28): 103–109.

Anand, R. K. 1981. "The Management of Breastfeeding in a Bombay Hospital." *Assignment Children* (55–56): 167–180.

Anderson, J. 1989. "Women's Community Service and Child Welfare in Urban Peru." In *Women, Work and Child Welfare in the Third World,* ed. J. Leslie and M. Paolisso. Boulder: Westview.

Anderson, M. A. 1989. "The Relationship between Maternal Nutrition and Child Growth in Rural India." Ph.D. diss., Tufts University School of Nutrition.

Anderson, M. A. 1986. "Targeting of Food Aid from a Field Perspective." In *Nutritional Aspects of Project Food Aid,* ed. M. Forman. Rome: United Nations ACC/SCN.

Anderson, M. A., J. Austin, J. Wray, and M. Zeitlin. 1981. "Supplementary Feeding." In *Nutrition Interventions in Developing Countries: Study I,* ed. J. Austin and M. Zeitlin. Cambridge, Mass.: Oelgeschlager, Gunn and Hain.

Anderson, P. 1989. *Interim Proposals for Re-Design of the Jamaican Food Stamp Programme.* Working Paper No. 2. Kingston: Jamaican Poverty Line Project, Planning Institute of Jamaica.

Anker, R., and J. C. Knowles. 1980. "An Empirical Analysis of Morbidity Differentials in Kenya at the Macro and Micro Levels." *Economic Development and Cultural Change* 29 (1): 165–185.

Anonymous 1. 1989. "Summary of Findings of USAID Assisted ICDS Impact Evaluation." Second follow-up survey 1987–1988 in Panchmahals (Gujarat) and Chandrapur (Maharashtra).

Anonymous 2. 1989. "The Family Nutrition Improvement Program (UPGK) in Indonesia: Program Comments." Fifth INPF International Conference on Crucial Elements of Successful Community Nutrition Programs, Seoul, Korea, 15–18 August.

Antle, J. M., and P. L. Pingali. 1992. "Pesticides, Farmer Health, and Productivity: A Philippine Case Study." Paper presented at a workshop on Measuring the Health and Environmental Effects of Pesticides, Bellagio, Italy, 30 March–3 April.

Antrobus, A. C. K. 1978. "Nutrition and Government Policy in Jamaica." In *Nutrition and National Policy,* ed. B. Winikoff. Cambridge, Mass.: Massachusetts Institute of Technology Press.

Arfaa, F., G. H. Sahba, I. Farahmandian, and H. Jalali. 1977. "Evaluation of the Effect of Different Methods of Control of Soil-Transmitted Helminths in

Khuzestan, Southwest Iran." *American Journal of Tropical Medicine and Hygiene* 26 (2): 230–233.

Arnauld, J., J. A. Alarcon, and M. D. C. Immink. 1990. "Food Security and Nutrition Surveillance in Central America: The Need for Functional Approaches." *Food and Nutrition Bulletin* 12 (1): 26–33.

Arole, M. 1988. "A Comprehensive Approach to Community Welfare: Growth Monitoring and the Role of Women in Jamkhed." *Indian Journal of Pediatrics* 55 (Supplement): S100–S105.

Ashworth, A. 1969. "Growth Rates in Children Recovering from Protein-Energy Malnutrition." *British Journal of Nutrition* 23 (4): 835–845.

Ashworth, A., and R. G. Feachem. 1986. "Interventions for the Control of Diarrhoeal Diseases among Young Children: Growth Monitoring Programmes." Unpublished document.

Austin, J. E., T. Belding, R. Brooks, R. Cahs, J. Fisher, R. Morrow, N. Pielemeyer, D. Pyle, J. Wray, and M. Zeitlin. 1981. "Integrated Nutrition and Primary Health Care Programs." In *Nutrition Intervention in Developing Countries, Study VII*, ed. J. E. Austin and M. Zeitlin. Cambridge, Mass.: Oelgeschlager, Gunn, and Hain.

Austin, J. E., M. Mahin, D. Pyle, and M. Zeitlin. 1978. *Annotated Directory of Nutrition Programs*. Cambridge, Mass.: Harvard Institute for International Development.

Austin, J. E., and M. F. Zeitlin. 1981. *Nutrition Intervention in Developing Countries*. Cambridge, Mass.: Oelgeschlager, Gunn, and Hain.

Babu, S. C., S. Thirumaran, and T. C. Mohanam. 1988. "Yield Variability, Nutritional Intake, and Gender Bias in Food Allocation: Some Evidence from South India." Paper presented at Women, Health, and Development Conference, East Lansing, Mich., October.

Bågenholm, G. C., and A. A. A. Nasher. 1989. "Mortality among Children in Rural Areas of the People's Democratic Republic of Yemen." *Annals of Tropical Paediatrics* 9 (2): 75–81.

Bailey, W. 1981. "Malnutrition among Babies Born to Adolescent Mothers." *West Indian Medical Journal* 30: 72–76.

Bairagi, R., M. K. Chowdhury, J. Kim, G. T. Curlin, and R. H. Gray. 1987. "The Association between Malnutrition and Diarrhoea in Rural Bangladesh." *International Journal of Epidemiology* 16 (3): 477–481.

Bairagi, R., M. K. Chowdhury, Y. J. Kim, and G. T. Curlin. 1985. "Alternative Anthropometric Indicators of Mortality." *American Journal of Clinical Nutrition* 42 (2): 296–306.

Bajaj, S. 1989. "The Nutrition Security System at the Household Level: Policy Implications." *Food and Nutrition Bulletin* 11 (4): 6–12.

Balderston, J., A. Wilson, M. Freire, and M. Simonen. 1981. *Malnourished Children of the Rural Poor*. Boston, Mass.: Auburn Press.

Bamberger, M. 1988. *The Role of Community Participation in Development Planning and Project Management*. EDI Seminar Policy Report No 13. Washington, D.C.: World Bank.

Barclay, A., A. Foster, and A. Sommer. 1987. "Vitamin A Supplementation and Measles-Related Mortality: A Randomized Clinical Trial." *British Medical Journal* 294: 294–296.

Barker, R., and R. Herdt. 1984. "Who Benefits from the New Technology?" In *The Rice Economy of Asia,* ed. R. Barker and R. Herdt. Washington, D.C.: Resources for the Future.

Barrell, R. A. E., and G. M. Rowland. 1979. "Infant Foods as a Potential Source of Diarrhoeal Illness in Rural West Africa." *Transactions of the Royal Society of Tropical Medicine and Hygiene* 73 (1): 85–90.

Barrera, A. 1990. "The Role of Maternal Schooling and Its Interaction with Public Health Programs in Child Health Production." *Journal of Development Economics* 32 (1): 69–92.

Barrera, A. 1987. "Maternal Schooling and Child Health." Ph.D. diss. Yale University.

Barth-Eide, W. 1980. "Rethinking Food and Nutrition Education under Changing Socio-Economic Conditions." *Food and Nutrition Bulletin* 2 (2): 23–28.

Bates, C. J., H. J. Powers, and D. I. Thurnham. 1989. "Vitamins, Iron, and Physical Work Capacity." *Lancet* 2: 313–314.

Bautista, A., P. A. Barker, J. T. Dunn, M. Sanchez, and K. L. Kaiser. 1982. "The Effects of Oral Iodized Oil on Intelligence, Thyroid Status, and Somatic Growth in School-Age Children from an Area of Endemic Goiter." *American Journal of Clinical Nutrition* 35 (1): 127–134.

Beaton, G. H. 1989. "Small but Healthy? Are We Asking the Right Question?" *Human Organization* 48 (1): 30–39.

Beaton, G. H., and H. Ghassemi. 1982. "Supplementary Feeding Programs for Young Children in Developing Countries." *American Journal of Clinical Nutrition* 35 (4): 864–916.

Beaton, G. H., A. Kelly, J. Kevany, R. Martorell, and J. Mason. 1990. *Appropriate Uses of Anthropometric Indices in Children.* ACC/SCN Nutrition Policy Discussion Paper No. 7. Geneva: World Health Organization.

Beaton, G. H., R. Martorell, K. J. Aronson, B. Edmonston, G. McCabe, A. C. Ross, and B. Harvey. 1993. *Effectiveness of Vitamin A Supplementation in the Control of Young Child Morbidity and Mortality in Developing Countries.* ACC/SCN Nutrition Policy Discussion Paper No. 13. Geneva: WHO.

Beaton, G. H., J. Milner, P. Corey, V. Mcguire, M. Cousins, E. Stewart, M. de-Ramos, D. Hewitt, P. V. Grambsch, N. Kassim, and J. A. Little. 1979. "Sources of Variance in 24-Hour Dietary Recall Data: Implications for Nutrition Study Design and Interpretation." *American Journal of Clinical Nutrition* 32: 2546–2559.

Becker, G. S. 1991. *A Treatise on the Family.* 2d ed. Cambridge, Mass.: Harvard University Press.

Becker, S., R. E. Black, and K. H. Brown. 1989. "Relative Effects of Diarrhea, Fever, and Food Intake on Weight Gain in Rural Bangladeshi Children." Johns Hopkins University, Baltimore, Md. Mimeographed.

Begg, C., and J. Berlin. 1988. "Publication Bias: A Problem in Interpreting Medical Data." *Journal of the Royal Statistical Society (A)* 151 (3): 419–463.

Behrman, J. R. Forthcoming. "Intrahousehold Distribution and the Family." In *Handbook of Population and Family Economics,* ed. Mark R. Rosenzweig and Oded Stark. Amsterdam: North-Holland.

Behrman, J. R. 1993. "The Economic Rationale for Investing in Nutrition in Developing Countries." *World Development,* 21 (11): 1749–1772.

Behrman, J. R. 1990a. "A Survey of Socioeconomic Development, Structural Adjustment, and Child Health and Mortality in Developing Countries." In *Child Survival Program: Issues for the 1990s,* ed. K. Hill. Baltimore: Johns Hopkins University, School of Hygiene and Public Health, Institute for International Programs.

Behrman, J. R. 1990b. *The Action of Human Resources and Poverty on One Another: What We Have Yet to Learn.* Washington, D.C.: Population and Human Resources Department, World Bank.

Behrman, J. R. 1990c. "Women's Schooling and Nonmarket Productivity: A Survey and a Reappraisal," University of Pennsylvania, Philadephia. Mimeographed. Prepared for the Women in Development Division of the Population and Human Resources Department of the World Bank.

Behrman, J. R. 1992. "Intra-household Allocation of Nutrients and Gender Effects: A Survey of Structural and Reduced-Form Estimates." In *Nutrition and Poverty,* ed. S. R. Osmani. Oxford: Clarendon Press.

Behrman, J. R. 1988a. "Nutrition, Health, Birth Order and Seasonality: Intrahousehold Allocation in Rural India." *Journal of Development Economics* 28 (1): 43–63.

Behrman, J. R. 1988b. "Intrahousehold Allocation of Nutrients in Rural India: Are Boys Favored? Do Parents Exhibit Inequality Aversion?" *Oxford Economic Papers* 40 (1): 32–54.

Behrman, J. R., and N. Birdsall. 1983. "The Quality of Schooling: Quantity Alone Is Misleading." *American Economic Review* 73 (5): 928–946.

Behrman, J. R., N. Birdsall, and R. Kaplan. 1994. "The Quality of Schooling and Labor Market Outcomes in Brazil: Some Further Explorations." Williams College, Williamstown, Mass.; and World Bank, Washington, D.C. Mimeographed (original 1990).

Behrman, J. R., and A. B. Deolalikar. 1990. "The Intrahousehold Demand for Nutrients in Rural South India: Individual Estimates, Fixed Effects and Permanent Income." *Journal of Human Resources* 25 (4): 665–696.

Behrman, J. R., and A. B. Deolalikar. 1988. "Health and Nutrition." In *Handbook of Development Economics,* Vol. 1, ed. H. Chenery and T. N. Srinivasan. New York: Elsevier Science Publishers B.V.

Behrman, J. R., and A. B. Deolalikar. 1987. "Will Developing Country Nutrition Improve with Income? A Case Study for Rural South India." *Journal of Political Economy* 95 (3): 108–138.

Behrman, J. R., A. Foster, and M. R. Rosenzweig. Forthcoming. "Stages of Agricultural Production and the Calorie-Income Relationship." *Journal of Econometrics.*

Behrman, J. R., and C. Sussangkarn. 1989. "Parental Schooling and Child Outcomes: Mother versus Father, Schooling Quality, and Interactions." University of Pennsylvania, Philadelphia. Mimeographed.

Behrman, J. R., and B. L. Wolfe. 1989. "Does More Schooling Make Women Better Nourished and Healthier? Adult Sibling Random Fixed Effect Estimates for Nicaragua." *Journal of Human Resources* 24 (4): 644–663.

Behrman, J. R., and B. L. Wolfe. 1987a. "How Does Mother's Schooling Affect the Family's Health, Nutrition, Medical Care Usage, and Household Sanitation?" *Journal of Econometrics* 36 (1–2): 185–204.

Behrman, J. R., and B. L. Wolfe. 1987b. "Investments in Schooling in Two Generations in Pre-Revolutionary Nicaragua: The Roles of Family Background and School Supply." *Journal of Development Economics* 27 (1–2): 395–420. Reprinted in *International Trade, Investment, Macro Policies and History: Essays in Memory of Carlos F. Diaz-Alejandro,* ed. P. Bardhan, J. R. Behrman, and A. Fishlow. Amsterdam: North-Holland, 1987.

Behrman, J. R., and B. L. Wolfe. 1984. "More Evidence on Nutrition Demand: Income Seems Overrated and Women's Schooling Underemphasized." *Journal of Development Economics* 14 (1–2): 105–128.

Bell, R. Q. 1971. "Stimulus Control of Parent or Caretaker Behavior by Offspring." *Developmental Psychology* 4 (63): 63–69.

Bentley, M. E. 1992. "Household Behaviors in the Management of Diarrhea and Their Relevance for Persistent Diarrhea." *Acta Pediatria Supplement* 381: 49–54.

Bentley, M. E. 1988. "The Household Management of Childhood Diarrhea in Rural North India." *Social Science and Medicine* 27 (1): 75–85.

Bentley, M. E., L. E. Caulfield, B. Torun, D. Schroeder, and E. Hurtado. 1992. "Maternal Feeding Behavior and Child Appetite during Acute Diarrheal Episodes and Subsequent Health in Guatemala." *FASEB Journal* 6 (5): A1648.

Bentley, M. E., K. A. Dettwyler, and L. Caulfield. 1993. "Child Anorexia and Its Management in Developing-Country Settings: Review and Recommendations." Paper prepared for the Workshop and Expert Meeting on the Guidelines for Nutrition and Feeding of Children 0–5 Years in the Latin American Region organized by PAHO-WHO/CAVENDES/UNU/CESNI, Porlamar, Venezuela, 14–19 March.

Bentley, M. E., K. L. Dickin, S. Mebrahtu, et al. 1991. "Development of a Nutritionally Adequate and Culturally Appropriate Weaning Food in Kwara State, Nigeria: An Interdisciplinary Approach." *Social Science and Medicine* 33: 1103–1111.

Bentley, M. E., G. Pelto, W. Straus, D. Schumann, C. Adegbola, E. de la Pena, G. Oni, K. Brown, and S. Huffman. 1988. "Rapid Ethnographic Assessment: Applications in a Diarrhea Management Program." *Social Science and Medicine* 27 (1): 107–116.

Bentley, M. E., R. Y. Stallings, M. Fukumoto, and J. A. Elder. 1991. "Maternal Feeding Behavior and Child Acceptance of Food during Diarrhea, Convalescence, and Health in the Central Sierra of Peru." *American Journal of Public Health* 81 (1): 43–47.

Berg, A. 1987a. *Malnutrition: What Can Be Done?* Baltimore: Johns Hopkins University Press.

Berg, A. 1987b. "Rejoinder: Nutrition Planning Is Alive and Well, Thank You." *Food Policy* 12 (4): 365–375.

Berg, A. 1985. *Results of an Assessment of the Communications Component of the Tamil Nadu Nutrition Project.* World Bank Internal Document. Washington, D.C.: World Bank.

Berg, A. 1981. *Malnourished People: A Policy View.* Poverty and Basic Needs Series. Washington, D.C.: World Bank.

Berg, A. 1973. *The Nutrition Factor: Its Role in National Development.* Washington, D.C.: Brookings Institution.

Berman, P. A. 1984. "Village Health Workers in Java, Indonesia: Coverage and Equity." *Social Science and Medicine* 19 (4): 411–422.

Berman, P. A., D. R. Gwatkin, and S. E. Berger. 1987. "Community-Based Health Worker: Head Start or False Start towards Health for All?" *Social Science and Medicine* 25 (5): 443–459.

Berman, S., and K. McIntosh. 1985. "Selective Primary Care: Strategies for Control of Disease in the Developing World. XXI. Acute Respiratory Infections." *Reviews of Infectious Diseases* 7 (5): 674–691.

Bhan, M. K., and S. Ghosh. 1986. *Successful Growth Monitoring: Some Lessons from India*. New Delhi, India: UNICEF ROSCA.

Bhandari, N., M. Bhan, S. Sazawal, J. Clemens, S. Bhatnagar, and V. Khoshoo. 1989. "Association of Antecedent Malnutrition with Persistent Diarrhoea: A Case-Control Study." *British Medical Journal* 298: 1284–1287.

Biggs, S., C. Edwards, and J. Griffin. 1977. "Irrigation in Bangladesh: Contradictions and Underutilized Potential." University of Chittagong, Department of Economics, Chittagong, Bangladesh. Mimeographed.

Bille, B., T. Mellbin, and F. Nordbring. 1964. "An Extensive Outbreak of Gastroenteritis Caused by Salmonella Newport, I—Some Observations on 795 Known Cases." *Acta Medica Scandinavica* 175 (May): 557–567.

Billewicz, W. Z., and I. A. McGregor. 1982. "A Birth-to-Maturity Longitudinal Study of Heights and Weights in Two West African (Gambian) Villages, 1951–1975." *Annals of Human Biology* 9 (4): 309–320.

Binswanger, H., and V. Ruttan, eds. 1978. *Induced Innovation: Technology, Institutions and Development*. Baltimore: Johns Hopkins University Press.

Binswanger, H. P., and S. V. R. Shetty. 1977. *Economic Aspects of Weed Control in Semi-Arid Tropical Areas in India*. Economics Program Occasional Paper No. 13. Patancheru, Andhra Pradesh, India: International Crops Research Institute for the Semi-Arid Tropics.

Binswanger, H., and J. von Braun. 1991. "Technological Change and Commercialization of Agriculture: The Effect on the Poor." *World Bank Research Observer* 6 (1): 57–80.

Birdsall, N. 1985. "Public Inputs and Child Schooling in Brazil." *Journal of Development Economics* 18 (1): 67–86.

Birdsall, N., and P. Chuhan. 1986. "Client Choice of Health Care Treatment in Mali." World Bank, Washington, D.C. Mimeographed.

Birdsall, N., and W. P. McGreevy. 1983. "Women, Poverty, and Development." In *Women and Poverty in the Third World*, ed. M. Buvinic, M. Lycette, and W. P. McGreevy. Baltimore: Johns Hopkins University Press.

Black, R. E., K. H. Brown, and S. Becker. 1984. "Malnutrition Is a Determining Factor in Diarrheal Duration, but Not Incidence, among Young Children in a Longitudinal Study in Rural Bangladesh." *American Journal of Clinical Nutrition* 37 (6) 87–94.

Black, R. E., L. C. Chen, O. Harkavy, M. M. Rahaman, and M. G. M. Rowland. 1983. "Prevention and Control of the Diarrheal Diseases." In *Diarrhea and Malnutrition: Interactions, Mechanisms, and Interventions*, ed. L. C. Chen and N. Scrimshaw. New York: Plenum Press.

Blaser, M. J., and L. S. Newman. 1982. "A Review of Human Salmonellosis: I—Infective Dose." *Reviews of Infectious Diseases* 4 (6): 1096–1106.

Blumberg, R. 1988. "Income under Female versus Male Control: Hypotheses from a Theory of Gender Stratification and Data from the Third World." *Journal of Family Issues* 9 (1): 51–84.

Blumenfeld, S. N. 1985. *Operations Research Methods: A General Approach in Primary Health Care.* PRICOR Monograph Series, Methods Paper 1. Bethesda: PRICOR, Center for Human Services.

Blyn, G. 1983. "The Green Revolution Revisited." *Economic Development and Cultural Change* 31 (4): 705–725.

Boerma, J. T., and G. T. Bicego. 1992. "Preceding Birth Intervals and Child Survival: Searching for Pathways of Influence." *Studies in Family Planning* 23 (4): 243–256.

Bogin, B., T. Sullivan, R. Hauspie, and R. B. MacVean. 1989. "Longitudinal Growth in Height, Weight, and Bone Age of Guatemalan, Latino, and Indian Schoolchildren." *American Journal of Human Biology* 1 (1): 103–113.

Bondad, M., L. Candelaria, L. Clark, J. G. Haaga, J. Haas, C. Henderson, F. Lisondra, G. Marks, J. B. Mason, and K. Test. 1984. *Philippine National School Survey of Nutritional Status: Interim Report of Methods and Results from Region VI.* Ithaca: Cornell Nutritional Surveillance Program.

Bongaarts, J. 1987. "Does Family Planning Reduce Infant Mortality Rates?" *Population and Development Review* No. 13: 323–334.

Bongaarts, J. 1982. "The Fertility-Inhibiting Effects of the Intermediate Fertility Variables." *Studies in Family Planning* No. 13: 179–186.

Boserup, E. 1970. *Women's Role in Economic Development.* New York: St. Martin's Press.

Bossert, T. J., and D. A. Parker. 1984. "The Political and Administrative Context of Primary Health Care in the Third World." *Social Science and Medicine* 18 (8): 693–702.

Bothwell, T. H., and R. W. Charlton. 1981. *Iron Deficiency in Women.* A report of the International Nutritional Anemia Consultive Group. New York: Nutrition Foundation.

Bouis, H. E. 1994. "The Effect of Income on Demand for Food in Poor Countries: Are Our Databases Giving Us Reliable Estimates?" *Journal of Development Economics* 43 (2).

Bouis, H. E., and L. J. Haddad. 1992. "Are Estimates of Calorie-Income Elasticities Too High? A Recalibration of the Plausible Range." *Journal of Development Economics* 39 (2): 333–364.

Bouis, H. E., and L. J. Haddad. 1990a. *Effects of Agricultural Commercialization on Land Tenure, Household Resource Allocation, and Nutrition in the Philippines.* Research Report No. 79. Washington, D.C.: International Food Policy Research Institute.

Bouis, H. E., and L. J. Haddad. 1990b. *Agricultural Commercialization, Nutrition, and the Rural Poor: A Study of Philippine Farm Households.* Boulder: Lynne Rienner.

Bray, F. 1986. *The Rice Economies: Technology and Development in Asian Societies.* New York: Blackwell.

Bray, R. S., and M. J. Anderson. 1979. "Falciparum Malaria and Pregnancy." Transactions of the Royal Society of Tropical Medicine and Hygiene No. 73: 427–431.

Brems, S. 1987. "Target Malnutrition: Results from Tamil Nadu." *Mothers and Children: Bulletin on Infant Feeding and Maternal Nutrition* (American Public Health Association) 6 (3): 1–5, 7.

Brems, S., and A. Berg. 1988. *'Eating Down' during Pregnancy: Nutrition, Obstetric, and Cultural Considerations in the Third World.* Discussion paper prepared for the ACC/SCN. Washington, D.C.: World Bank, Population, Health, and Nutrition Division.

Breznitz, Z., and S. L. Friedman. 1988. "Toddler's Concentration: Does Maternal Depression Make a Difference?" *Journal of Child Psychology and Psychiatry* 29 (3): 267–279.

Briend, A. 1985. "Normal Fetal Growth Regulation: Nutritional Aspects." In *Nutritional Needs and Assessment of Normal Growth,* ed. M. Gracey and F. Falkner. Nestle Nutrition Workshop Series 7: 1–22. New York: Raven Press.

Briend, A., and A. Bari. 1989. "Critical Assessment of the Use of Growth Monitoring for Identifying High Risk Children in Primary Health Care Programmes." *British Medical Journal* 298 (6688): 1607–1611.

Briend, A., K. Z. Hanson, K. M. A. Aziz, et al. 1989. "Are Diarrhoea Control Programs Likely to Reduce Childhood Malnutrition? Observations from Rural Bangladesh." *Lancet* 2: 319–322.

Briend, A., B. Wojtyniak, and M. G. M. Rowland. 1988. "Breastfeeding, Nutritional State and Child Survival in Rural Bangladesh." *British Medical Journal* No. 296: 879–882.

Briscoe, J. 1984. "Intervention Studies and the Definition of Dominant Transmission Routes." *American Journal of Epidemiology* 120 (3): 449–455.

Brooks, R. M., D. Abunain, D. Karyadi, I. Sumarno, D. Williamson, M. C. Latham, and J.-P. Habicht. 1985. "A Timely Warning and Intervention System for Preventing Food Crises in Indonesia: Applying Guidelines for Nutritional Surveillance." *Food and Nutrition Bulletin* 11 (2): 37–43.

Brown, J. E., and R. C. Brown. 1982. "Tackling Child Malnutrition in the Community." *Contact* (69): 1–15.

Brown, K. H., N. A. Akhtar, A. D. Robertson, and M. G. Ahmed. 1986. "Lactational Capacity of Marginally Nourished Mothers: Relationships between Maternal Nutritional Status and Quantity and Proximate Composition of Milk." *Pediatrics* 78 (5): 909–919.

Brown, K. H., and M. E. Bentley. 1988. *Improved Nutritional Therapy of Diarrheal Diseases: A Guide for Managers of Diarrheal Disease Control Programs.* Baltimore: Division of Human Nutrition, Department of International Health, Johns Hopkins University.

Brown, K. H., R. E. Black, S. Becker, S. Nahar, and J. Sawyer. 1982. "Consumption of Foods and Nutrients by Weanlings in Rural Bangladesh." *American Journal of Clinical Nutrition* 36 (5): 878–889.

Brown, K. H., R. E. Black, A. D. Robertson, and S. Becker. 1985. "Effects of Season and Illness on the Dietary Intake of Weanlings during Longitudinal Studies in Rural Bangladesh." *American Journal of Clinical Nutrition* (41): 343–355.

Brown, K. H., K. L. Dickin, M. E. Bentley, G. A. Oni, V. T. Obassaju, S. A. Esrey, S. Mebrahtu, I. Alade, and R. Y. Stallings. 1988. "Consumption of Weaning Foods from Fermented Cereals in Kwara State, Nigeria." In *Improving Young*

Child Feeding in Eastern and Southern Africa, Household Level Food Technology: Proceedings of a Workshop Held in Nairobi, Kenya, 12 Oct. 1987, ed. D. Alnwick, S. Moses, and O. G. Schmidt. Ottawa: IDRC.

Brown, L., B. L. Rogers, M. F. Zeitlin, S. N. Gershoff, N. Huq, and K. E. Peterson. 1993. "Comparison of the Costs of Compliance with Nutrition Education Messages to Improve the Diets of Bangladeshi Breastfeeding Mothers and Weaning-Age Children." *Ecology of Food and Nutrition* 30: 99–126.

Brown, L. V., M. F. Zeitlin, K. E. Peterson, A. M. R. Chowdhury, B. L. Rogers, L. H. Weld, and S. N. Gershoff. 1992. "Evaluation of the Impact of Weaning Food Messages on Infant Feeding Practices and Child Growth in Rural Bangladesh." *American Journal of Clinical Nutrition* 56: 994–1003.

Brownlea, A. 1987. "Participation: Myths, Realities, and Prognosis." *Social Science and Medicine* 25 (6): 605–614.

Brun, T. A., C. Geissler, and E. Kennedy. 1990. "Evaluation of the Impact of Agricultural Projects on Food, Nutrition, and Health." In *World Food Issues: Maldevelopment and Malnutrition,* Vol. 2, ed. T. A. Brun and M. C. Latham. Ithaca: Center for Analysis of World Food Issues, Program in International Agriculture, College of Agriculture and Life Sciences, Cornell University.

Burkhalter, B. R. 1986. *Summary Evaluation: Egypt Nutrition Education in Health Centers Project.* Ann Arbor: Community Systems Foundation.

Butte, N. F., C. Garza, E. O. Smith, and B. L. Nichols. 1984. "Human Milk Intake and Growth Performance of Exclusively Breast-Fed Infants." *Journal of Pediatrics* 104 (2): 187–195.

Butz, W. P., J.-P. Habicht, and J. DaVanzo. 1984. "Environmental Factors in the Relationship between Breastfeeding and Infant Mortality: The Role of Sanitation and Water in Malaysia." *American Journal of Epidemiology* 119:516–525.

Cairncross, S., and J. L. Cliff. 1987. "Water Use and Health in Mueda, Mozambique." *Transactions of the Royal Society of Tropical Medicine and Hygiene* 81 (1): 51–54.

Caldwell, J. C., and P. Caldwell. 1987. "The Cultural Context of High Fertility in Sub-Saharan Africa." *Population and Development Review* 13 (3): 409–437.

Caldwell, J. C., and H. Raven. 1977. "The Evolution of Family Planning in an African City: Ibadan, Nigeria." *Population Studies* No. 31: 487–507.

Caldwell, J. C., P. H. Reddy, and P. Caldwell. 1983. "The Social Component of Mortality Decline: An Investigation in South India Employing Alternative Methodologies." *Population Studies* 37 (2): 185–205.

Calkins, P. J., and D. G. Sisler. 1978. *The Impact of Horticultural Development on Income, Employment, and Nutrition in Nuwakot District, Nepal.* Ithaca: Cornell University.

Calloway, D. H., S. Murphy, J. Balderstone, O. Receveur, D. Lein, and M. Hudes. 1992. "Village Nutrition in Egypt, Kenya, and Mexico: Looking across the CRSP Projects." University of California, Berkeley. Mimeographed.

Cape, N. 1988. "Growth Charts: Help or Hindrance?" *Health Policy and Planning* 3 (2): 167–170.

Capone, C. 1977. "Integrating Title II Program with Locally Operated Nutrition, Socio-Economic, and Humanitarian Activities." A Proposal for Structuring and Expanding the Title II Supported Food and Nutrition Program. Paper presented at the CRS Regional Conference, Dakar, Senegal, 8–19 February.

Cash, R. A., R. A. Music, J. P. Liborati, M. J. Snyder, R. P. Wenzel, and R. B. Hornick. 1974. "Response of Man to Infection with Vibrio Cholerai: I—Clinical, Serologic and Bacteriologic Responses to Known Inoculum." *Journal of Infectious Diseases* 129 (1): 45–52.

Cassidy, C. M. 1980. "Benign Neglect and Toddler Malnutrition." In *Social and Biological Predictors of Nutritional Status, Physical Growth, and Neurological Development,* ed. F. E. Johnston and L. S. Greene. New York: Academic Press.

Castañeda, T. 1985. "Determinantes del descenso de la mortalidad infantil en Chile, 1975–1983." *Cuadernos de Economía* 22 (66): 195–214.

Cernea, M. M. 1983. *A Social Methodology for Community Participation in Local Investments: The Experience of Mexico's PIDER Program.* Staff Working Paper No. 598. Washington, D.C.: World Bank.

Cernea, M. M. 1979. *Measuring Project Impact: Monitoring and Evaluation in PIDER.* Washington, D.C.: IBRD.

Cerqueira, M. T., E. Casanueva, A. M. Ferrer, G. Fontanot, A. Chavez, and R. Flores. 1979. "A Comparison of Mass Media Techniques and a Direct Method for Nutrition Education in Rural Mexico." *Journal of Nutrition Education* 11 (3): 133–137.

Chabot, H. T. J. 1984. "Primary Health Care Will Fail If We Do Not Change Our Approach." *Lancet* 2: 340–341.

Chambers, R., and J. Morris, eds. 1973. *MWEA: An Irrigated Rice Settlement in Kenya.* Munich: Welform Verlag.

Chan, G. M., M. McMurry, K. Westover, K. Engelbert-Fenton, and M. R. Thomas. 1987. "Effects of Increased Dietary Calcium Intake upon the Calcium and Bone Mineral Status of Lactating Adolescent and Adult Women." *American Journal of Clinical Nutrition* 46 (2): 319–323.

Chan, G. M., P. Slater, N. Ronald, C. C. Roberts, M. R. Thomas, D. Folland, and R. Jackson. 1982. "Bone Mineral Status of Lactating Mothers of Different Ages." *American Journal of Obstetrics and Gynecology* 144 (4): 438–441.

Chatterjee, M. 1989. *Indian Women, Health, and Productivity.* Washington, D.C.: World Bank, Women in Development Division.

Chatterjee, M., and J. Lambert. 1989. "Women and Nutrition: Reflections from India and Pakistan." *Food and Nutrition Bulletin* 11 (4): 13–28.

Chaudhuri, S. N. 1988. "Growth Monitoring in the Evolution of Clinic Based Health Care through a Community Based Action Program." *Indian Journal of Pediatrics* 55 (1, Suppl.): S84–S87.

Chaudhury, R. H. 1984. "Determinants of Dietary Intake and Dietary Adequacy for Pre-School Children in Bangladesh." *Food and Nutrition Bulletin* 6 (4): 24.

Chávez, A., C. Martinez, and L. Schlaepfer. 1981. "Health Effects of Supplementary Feeding Programs." In *Nutrition in the 1990s: Constraints on our Knowledge,* ed. N. Selvey and P. L. White. New York: Alan R. Liss.

Chávez, A., C. Martinez, and T. Yaschine. 1975. "Nutrition, Behavioral Development, and Mother-Child Interaction in Young Rural Children." *Federation of American Societies for Experimental Biology* 34 (7): 1574–1582.

Chen, L. C. 1983. "Interactions of Diarrhea and Malnutrition: Mechanisms and Interventions." In *Diarrhea and Malnutrition: Interactions, Mechanisms, and Interventions,* ed. L. C. Chen and N. Scrimshaw. New York: Plenum Press.

Chen, L. C., A. Chowdhury, and S. L. Huffman. 1980. "Anthropometric Assessment of Energy Protein Malnutrition and Subsequent Rigs of Mortality among Preschool Aged Children." *American Journal of Clinical Nutrition* 33 (8): 1836–1845.

Chen, L. C., E. Huq, and S. D'Souza. 1981. "Sex Bias in the Family Allocation of Food and Health Care in Rural Bangladesh." *Population and Development Review* 7 (1): 55–70.

Chen, L. C., and N. S. Scrimshaw, eds. 1983. *Diarrhea and Malnutrition: Interactions, Mechanisms, and Interventions.* New York: Plenum Press.

Cherias, J. 1990. "Greenpeace and Science: Oil and Water?" *Science* 247: 1288–1290.

Chernichovsky, D., and L. Zangwill. 1988. "Microeconomic Theory of the Household and Nutrition Program." Policy, Planning and Research Working Papers No. 82 on Population, Health, and Nutrition, Population and Human Resources. Washington, D.C.: World Bank.

Cherry, F. F., F. Mather, and N. Mock. 1987. "Long-Term Effect of Gynecologic Age on Somatic Growth of Children." *Journal of Community Health* No. 12: 108–116.

Chidambaram, G. 1989. *Terminal Evaluation of Tamil Nadu Integrated Nutrition Project.* Washington, D.C.: Government of Tamil Nadu and the World Bank.

Church, M. A. 1982. "Evaluation as an Integral Aspect of Nutrition Education." In *Evaluation of Nutrition Education in Third World Communities,* ed. B. Schurch. Vienna: Hans Huber.

CIMMYT. 1984. *Report on Wheat Improvement 1981.* El Batan: CIMMYT.

CIMMYT. 1983. *Report on Wheat Improvement 1980.* El Batan: CIMMYT.

Clark, B. A. 1975. "The Work Done by Rural Women in Malawi." *East African Journal of Rural Development* 8 (1–2): 80–91.

Clark, C. 1981. *Demographic and Socioeconomic Correlates of Infant Growth in Guatemala.* N1702–AID/RF. Santa Monica, Calif.: RAND Corporation.

Clavano, N. R. 1982. "Mode of Feeding and Its Effect on Infant Mortality and Morbidity." *Journal of Tropical Pediatrics* No. 28: 287–293.

Clay, E. 1974. "Planners' Preferences and Tubewell Irrigation Technology in North East India." Ph.D. diss., University of Sussex.

Cleland, J., and J. van Ginneken. 1988. "Maternal Education and Child Survival in Developing Countries: The Search for Pathways of Influence." *Social Science and Medicine* 27: 1357–1368.

Clemens, J. D., B. Stanton, B. Stoll, N. Shahid, H. Banu, and A. K. M. Chowdhury. 1986. "Breastfeeding as a Determinant of Severity of Shigellosis." *American Journal of Epidemiology* No. 123: 710–720.

Cobb, R., J. Ross, and M. Ross. 1976. "Agenda Building as a Comparative Political Process." *American Political Science Review* 70 (1): 126–137.

Cochrane, S., J. Leslie, and D. J. O'Hara. 1982. "Parental Education and Child Health: Intracountry Evidence." *Health Policy and Education* 2 (3–4): 213–250.

Cohen, J. M., and N. T. Uphoff. 1980. "Participation's Place in Rural Development: Seeking Clarity through Specificity." *World Development* 8: 213–235.

Cohen, S. E., and A. H. Parmelee. 1983. "Prediction of Five-Year Stanford-Binet Scores in Preterm Infants." *Child Development* 54 (5): 1242–1253.

Colclough, C. 1982. "The Impact of Primary Schooling on Economic Development: A Review of the Evidence." *World Development* 10: 167–185.

Cole, T. J., and J. M. Parkin. 1977. "Infection and Its Effect on the Growth of Young Children: A Comparison of the Gambia and Uganda." *Transactions of the Royal Society of Tropical Medicine and Hygiene* 71 (3): 196–198.

Colle, R. D. 1977. "The Traditional Laundering Place as a Non-Formal Health Education Setting." *Convergence* 10 (2): 32–40.

Committee on Nutritional Status during Pregnancy and Lactation. 1970. *Nutrition during Pregnancy.* Washington, D.C.: Institute of Medicine.

Committee on Population, National Research Council. 1989. *Contraception and Reproduction: Health Consequences for Women and Children in the Developing World.* Washington, D.C.: National Academy Press.

Cook, F. 1981. "Crime and the Elderly: The Emergence of a Political Issue." In *Reactions to Crime,* ed. D. Lewis. Beverly Hills, Calif.: Sage.

Cornia, G., R. Jolly, and F. Stewart. 1988. *Adjustment with a Human Face.* Oxford: Oxford University Press.

Costello, A. M. 1988. "GOBI and Infant Mortality." *Lancet* 1:186.

Cowan, B. 1988. "Growth Monitoring as a Critical Means to Provide Primary Health Care." *Indian Journal of Pediatrics* 55 (1, Suppl.): S74–S77.

Crockenberg, S. 1988. "Social Support and Parenting." In *Theory and Research in Behavioral Pediatrics,* Vol. 4, ed. H. E. Fitzgerald, B. M. Lester, and M. W. Yogman. New York: Plenum Press.

Crowther, C. A. 1986. "A Prospective Study of Hypertension in Pregnancy at Harare Maternal Hospital." *Central African Journal of Medicine* No. 32: 175–180.

CRS-Africa Regional Office. 1979. *Instructions for the Use of the Master Chart and the Growth Surveillance Chart.* Nairobi: Catholic Relief Services–USCC–Africa Regional Office.

CRS-USCC-The Gambia. 1989. "Program Summary." In Workshop on Managing Successful Nutrition Programmes, Korea, August.

Curtis, V. 1986. *Women and the Transport of Water.* London: Intermediate Technology Publications.

DaVanzo, J., and D. S. Levy. 1989. "Influences on Breastfeeding Decisions in Peninsular Malaysia." RAND Corporation, Santa Monica, Calif. Mimeographed.

DaVanzo, J., and E. H. Starbird. 1990. "Correlates of Short Inter-Birth Intervals in Peninsular Malaysia: Their Pathways of Influence through Breast-Feeding and Contraceptive Use." Paper presented to Population Association of America, May.

David, P. 1985. "Clio and the Economics of QWERTY." *American Economic Review* 75 (2): 1332–1337.

Davies, A. M., and W. Dunlop. 1983. "Hypertension in Pregnancy." In *Obstetrical Epidemiology,* ed. S. L. Barron and A. M. Thompson. London: Academic Press.

Deboeck, G., and D. Rubin, eds. 1980. *Selected Case Studies on Monitoring and Evaluation of Rural Development Projects,* Vols. 1 and 2. Washington, D.C.: World Bank.

De Janvry, A. 1978. "Social Structure and Biased Technical Change in Argentine Agriculture." In *Induced Innovation: Technology, Institutions and Develop-*

ment, ed. H. Binswanger and V. Ruttan. Baltimore: Johns Hopkins University Press.

DeKlerk, N. H., D. R. English, and B. K. Armstrong. 1989. "A Review of the Effects of Random Measurement Error on Relative Risk Estimates in Epidemiological Studies." *International Journal of Epidemiology* 18 (3): 705–712.

DeMaeyer, E., and M. Adiels-Tegman. 1985. "The Prevalence of Anemia in the World." *World Health Statistics Quarterly* 38: 302–316.

Deolalikar, A. B. 1988. "Nutrition and Labor Productivity in Agriculture: Estimates for Rural South India." *Review of Economics and Statistics* 70 (3): 406–413.

Dervin, B. 1984. "Mass Communicating: Changing Conceptions of the Audience." In *Public Communications Campaigns,* ed. R. Rice and W. Paisley. Newbury Park, Calif.: Sage.

De Schryver, A., and A. Meheus. 1989. "International Travel and Sexually Transmitted Diseases." *World Health Statistics Quarterly* No. 42: 90–99.

Dettwyler, K. A. 1987. "Breastfeeding and Weaning in Mali: Cultural Context and Hard Data." *Social Science and Medicine* 24 (8): 633–644.

Dettwyler, K. A. 1986. "Infant Feeding in Mali, West Africa: Variations in Belief and Practice." *Social Science and Medicine* 23 (7): 651–664.

DeWalt, K. M. 1989. "Agricultural Change as Nutrition Intervention in Rural Areas." Paper presented at the Annual Meetings of the American Anthropological Association, Washington, D.C., 15–20 November.

Dewey, K. G. 1989. "Nutrition and the Commoditization of Food Systems in Latin America and the Caribbean." *Social Science and Medicine* 28 (5): 415–424.

Dewey, K. G. 1981. "Nutritional Consequences of the Transformation from Subsistence to Commercial Agriculture, Mexico." *Human Ecology* 9: 151–187.

Dewey, K. G. 1979. "Commentary: Agricultural Development, Diet and Nutrition." *Ecology of Human Nutrition* 8: 265–273.

Dewey, K. G., M. J. Heinig, L. A. Nommsen, J. M. Peerson, and B. Zonnerdal. 1992. "Growth of Breast-fed and Formula-fed Infants from 0 to 18 months: The DARLING Study." *Pediatrics* 89: 1035–1041.

Dey, J. 1985. "Women in African Rice Farming Systems." In *Women in Rice Farming.* Westmead, N.H.: Gower.

DHS. 1988. *Demographic and Health Surveys Newsletter.* Columbia, Md.: Institute for Resource Development/Westinghouse, Summer.

Dibley, M. J., J. B. Goldsby, N. W. Staehling, and F. L. Trowbridge. 1987a. "Development of Normalized Curves for the International Growth Reference: Historical and Technical Considerations." *American Journal of Clinical Nutrition* 46 (5): 736–748.

Dibley, M. J., N. W. Staehling, P. Nieburg, and F. L. Trowbridge. 1987b. Interpretation of Z-Score Anthropometric Indicators Derived from the International Growth Reference." *American Journal of Clinical Nutrition* 46 (5): 749–762.

Dillon, B., and M. Stiefel. 1987. *Making the Concept Concrete: The UNRISD Participation Program.* Bulletin 21. Reading, U.K.: Reading Rural Development Communications.

Dixon, R. B. 1982. "Women in Agriculture: Counting the Labor Force in Developing Countries." *Population and Development Review* 8 (3): 539–566.

Dobbing, J., ed. 1988. *Infant Feeding: Anatomy of a Controversy, 1973–1984.* New York: Springer-Verlag.

Dreze, J. 1988. *Famine Prevention in India.* Development Economics Paper No. 3 (February). London: London School of Economics.

Drosin, J. 1989. "The Mamans Bongisa Program." Presentation at U.S. Agency for International Development, Food for Peace Office Conference on Targeted Consumer Food Subsidy Schemes and the Role of U.S. Food Aid Programming in Africa, Arlington, Va., November.

Drummond, T. 1977. "Rethinking Nutrition Education." In *Teaching Nutrition in Developing Countries,* ed. K. Shack. Santa Barbara: Meals for Millions Foundation.

D'Souza, S., and L. C. Chen. 1980. "Sex Differentials in Mortality in Rural Bangladesh." *Population and Development Review* 6 (2): 257–270.

Dupont, H. L., S. B. Formal, R. B. Hornick, M. J. Snyder, J. P. Libonati, D. G. Sheahan, E. H. LaBrec, and J. P. Kalas. 1971. "Pathogenesis of Escherichia Coli Diarrhea." *New England Journal of Medicine* 285 (1): 1–9.

Durnin, J. V. G. A. 1987. "Energy Requirements of Pregnancy: An Integration of the Longitudinal Data from the Five-Country Study." *Lancet* 2: 1131–1133.

Durnin, J. V. G. A., and R. Passmore. 1967. *Energy, Work and Leisure.* London: Heinemann Educational Books.

Dworkin, D., B. Pillsbury, R. Thatsanatheb, and S. Satchakul. 1980. *The Potable Water Project of Rural Thailand.* Project Impact Evaluation No. 3. Washington, D.C.: United States Agency for International Development.

Edgerton, V. R., G. W. Gardner, Y. Ohira, K. A. Gunawardena, and B. Senewiratne. 1979. "Iron Deficiency Anaemia and Its Effect on Worker Productivity and Activity Patterns." *British Medical Journal* 2: 1546–1549.

Edirisinghe, N. 1987. *The Food Stamp Scheme in Sri Lanka: Costs, Benefits, and Options for Modification.* IFPRI Research Report No. 58. Washington, D.C.: IFPRI.

Edmundson, W. C., and P. V. Sukhatme. 1990. "Food and Work: Poverty and Hunger?" *Economic Development and Cultural Change* 38: 263–280.

Efiong, E. I., and M. O. Banjoko. 1975. "The Obstetric Performance of Nigerian Primigravidae Aged 16 and Under." *British Journal of Obstetrics and Gynecology* No. 82: 228–233.

Eisemon, T. O. 1988. "The Consequences of Schooling: A Review on the Outcomes of Primary Schooling in Developing Countries." Harvard University, Cambridge, Mass. Mimeographed.

Elliot, T., K. O. Agunda, J. Kigondu, S. Kinoti, and M. Latham. 1985. "Breastfeeding versus Infant Formula: The Kenyan Case." *Food Policy* 10 (1): 7–10.

Elmore, R. F. 1982. "Backward Mapping: Implementation Research and Policy Decisions." In *Studying Implementation: Methodological and Administrative Issues,* ed. W. Williams. Chatham: Chatham House.

El Samani, E. F. Z., W. C. Willett, and J. H. Ware. 1988. "Association of Malnutrition and Diarrhea in Children Aged under Five Years: A Prospective Follow-Up Study in a Rural Sudanese Community." *American Journal of Epidemiology* 128 (1): 93–105.

Engle, P. L. Forthcoming. "Mother's Money, Father's Money, and Parental Commitment: Guatemala and Nicaragua." In *Engendering Wealth and Well-Being,* ed. R. Blumberg. Boulder, Colo.: Westview.

Engle, P. L. 1994. *An Interactive Model of Child Care and Implications for Programs.* UNICEF/Cornell Lecture Series on Food and Nutrition Policy. Ithaca: Cornell Food and Nutrition Policy Program, Cornell University.

Engle, P. L. 1992. "Care and Child Nutrition." Theme paper for the International Conference on Nutrition (ICN). New York: Nutrition Section of UNICEF, March.

Engle, P. L. 1991. "Maternal Work and Child Care Strategies in Peri-Urban Guatemala: Nutritional Effects." *Child Development* 62: 954–965.

Engle, P. L. 1989. "Mother's Income Control: Consequences for Mothers and for Their Children." Paper presented at the Association for Women in Development, Washington, D.C.

Engle, P. L., and C. Breaux. 1994. *Is There a Father Instinct? Fathers' Responsibilities for Children.* New York: Population Council/International Center for Research on Women Series.

Engle, P. L. and M. Garcia de Sanchez. 1989. "Options to Mother Care: A Report on Day Center Programs in Guatemala." Report to UNICEF/Guatemala.

Engle, P. L., J. La Montagne, and M. Zeitlin. 1993. "Caring Behaviors and Nutritional Status of Weaning Age Children in Managua, Nicaragua." Report to UNICEF, New York.

Engle, P. L., and J. B. Lumpkin. 1992. "How Accurate Are Time Reports? Effects of Cognitive Enhancement and Culture on Recall Accuracy." *Applied Cognitive Psychology* 6: 141–159.

Engle, P. L., and I. Nieves. 1993. "Intrahousehold Food Distribution Patterns among Guatemalan Families in a Supplementary Feeding Program: Behavior Patterns." *Social Science and Medicine* 36 (12): 1605–1612.

Engle, P. L., I. Nieves, M. Zeitlin, J. La Montagne, and Y. Medrano. 1990. "Active Feeding Behavior: Guatemala and Nicaragua." Paper presented at the Society for Cross-Cultural Research, Claremont, Calif.

Engle, P. L., and M. Pedersen. 1989. "Maternal Work for Earnings and Children's Nutritional Status in Urban Guatemala." *Ecology of Food and Nutrition* 22 (1): 211–223.

Engle, P. L., M. Zeitlin, and Y. Medrano. Forthcoming. "Growth Consequences of Low-Income Nicaraguan Mothers' Theories about Feeding One-Year Olds." In *Parents' Cultural Belief Systems,* ed. S. Harkness and C. Super, New York: Guilford Press.

Esrey, S. A. 1993. "Multi-Country Study to Examine Relationships between the Health and Children and the Level of Water and Sanitation Service, Distance to Water, and Type of Water Used." Report prepared for CIDA, Water Sector, Ottawa.

Esrey, S. A. 1987. "The Effect of Improved Water Supplies and Sanitation on Child Growth and Diarrheal Rates in Lesotho." Ph.D. diss., Cornell University.

Esrey, S., and M. Bentley. 1989. *Nutrition and Diarrhea.* PRITECH CDD Action Strategy Paper. Arlington, Va.: Information Center, PRITECH Project.

Esrey, S. A., H. Creed, K. Brown, M. Bentley, and G. Lopez de Romona. 1989. "Energy Intake during Diarrhea, Convalescence, and Health by Rural Peruvian Children (Abstract)." *Federation of American Societies for Experimental Biology Journal* 2 (5): A1194.

Esrey, S. A., and R. G. Feachem. 1989. *Interventions for the Control of Diarrhaeal Diseases among Young Children: Promotion of Food Hygiene.* Geneva: World Health Organization.

Esrey, S. A., R. G. Feachem, and J. M. Hughes. 1985. "Interventions for the Control of Diarrhoeal Disease among Young Children: Improving Water Supplies and Excreta Disposal Facilities." *Bulletin of the World Health Organization* 63 (4): 757–772.

Esrey, S. A., and J.-P. Habicht. 1988. "Maternal Literacy Modifies the Effect of Toilets and Piped Water on Infant Survival in Malaysia." *American Journal of Epidemiology* 127 (5): 1079–1087.

Esrey, S. A., and J.-P. Habicht. 1986. "Epidemiologic Evidence for Health Benefits from Improved Water and Sanitation in Developing Countries." *Epidemiologic Reviews* 8:117–128.

Esrey, S. A., and J.-P. Habicht. 1985. "The Impact of Improved Water Supplies and Excreta Disposal Facilities on Diarrheal Morbidity, Growth and Mortality among Children." In *A Methodology to Review Public Health Interventions: Results from Nutrition Supplementation and Water and Sanitation Projects,* ed. S. A. Esrey, J.-P. Habicht, and W. P. Butz. Cornell International Nutrition Monograph Series No. 15. Ithaca: Cornell University.

Esrey, S. A., J.-P. Habicht, and G. Casella. 1992. "The Complementary Effect of Latrines and Increased Water Usage on the Growth of Infants in Rural Lesotho." *American Journal of Epidemiology* 135: 659–666.

Esrey, S. A., J. B. Potash, L. Roberts, and C. Shiff. 1991. "Effects of Improved Water Supply and Sanitation on Ascariasis, Diarrhoea, Dracunculiasis, Hoodwork Infection, Schistosomiasis, and Trachoma." *Bulletin of the World Health Organization* 69 (5): 609–621.

Eveleth, P. B., and J. M. Tanner. 1976. *Worldwide Variation In Human Growth.* Cambridge, Eng.: Cambridge University Press.

Evenson, R., and Y. Kislev. 1976. *Agricultural Research and Productivity.* New Haven: Yale University Press.

Ewbank, D. C., and S. H. Preston. 1990. "Personal Health Behavior and the Decline in Infant and Child Mortality: The United States, 1900–1930." In *What We Know about the Health Transition: The Cultural, Social, and Behavioural Determinants of Health,* Vol. 1, ed. John Caldwell, Sally Findley, Pat Caldwell, Daphne Broers-Freeman, and Wendy Cosford. Canberra: Australian National University.

FAO. 1987. *Health and Nutritional Aspects of Agriculture and Rural Development Projects.* Proceedings of the Ad Hoc FAO/WHO Consultation, 10–14 November. Rome: FAO.

FAO. 1984. "Integrating Nutrition into Agricultural and Rural Development Projects: Six Case Studies." *Nutrition in Agriculture* No. 2. Rome: FAO.

FAO/WHO/UNU. 1985. *Energy and Protein Requirements.* Report of a Joint FAO/WHO/UNU Expert Consultation. WHO Technical Report Series No. 724. Geneva: WHO.

Farrington, J. 1989. "Farmer Participation in Agricultural Research." *Food Policy* 14 (2): 97–100.

Faruqee, R., and E. Johnson. 1982. *Health, Nutrition, and Family Planning in*

India: A Survey of Experiments and Special Projects. Working Paper No. 507. Washington, D.C.: World Bank.

Feachem, R. G. 1986. "Preventing Diarrhoea: What Are the Policy Options?" *Health Policy and Planning* 1 (2): 109–117.

Feachem, R. G., E. Burns, S. Cairncross, A. Cronin, P. Cross, D. Curtis, M. K. Khan, D. Lamb, and H. Southall. 1978. *Water, Health and Development: An Interdisciplinary Evaluation.* London: Tri-Med Books.

Ferraz, E. M., R. H. Gray, P. L. Fleming, and T. M. Maria. 1988. "Interpregnancy Interval and Low Birth Weight: Findings from a Case-Control Study." *American Journal of Epidemiology* No. 128: 1111–1116.

Field, J. O. 1987. "Multisectoral Nutrition Planning: A Post-Mortem." *Food Policy* 12 (1): 15–28.

Field, J. O. 1985. "Implementing Nutrition Programs: Lessons from an Unheeded Literature." *Annual Reviews of Nutrition* 5: 143–172.

Filstead, W. J. 1979. "Qualitative Methods: A Needed Perspective in Evaluation Research." In *Quantitative and Qualitative Methods in Evaluation Research,* ed. T. D. Cook and C. S. Reighardt. Beverly Hills, Calif.: Sage.

Fleming, P. L. 1987. "The Influence of Birth Spacing on Child Growth." Ph.D. diss., Johns Hopkins University.

Fleuret, P., and A. Fleuret. 1980. "Nutrition, Consumption and Agricultural Change." *Human Organization* 39 (3): 250–260.

Florentino, R., C. Adorno, and F. Solon. 1982. "Interface Problems between Nutrition Policy and Its Implementation: The Philippine Case Study." In *Nutrition Policy Implementation: Issues and Experience,* ed. M. B. Wallerstein. New York: Plenum Press.

Folbre, N. 1989. Presentation at the Fourth Seminar on Female Headed Households Sponsored by the International Center for Research on Women and the Population Council, New York City, 28 November.

Folbre, N. 1986. "Cleaning House: New Perspectives on Households and Economic Development." *Journal of Development Economics* 22 (1): 5–40.

Folbre, N. 1984. "Market Opportunities, Genetic Endowments, and Intrafamily Resource Distribution: Comment." *American Economic Review* 74 (3): 518–520.

Fortney, J., J. E. Higgins, A. Diaz-Infante, F. Hefnawi, L. G. Lanpe, and I. Batar. 1983. "Childbearing after Age 35: Its Effect on Early Perinatal Outcome." In *Childbirth in Developing Countries,* ed., M. Potts, B. Janowitz, and J. A. Fortney. Boston: MTP Press.

Fraker, T. 1990. *The Effects of Food Stamps on Food Consumption: A Review of the Literature.* Washington, D.C.: USDA, Food and Nutrition Service, Office of Analysis and Evaluation.

Freire, P. 1974. *The Pedagogy of the Oppressed.* New York: Seabury Press.

Freire, P. 1973. *La concienciación en el medio rural.* Mexico, DF.: Siglo XXI Ed.

Freire, P. 1971. *La educación como práctica de la libertad.* Mexico, DF.: Siglo XXI Ed.

Frisancho, A. R., J. Matos, W. R. Leonard, and L. A. Yaroch. 1985. "Developmental and Nutritional Determinants of Pregnancy Outcome among Teenagers." *American Journal of Physical Anthropology* 66: 247–261.

Fuerstein, M.-T. 1986. *Partners in Evaluation: Evaluating Development and Community Programs with Participants.* London: Macmillan.

Funnell, D. C. 1982. "Changes in Farm Income and the Rural Development Program in Swaziland." *Journal of Developing Areas* 16: 271–290.

Gadomski, A., and R. Black. 1988. *Child Survival Programs: Issues for the 1990s, Impact of the Direct Interventions.* Baltimore: Department of International Health, School of Hygiene and Public Health, Johns Hopkins University.

Gailbraith, J. 1988. "The Grammar of Political Economy." In *The Consequences of Economic Rhetoric,* ed. A. Klamer, D. McCloskey, and R. Solow. Cambridge, Eng.: Cambridge University Press.

Galbraith, R. 1976. "Evaluation of Health Care in an African Village." *Journal of Tropical Pediatrics and Environmental Child Health* 22: 153–155.

Galler, J. R., H. N. Ricciuti, M. A. Crawford, and L. T. Kucharski. 1984. "The Role of the Mother-Infant Interaction in Nutritional Disorders." In *Human Nutrition: A Comprehensive Treatise (Nutrition and Behaviour),* Vol. 5, ed. J. R. Galler. New York: Plenum.

Garcia, M. 1988. "Food Subsidies in the Philippines: Preliminary Results." In *Food Subsidies in Developing Countries,* ed. P. Pinstrup-Andersen. Baltimore: Johns Hopkins University Press.

Garcia, M., and P. Pinstrup-Andersen. 1987. *The Pilot Food Price Subsidy Scheme in the Philippines: Its Impact on Income, Food and Consumption, and Nutritional Status.* Research Report No. 61. Washington, D.C.: International Food Policy Research Institute.

Garcia, S. E., L. L. Kaiser, and K. G. Dewey. 1990a. "The Relationship of Eating Frequency and Caloric Density to Energy Intake among Rural Mexican Preschool Children." *Journal of Clinical Nutrition* 44: 381–387.

Garcia, S. E., L. L. Kaiser, and K. G. Dewey. 1990b. "Self-Regulation of Food Intake among Rural Mexican Preschool Children." *European Journal of Clinical Nutrition* 44: 371–380.

Garn, S. M., and D. C. Clark. 1976. "Problems in the Nutritional Assessment of Black Individuals." *American Journal of Physical Anthropology* 66 (3): 262–267.

Geervani, P., and G. Jayashree. 1988. "A Study of Nutritional Status of Adolescent and Adult Pregnant and Lactating Women and Growth of Their Infants." *Journal of Tropical Pediatrics* 34: 234–237.

Genece, E., and J. E. Rohde. 1988. "Growth Monitoring as an Entry Point for Primary Health Care." *Indian Journal of Pediatrics* 55 (1, Suppl.): S78–S83.

George, S. 1977. *How the Other Half Dies.* Montclair, N.J.: Allanheld, Ormun.

George S. M., M. C. Latham, and R. Abel. 1992. "Successful Growth Monitoring in South Indian Villages." In *Growth Promotion for Child Development,* ed. J. Cervinskas et al., eds. Ottawa, Canada: International Development Research Centre (IDRC). Proceedings of a Colloquium held in Nyeri, Kenya, 12–13 May 1992.

Gerein, N. M. 1988. "Is Growth Monitoring Worthwhile? Review Article." *Health Policy and Planning* 3 (3): 181–194.

Gerein, N. M., and D. A. Ross. 1991. "Is Growth Monitoring Worthwhile? An Evaluation of Its Use in Three Child Health Programmes in Zaire." *Social Science and Medicine* 32 (6): 667–675.

Gertler, P. J. 1990. *Gender Differences in the Utilization of Medical Care in Peru: Implications for User Fee Policy.* Report No. 13B, Maternal Nutrition and Health Care Program. Washington, D.C.: International Center for Research on Women.

Gertler, P., and H. Alderman. 1989. "Family Resources and Gender Differences in Human Capital Investments: The Demand for Children's Medical Care in Pakistan." Rand Corporation, Santa Monica, Calif. Mimeographed.

Gertler, P., L. Locay, and W. Sanderson. 1987. "Are User Fees Regressive? The Welfare Implications of Health Care Financing Proposals in Peru." *Journal of Econometrics* 36 (1–2): 67–88.

Gertler, P., and J. van der Gaag. 1988. *The Willingness-to-Pay for Medical Care: Evidence from Two Developing Countries.* Washington, D.C.: World Bank.

Ghai, D. 1988. "Participatory Development: Some Perspectives from Grass-Roots Experiences." *Journal of Development Planning* No. 19: 215.

Ghassemi, H. 1989. "Supplementary Feeding Revisited." Paper prepared for the Food Policy and Nutrition Division, Food and Agriculture Organization of the United Nations, Rome, September.

Ghosh, S. 1988. "Growth Monitoring: Lessons from India." *Indian Journal of Pediatrics* 55 (1, Suppl.): S67–S73.

Gillespie, S., J. Kevany, and J. Mason. 1991. *Controlling Iron Deficiency: A Report Based on an ACC/SCN Workshop.* ACC/SCN State-of-the-Art Series Nutrition Discussion Policy Discussion Paper No. 9. Geneva, Switzerland: World Health Organization.

Glewwe, P. 1986. *The Distribution of Welfare in the Republic of Côte d'Ivoire.* LSMS Working Paper No. 29. Washington, D.C.: World Bank.

Gokulanathan, K. S., and K. P. Verghese. 1969. "Sociocultural Malnutrition (Growth Failure in Children Due to Socio-Cultural Factors)." *Journal of Tropical Pediatrics* 15 (3): 118–124.

Goldman, R. H., and C. A. Overholt. 1981. "Agricultural Production, Technical Change, and Nutrition Goals: Study IV." In *Nutrition in Developing Countries,* ed. J. E. Austin and M. Zeitlin. Cambridge, Mass.: Oelgeschlager, Gunn and Hain.

Goldman, R. H., and L. Squire. 1978. "Technical Change, Labor Use and Income Distribution in the Muda Irrigation Project." Discussion Paper 35. Cambridge, Mass.: Harvard Institute for International Development.

Goldsmith, A., B. Pillsbury, and D. Nicholas. 1985. *Community Organization.* Monograph Series Issues Paper No. 3. Chevy Chase, Md.: PRICOR.

Goldstein, H., and J. M. Tanner. 1980. "Ecological Considerations in the Creation and the Use of Child Growth Standards." *Lancet* 1: 582–588.

Gomez de Leon, J., and J. E. Potter. 1989. "Modelling the Inverse Association between Breastfeeding and Contraceptive Use." *Population Studies* No. 43: 69–93.

Gopalan, C. 1987. "Growth Monitoring: Some Basic Issues." *Bulletin of the Nutrition Foundation of India* 8 (2): 1–4.

Gopalan, C. 1983. "Small Is Healthy? For the Poor, Not for the Rich." *Nutrition Foundation of India Bulletin* 4 (4): 1–5.

Gopalan, C., and M. Chatterjee. 1985. *Use of Growth Charts for Promoting*

Child Nutrition: A Review of Global Experience. Special Publication Series No. 2. New Delhi: Nutrition Foundation of India.

Gopaldas, T. 1988. "Field Level Health Workers' Skills in Detection of Growth Retardation and Faltering of Young Children." *Indian Journal of Pediatrics* 55 (1, Suppl.): S55–S58.

Gordon, J. E., J. B. Wyon, and W. Ascoli. 1967. "The Second Year Death Rate in Less Developed Countries." *American Journal of Medical Sciences* 254: 357–380.

GOT/WHO/UNICEF (Government of Tanzania/World Health Organization/United Nations Children's Fund). 1988. *The Joint WHO/UNICEF Nutrition Support Programme in Iringa, Tanzania: 1983–88 Evaluation Report.* Dar es Salaam: Government of the United Republic of Tanzania.

Gould, S. J. 1981. *The Mismeasurement of Man.* New York: Norton.

Gow, D. D., and J. Vansant. 1983. "Beyond the Rhetoric of Rural Development Participation: How Can It Be Done?" *World Development* 11 (5): 427–446.

Graham, G. G., and T. B. Adrainzen. 1972. "Late 'Catch-up' Growth after Severe Infantile Malnutrition." *Johns Hopkins Medical Journal* 131: 204–211.

Graitcer, P. L., and E. M. Gentry. 1981. "Measuring Children: One Reference for All." *Lancet* 2: 297–299.

Grant, J. P. 1987. *The State of the World's Children 1987.* New York: UNICEF.

Grantham-McGregor, S., C. Powell, and S. Walker. 1989. "Nutritional Supplements, Stunting, and Child Development." *Lancet* 2: 809–810.

Grantham-McGregor, S. M., W. Schofield, and D. Haggard. 1989. "Maternal-Child Interaction in Survivors of Severe Malnutrition Who Received Psychosocial Stimulation." *European Journal of Clinical Nutrition* 43 (1): 45–52.

Grantham-McGregor, S. M., W. Schofield, and C. Powell. 1987. "The Development of Severely Malnourished Children Who Received Psychosocial Stimulation: Six Year Follow-up." *Pediatrics* 79 (2): 247–254.

Gratz, N. G. 1987. *The Effect of Water Development Programmes on Malaria and Malaria Vectors in Turkey.* PEEM/7/WP/87.6b. Rome: Joint WHO/FAO/UNEP Panel of Experts on Environmental Management for Vector Control.

Graves, P. L. 1978. "Nutrition and Infant Behavior: A Replication Study in the Katmandu Valley, Nepal." *American Journal of Clinical Nutrition* 31 (3): 541–551.

Gray, C. S. 1986. "State-Sponsored Primary Health Care in Africa: The Recurrent Cost of Performing Miracles." *Social Science and Medicine* 22 (3): 361–368.

Greeley, M., and S. Begum. 1983. "Women's Employment and Agriculture: Extracts from a Case Study." In *Women in Bangladesh: Some Socio-Economic Issues,* ed. J. Huq, H. A. Begum, K. Salahuddin, and S. R. Qadir. Dhaka: Women for Women.

Greene, J. 1989. "Tamil Nadu: Where Do We Go from Here?" International Nutrition Seminar. Ithaca: Cornell University, 5 October.

Greene, J. G., N. A. Fox, and M. Lewis. 1983. "The Relationship between Neonatal Characteristics and Three-Month Mother-Infant Interaction in High-Risk Infants." *Child Development* 54 (5): 1286–1296.

Greenwood, B., A. Greenwood, and S. Bradley. 1987. "Deaths in Infancy and Early Childhood in a Well-Vaccinated Rural West African Population." *Annals of Tropical Pediatrics* No. 2: 91–99.

Greer, J., and E. Thorbecke. 1986. "Food Poverty Profile Applied to Kenyan Smallholders." *Economic Development and Cultural Change* 35 (1): 115–141.

Greiner, T. 1975. *The Promotion of Bottle Feeding by Multinational Corporations: How Advertising and the Health Professions Have Contributed.* Cornell International Monograph Series 2. Ithaca: Cornell University.

Greiner, T., and M. C. Latham. 1981. "Factors Associated with Nutritional Status among Young Children in St. Vincent." *Ecology of Food and Nutrition* 10 (2): 135–141.

Gribble, J. N. 1993. "Birth Intervals, Gestational Age, and Low Birth Weight: Are the Relationships Confounded?" *Population Studies* 47 (1): 133–146.

Griffiths, M. 1991. "The Weaning Project: Improving Young Child Feeding Practices. Indonesia: Project Overview." Washington, D.C.: Manoff Group.

Griffiths, M. 1988a. "Growth Monitoring: Making It a Tool for Education." *Indian Journal of Pediatrics* 55 (1, Suppl.): S59–S66.

Griffiths, M. 1988b. "Maternal Confidence and Child Well-Being." Paper presented at the Annual Meeting of the Society for Applied Anthropology, Tampa, Fl.

Griffiths, M. 1985a. "Growth Monitoring of Preschool Children: Practical Considerations for Primary Health Care Projects." Information for Action Issue Paper. Washington, D.C.: World Federation of Public Health Associations, Prepared for UNICEF.

Griffiths, M. 1985b. "Healthy Children: Strong Communities. CARITAS Dominicana. ANEP." *Mothers and Children, Bulletin on Infant Feeding and Maternal Nutrition (American Public Health Association)* 4 (3): 1–3.

Griffiths, M. 1984. *A Nutrition Education Strategy for the Applied Nutrition Education Project (ANEP) CRS/CARITAS, Dominican Republic.* Consultant Report Series. Newton, Mass.: International Nutrition Communication Service, Education Development Center.

Griffiths, M., E. Piwoz, M. Favin, and J. Rosso. 1988. *Improved Young Child Feeding during Diarrhea: A Guide for Investigators and Program Managers.* Rosslyn, Va.: PRITECH.

Grosh, M. 1991. "The Household Survey as a Tool for Policy Change." Living Standards Measurement Study Working Paper No. 80. Washington, D.C.: World Bank, May.

Gross, D. R., and B. A. Underwood. 1971. "Technological Change and Caloric Costs: Sisal Agriculture in Northeast Brazil." *American Anthropologist* 73: 725–740.

Gross, R., M. Stange, N. W. Solomons, U. Oltersdorf, and I. R. Esquivel. 1987. "The Influence of Economic Deterioration in Brazil on the Nutritional Status of Children in Rio de Janeiro, Brazil." *Ecology of Food and Nutrition* 19: 265–279.

Guerrant, R. L., L. V. Kirchhoff, D. S. Shields, M. K. Nations, J. Leslie, M. A. DeSousa, J. G. Araujo, L. L. Correia, K. T. Sauer, K. E. McClelland, R. L. Trowbridge, and J. M. Hughes. 1983. "Prospective Study of Diarrheal Illnesses in Northeastern Brazil: Patterns of Disease, Nutritional Impact, Etiologies and Risk Factors." *Journal of Infectious Diseases* 148 (6): 986–997.

Gussow, J. D., and I. Contento. 1984. "Nutrition in a Changing World." *World Review of Nutrition and Dietetics* 44: 1–56.

Guyer, J. L. 1980 *Household Budgets and Women's Incomes.* Working Paper No. 28. Boston: Boston University.

Gwatkin, D. R., J. R. Wilcox, and J. D. Wray, eds. 1980. *Can Health and Nutrition Interventions Make a Difference?* Overseas Development Council Monograph No. 13. Washington, D.C.: Overseas Development Council.

Haaga, J. 1989. "Mechanisms for the Association of Maternal Age, Parity, and Birthspacing with Infant Health." In *Contraceptive Use and Controlled Fertility: Health Issues for Women and Children,* ed. A. M. Parnell. Washington, D.C.: National Academy Press.

Haaga, J., C. Kenrick, K. Test, and J. Mason. 1985. "An Estimate of the Prevalence of Malnutrition in Developing Countries." *World Health Statistics Quarterly* 38 (3): 331–347.

Haaga, J., J. Mason, F. Z. Omoro, V. Quinn, A. Rafferty, K. Test, and L. Wasonga. 1986. "Child Malnutrition in Rural Kenya: A Geographic and Agricultural Classification." *Ecology of Food and Nutrition* 18: 297–307.

Haas, E. 1990. *When Knowledge Is Power: Three Models of Change in International Organizations.* Berkeley: University of California Press.

Haas, J. D., H. Balcazar, and L. Caulfield. 1987. "Variation in Early Neonatal Mortality for Different Types of Fetal Growth Retardation." *American Journal of Physical Anthropology* No. 73: 467–473.

Habicht, J.-P. 1990. *Nutritional Surveillance for Policy Decisions.* Pew/Cornell Lecture Series on Food and Nutrition Policy. Ithaca: CFNPP.

Habicht, J.-P., and W. P. Butz. 1985. "Measurement of Health and Nutrition Effects of Large-Scale Nutrition Intervention Projects." Cornell University, Ithaca, N.Y. Mimeographed.

Habicht, J.-P., and W. P. Butz. 1983. "Measurement of Health and Nutrition Effect of Large-Scale Nutrition Projects." In *A Methodology to Review Public Health Interventions: Results from Nutrition Supplementation and Water and Sanitation Projects.* Cornell International Nutrition Monograph Series No. 15. Ithaca: Cornell University.

Habicht, J.-P., J. DaVanzo, and W. P. Butz. 1988. "Mother's Milk and Sewage: Their Interactive Effects on Infant Mortality." *Pediatrics* 81 (3): 456–520.

Habicht, J.-P., J. DaVanzo, and W. P. Butz. 1985. "Does Breastfeeding Really Save Lives or Are Apparent Benefits Due to Biases?" *American Journal of Epidemiology* 123 (2): 279–290.

Habicht, J.-P., J. M. Lane, and A. J. McDowell. 1978. "National Nutrition Surveillance." *Federation Proceedings* 37 (5): 1181–1187.

Habicht, J.-P., J. B. Mason, and H. Tabatabai. 1984. "Basic Concepts for the Design of Evaluation during Program Implementation." In *Methods for the Evaluation of the Impact of Food and Nutrition Programmes,* ed. D. E. Sahn, R. Lockwood, and N. S. Scrimshaw. Cambridge: United Nations University.

Haddad, L., and H. E. Bouis. 1990. *The Impact of Nutritional Status on Agricultural Productivity: Wage Evidence from the Philippines.* Discussion Paper 97. Warwick, Eng.: Development Economics Research Centre, University of Warwick.

Haddad, L., and J. Hoddinott. 1991. *Gender Aspects of Household Expenditures and Resource Allocation in the Côte d'Ivoire.* Applied Economics Discussion

Paper No. 112, Institute of Economics Studies Working Paper. Oxford: Oxford University.

Haines, M. R., and R. C. Avery. 1982. "Differential Infant and Child Mortality in Costa Rica: 1968–1973." *Population Studies* 36 (3): 31–44.

Hakim, P., and G. Solimano. 1976. "Nutrition and National Development: Establishing the Connection." *Food Policy* 1 (3): 249–259.

Hamill, P. V. V., T. A. Drizd, C. L. Johnson, R. B. Reed, A. F. Roche, and W. M. Moore. 1979. "Physical Growth: National Center for Health Statistics." *American Journal of Clinical Nutrition* 32 (3): 607–629.

Hamilton, S., B. Popkin, and D. Spicer. 1984. *Women and Nutrition in Third World Countries*. New York: Praeger Special Studies, Begin and Garvey Publishers.

Han, A. M., K. N. Oo, T. Aye, and T. Hliang. 1986. "Personal Toilet after Defecation and the Degree of Hand Contamination according to Different Methods Used." *Journal of Tropical Medicine and Hygiene* 89 (5): 237–241.

Hansen, J. P. 1986. "Older Maternal Age and Pregnancy Outcome: A Review of the Literature." *Obstetrical and Gynecological Survey* No. 41: 726–742.

Haratani, J., A. M. Viveros-Long, and A. M. Becerra Marzano de Gonzales. 1981. *Peru: CARE OPG Water Health Services Project*. Project Impact Evaluation No. 24. Washington, D.C.: United States Agency for International Development.

Harbert, L., and P. Scandizzo. 1982. *Food Distribution and Nutrition Intervention: The Case of Chile*. Staff Working Paper No. 512. Washington, D.C.: World Bank.

Harkness, R. M. 1983. "Village Women, Water and Development: An Evaluative Study of the Upper Region Water Supply Project in Bolgatanga District, Ghana." M.A. thesis, Carleton University.

Harrell, M. W., C. Parillon, and R. L. Franklin. 1989. "Nutritional Classification Study of Peru: Who and Where Are the Poor?" *Food Policy* 4: 313–329.

Harris, M. 1978. *Cannibals and Kings: The Origins of Culture*. New York: Random House.

Harrison, K. A. 1985. "Child-Bearing, Health and Social Priorities: A Survey of 22,774 Consecutive Births in Zaria, Northern Nigeria." *British Journal of Obstetrics and Gynecology* No. 92 (Suppl.): 1–22.

Harriss, B. 1987. "Nutrition and International Agricultural Research." *Food Policy* 12 (1): 29–34.

Hauspie, R. C., S. R. Das, M. A. Preece, and J. M. Tanner. 1980. "A Longitudinal Study of the Growth in Height of Boys and Girls of West Bengal (India) Aged Six Months to 20 Years." *Annals of Human Biology* 7 (5): 429–441.

Hazell, P. B. R. 1987. "Changing Patterns of Variability in Cereal Prices and Production." In *Agricultural Price Policy for Developing Countries*, ed. J. W. Mellor and R. Ahmed. Baltimore: Johns Hopkins University Press.

Hendrata, L. 1987. "Growth Monitoring and Promotion." Guideline for Programming. Unpublished.

Hendrata, L. 1985. "Growth Monitoring: Basic Concept, Management and Operational Issues." In *Growth Monitoring as a Primary Health Care Activity*. Workshop Proceedings, Yogyakarta, Indonesia, 20–24 August 1984.

Henry, F. J., A. Briend, and E. S. Cooper. 1989. "Targeting Nutritional Interventions: Is There a Role for Growth Monitoring?" *Health Policy and Planning* 4 (4): 295–300.

Hepinstall, E., C. Puckering, D. Skuse, K. Start, S. Zur–Spiro, and L. Dowdney. 1987. "Nutrition and Mealtime Behavior in Families of Growth-Retarded Children." *Human Nutrition: Applied Nutrition* 41A: 390–402.

Hepner, R., and N. C. Maiden. 1971. "Growth Rate, Nutrient Intake and Mothering as Determinants of Malnutrition in Disadvantaged Children." *Nutrition Review* 29 (10): 219–223.

Herdt, R. W., and C. Capule. 1983. *Adoption Spread and Production Impact of Modern Rice Varieties in Asia.* Los Baños, Philippines: International Rice Research Institute.

Hernandez, M. 1974. "Effect of Economic Growth on Nutrition in a Tropical Community." *Ecology of Food and Nutrition* 3: 283–291.

Herrera, M. G., J. O. Mora, B. de Paredes, and M. Wagner. 1980. "Maternal Weight/Height and the Effect of Food Supplementation during Pregnancy and Lactation." In *Maternal Nutrition during Pregnancy and Lactation,* ed. H. Aebi and R. Whitehead. Bern: Hans Huber.

Hetzel, B. S. 1988. *The Prevention and Control of Iodine Deficiency Disorders.* ACC/SCN State-of-the-Art Series Nutrition Policy Discussion Paper No. 3. Rome: United Nations Food and Agriculture Organization.

Heywood, P. 1982. "The Functional Significance of Malnutrition: Growth and Prospective Risk of Death in the Highlands of Papua New Guinea." *Journal of Food and Nutrition* 39 (1): 1–19.

Himes, J. H. 1984. "Appropriateness of Parent-Specific Stature Adjustment for U.S. Black Children." *Journal of National Medical Association* 76 (1): 55–57.

Himes, J. R., C. Landers, and J. Leslie. 1992. *Women, Work, and Child Care.* Florence, Italy: UNICEF, International Child Development Centre.

Hirshhorn, N. 1985. "Oral Rehydration Therapy: The Program and the Promise." Paper prepared for the Harvard School of Public Health and UNICEF Joint Conference by the John Snow Public Health Group, May.

Hobcraft, J. 1987. "Does Family Planning Save Children's Lives?" Paper prepared for the International Conference on Better Health for Women and Children through Family Planning, Nairobi, Kenya, 5–9 October.

Hoben, A. 1979. *Lessons from a Critical Examination of Livestock Projects in Africa.* USAID Program Evaluation Working Paper 26. Washington, D.C.: USAID.

Holland, C. 1987. "Hookworm Infection." In *The Impact of Helminth Infections on Human Nutrition: Schistosomes and Soil-Transmitted Helminths,* ed. L. S. Stephenson. Philadelphia: Taylor and Francis.

Hollis, C. 1986. *Using Communications to Solve Nutrition Problems: A Compendium.* Washington, D.C.: International Nutrition Communication Service and USAID.

Hollnsteiner, M. R. 1982. "Government Strategies for Urban Areas and Community Participation." *Assignment Children* Nos. 57–58: 44–64.

Holmboe-Ottesen, G., O. Mascarenhas, and M. Wandel. 1989. *Women's Role in Food Chain Activities and the Implications for Nutrition.* ACC/SCN State-of-the-Art Series Nutrition Policy Discussion Paper No. 4. Geneva: World Health Organization.

Holt, E. A. 1987. "Evaluation of the Impact of Measles Vaccination on Mortality and Nutritional Status in Haitian Children." Ph.D. diss., Tulane University.

Holt, E. A., R. Boulos, N. Halsey, L. M. Boulos, and C. Boulos. 1990. "Child Survival in Haiti: The Protective Effect of Measles Vaccination." *Pediatrics* 85 (2): 188–190.

Hook, E. B. 1985. "Maternal Age, Parental Age, and Human Chromosome Abormality: Nature, Magnitude, Etiology, and Mechanism of Effects." *Basic Life Sciences* No. 36: 117–132.

Hoorweg, J. and I. McDowell. 1979. *Evaluation of Nutrition Education in Africa.* New York: Mouton.

Hoorweg, J., and R. Niemeijer. 1989. *Intervention in Child Nutrition.* London: Kegan Paul International.

Hoorweg, J., and R. Niemeijer. 1980a. *The Impact of Nutrition Education at Three Centres in Central Province, Kenya.* Research Report No. 10. Leiden: African Studies Centre.

Hoorweg, J., and R. Niemeijer. 1980b. *The Nutritional Impact of the Pre-School Health Program at Three Clinics in Central Province, Kenya.* Research Report No. 11. Leiden: African Studies Centre.

Hopkins, R. 1987. "Interests and Regimes: The Subjective Dimension of International Politics." Paper presented at the Annual Meeting of the American Political Science Association, September.

Hornik, R. 1989. *Channel Effectiveness in Development Communication Programs.* Working Paper 111. Annenberg School of Communications, University of Pennsylvania. In *Public Communication Campaigns,* ed., R. Rice and C. Atkin. Newbury Park, Calif.: Sage.

Hornik, R. 1988. *Development Communication. Part Three: Communication and Nutrition.* Chapters 7, 8, and 9. New York: Longman.

Hornik, R. 1987. "Nutrition Education: An Overview." In *Food Policy,* ed. J. P. Gittinger, J. Leslie, and C. Hoisington. Baltimore: Johns Hopkins University Press.

Hornik, R. 1985. *Nutrition Education: A State of the Art Review.* ACC/SCN Nutrition Policy Discussion Paper No. 1. Rome: United Nations Food and Agriculture Organization.

Hoyle, B., M. Yunus, and L. Chen. 1980. "Breast-Feeding and Food Intake among Children with Acute Diarrheal Disease." *American Journal of Clinical Nutrition* No. 33: 2365–2371.

Huffman, S. L., G. Lopez de Romano, S. Madrid, K. Brown, M. Bentley, and R. Black. 1988. "Do Child Feeding Practices Change Due to Diarrhea in the Central Peruvian Highlands?" Center to Prevent Childhood Malnutrition, Bethesda, Md. Mimeographed.

Huffman, S. L., E. Piwoz, and M. Griffiths. 1985. "Effectiveness of a Community Based Growth Monitoring Project: Comparison of Weight-for-Age and Arm Circumference." Research Proposal. Baltimore and Washington, D.C.: Johns Hopkins University Press and Manoff International.

Huffman, S. L., M. Wolff, and S. Lowell. 1985. "Nutrition and Fertility in Bangladesh: Nutritional Status of Nonpregnant Women." *American Journal of Clinical Nutrition* 42(4):725–738.

Hughes, C. C., and J. M. Hunter. 1970. "Disease and 'Development' in Africa." *Social Science and Medicine* 3:443–493.

Hussain, M. A., C. N. Nwaka, and A. Omololu. 1985. "Effect of Early Malnutrition on Subsequent Growth in a Group of Nigerian Village Children." *Nutrition Reports International* 32 (4):885–891.

Huttly, S. R. A., D. Blum, B. R. Kirkwood, R. M. Emeh, N. Okeke, M. Ajala, G. S. Smith, D. C. Carson, O. Dosunmu-Ognbi, and R. G. Feachem. 1990. "The Imo State (Nigeria) Drinking Water Supply and Sanitation Project II: Impact on Dracunculiasis, Diarrhoea and Nutritional Status." *Transactions of the Royal Society of Tropical Medicine and Hygiene* 84 (2):316–321.

ICN (International Conference on Nutrition). 1992. *World Declaration and Plan of Action for Nutrition.* Papers presented at the International Conference on Nutrition held at the Food and Agriculture Organization of the United Nations, Rome, December 1992. Geneva: World Health Organization.

ICRW (International Center for Research on Women). 1989. *Strengthening Women: Health Research Priorities for Women in Developing Countries.* Washington, D.C.: International Center for Research on Women.

Imong, S. M., K. Rungruengthanakit, C. Ruangyuttikarn, L. Wongsawasdi, D. A. Jackson, and R. F. Drewett. 1989. "The Bacterial Content of Infant Weaning Foods and Water in Rural Northern Thailand." *Journal of Tropical Pediatrics* 35 (1):14–18.

Institute for Resource Development. 1989. *Burundi Demographic and Health Survey.* Columbia, Md.: Institute for Resource Development/Westinghouse.

Institute for Resource Development. 1980. *Published Reports in DHS Series.* Columbia, Md.: Institute for Resource Development/Westinghouse.

International Child Health Foundation. 1987. *Symposium Proceedings, Cereal-Based Oral Rehydration Therapy: Theory and Practice,* ed. C. B. Dale and R. S. Northrup. Columbia, Md.: International Child Health Foundation.

IFPRI (International Food Policy Research Institute). 1993. "Food Policy and Agricultural Technology to Improve Diet Quality and Nutrition: A Proposal for Strengthened Research Cooperation on Nutrition in the CGIAR and with National Institutions." IFPRI, Washington, D.C. Mimeographed.

International Vitamin A Consultative Group. 1992. *Nutrition Communications in Vitamin A Programs: A Resource Book.* Washington, D.C.: Nutrition Foundation.

IRRI (International Rice Research Institute). 1978. *Economic Consequence of the New Rice Technology.* Los Baños: International Rice Research Institute.

Irwin, D. 1989. "Political Economy and Peel's Repeal of the Corn Laws." *Economics and Politics* 1 (1):41–59.

Israel, R., and J. P. N. Tighe. 1984. *Nutrition Education, Review and Analysis of the Literature.* Nutrition Education Series No. 7. Paris: UNESCO.

Jayasuriya, S. K., and R. T. Shand. 1986. "Technical Change and Labour Absorption in Asian Agriculture: Some Emerging Trends." *World Development* 14 (3):415–428.

Jelliffe, D. B. 1966. *The Assessment of the Nutritional Status of the Community.* Geneva: WHO.

Jelliffe, D. B., and E. Jelliffe. 1978. *Human Milk in the Modern World.* Oxford: Oxford University Press.

Jelliffe, D. B., and I. Maddocks. 1964. "Ecological Malnutrition in the New Guinea Highlands." *Clinical Pediatrics* 3 (7):432–438.

Jiggins, J. 1986. *Gender-Related Impacts and the Work of the International Agricultural Research Centers.* CGIAR Study Paper No. 17. Washington, D.C.: World Bank.

Jimenez. E. 1990. "Social Sector Pricing Policy Revisited: A Survey of Some Recent Controversies." *Proceedings of the World Bank Annual Conference on Development Economics 1989* (Supplement to *World Bank Economic Review* and *World Bank Research Observer*), pp. 109–138.

Jobert. B. 1985. "Populism and Health Policy: The Case of Community Health in India." *Social Science and Medicine* 20 (1):1–28.

Joekes, S. 1989. "Women's Work and Social Support for Child Care in the Third World." In *Women, Work and Child Welfare in the Third World,* ed. J. Leslie and M. Paolisso. Boulder: Westview Press.

Johnson, D. W., and R. T. Johnson. 1985. "Nutrition Education: A Model for Effectiveness, a Synthesis of Research." *Journal of Nutrition Education* 17 (2, Suppl.): S1–S24.

Johnston, B. F., and W. C. Clark, eds. 1982. *Redesigning Rural Development: A Strategic Perspective.* Baltimore: Johns Hopkins University Press.

Johnston, F. E., B. Newman, J. Cravioto, E. DeLicardie, and T. Scholl. 1980. "A Factor Analysis of Correlates of Nutritional Status in Mexican Children, Birth to 3 Years." In *Social and Biological Predictors of Nutritional Status, Physical Growth, and Neurological Development,* ed. L. S. Greene and F. E. Johnston. New York: Academic.

Jones, C. 1983. "The Mobilization of Women's Labor for Cash Crop Production: A Game Theoretic Approach." *American Journal of Agricultural Economics* 65 (5):1049–1054.

Jones, C. D. R., M. S. Jarjou, R. G. Whitehead, and E. Jequier. 1987. "Fatness and the Energy Cost of Carrying Loads in African Women." *Lancet* 2:1331–1332.

Jonsson, U. 1989. Personal communication about the nature of nutrition education in the Iringa Nutrition Programme. Cornell University, Ithaca, N.Y.

Jonsson, U. 1988. "A Conceptual Approach to the Understanding and Explanation of Hunger and Malnutrition in Society." In *Hunger and Society,* Vol. 1, *Understanding of the Causes.* Cornell International Nutrition Monograph Series No. 17. Ithaca: Cornell University.

Jonsson, U., M. C. Latham, L. L. Bondestam, and R. Chorlton. 1988. *Causes and Strategies in Tanzania.* Cornell International Nutrition Monograph Series No. 19. Ithaca: Cornell University.

Joseph, S. 1985. "The Case for Clinical Services." In *Good Health at Low Cost,* ed. S. B. Halstead, J. A. Walsh, and K. S. Warren. New York: Rockefeller Foundation.

Joy, L. 1973. "Food and Nutrition Planning." *Journal of Agricultural Economics* 24 (1):165–193.

Juster, F. T., and F. P. Stafford. 1991. "The Allocation of Time: Empirical Findings, Behavioral Models, and Problems of Measurement." *Journal of Economic Literature* 39:471–522.

Kadt, E. 1982. "Community Participation for Health: The Case of Latin

America." In *Practicing Health for All*, ed. D. Morley, J. Rohde, and G. Williams. Oxford: Oxford Medical Publications.

Kakwani, N. 1986. *Is Sex Bias Significant?* Working Paper No. 9. Helsinki: World Institute for Development Economics Research.

Kanaaneh. H. 1972. "The Relationship of Bottle Feeding to Malnutrition and Gastroenteritis in a Pre-industrial Setting." *Journal of Tropical Pediatrics and Child Health* No. 18:302–306.

Karlin, B. 1976. *Summary: The State of the Art of Delivering Low-Cost Health Services in Less-Developed Countries.* Washington, D.C.: American Public Health Association.

Kasarda, J. O., J. O. G. Billy, and K. West. 1986. *Status Enhancement and Fertility.* Orlando: Academic Press.

Kasongo Project Team. 1986. "Growth Decelerations among Under-5-Year-Old Children in Kasongo (Zaire). II. Relationship with Subsequent Risk of Dying, and Operational Consequences." *Bulletin of the World Health Organization* 64 (5):703–709.

Kasongo Project Team. 1983. "Anthropometric Assessment of Young Children's Nutritional Status as an Indicator of Subsequent Risk of Dying." *Journal of Tropical Pediatrics* 29 (1):69–75

Kasongo Project Team. 1981. "Influence of Measles Vaccination on Survival Pattern of 7- to 35-Month-Old Children in Kasongo, Zaire." *Lancet* 1:764–767.

Katz, J., K. P. West, I. Tarwotjo, and A. Sommer. 1989. "The Importance of Age in Evaluating Anthropometric Indices for Predicting Mortality." *American Journal of Epidemiology* 130 (6):1219–1226.

Kebede, H. 1978. *Improving Village Water Supplies in Ethiopia: A Case Study of the Socio-Economic Implication.* Addis Ababa: United Nations Economic Commission for Africa, UNICEF.

Kennedy, E. T. 1993. "The Effects of the Commercialization of Agriculture on Women's Control of Income and Health and Nutritional Status: The Case of Sugarcane in Kenya." In *Effects of Selected Policies and Programs on Women's Health and Nutritional Status.* Washington, D.C.: International Food Policy Research Institute.

Kennedy, E. T. 1988. "Alternatives to Consumer-Oriented Food Subsidies for Achieving Nutritional Objectives." In *Food Subsidies in Developing Countries,* ed. P. Pinstrup-Andersen. Baltimore: Johns Hopkins University Press.

Kennedy, E. T., and H. Alderman. 1987. *Comparative Analyses of Nutritional Effectiveness of Food Subsidies and Other Food-Related Interventions.* Washington, D.C.: International Food Policy Research Institute with Joint WHO/UNICEF Nutrition Support Programme.

Kennedy, E. T., and H. E. Bouis. 1993. *Linkages between Agriculture and Nutrition: Implications for Policy and Research.* Washington, D.C.: International Food Policy Research Institute.

Kennedy, E. T., and B. Cogill. 1988. *The Case of Sugarcane in Kenya: Part I, Effects of Cash Crop Production on Women's Income, Time Allocation, and Child Care Practices.* MSU/WID Working Paper No. 167. East Lansing: Michigan State University.

Kennedy, E. T., and B. Cogill. 1987. *Income and Nutritional Effects of the Com-*

mercialization of Agriculture in Southwestern Kenya. Research Report No. 63. Washington, D.C.: International Food Policy Research Institute.

Kennedy, E. T., and M. Garcia. 1993. "Effects of Selected Policies and Programs on Women's Health and Nutritional Status." International Food Policy Research Institute, Washington, D.C. Mimeographed.

Kennedy, E. T., S. Gershoff, R. Reed, and J. Austin. 1982. "Evaluation of the Effects of WIC Supplement Feeding on Birth Weight." *Journal of American Dietetic Association* 80 (3):220.

Kennedy, E. T., and O. Knudsen. 1985. "A Review of Supplementary Feeding Programmes and Recommendations on Their Design." In *Nutrition and Development,* ed. M. Biswas and P. Pinstrup-Andersen. Oxford: United Nations University and Oxford University Press.

Kennedy, E. T., and P. Peters. 1992. "Household Food Security and Child Nutrition: The Interaction of Income and Gender of Household Head." *World Development* 20(8):1077–1085.

Kennedy, E. T., and P. Pinstrup-Andersen. 1983. *Nutrition-Related Policies and Programs: Past Performances and Research Needs.* Washington, D.C.: International Food Policy Research Institute.

Kenya, P. R., O. W. Oddongo, G. Ounda, K. Waswa, J. Muttunga, A. Molla, S. Nath, A. Molla, W. Greenough, R. Juma, and B. Were. 1989. "Cereal Based Oral Rehydration Solutions." *Archives of Disease in Childhood* No. 64:1032–1035.

Kerkvliet, B. J. 1976. "Land Reform in the Philippines since the Marcos Coup." Paper presented at meeting of the Association of Asian Studies, Boston, April.

Kessel, E., S. Sastrinawata, and S. D. Mumford. 1985. "Correlates of Fetal Growth and Survival." *Acta Paediatrica Scand* 319 (Suppl.):120–127.

Keynes, G. M. 1935. *General Theory of Employment, Interest, and Money.* New York: Harcourt, Brace.

Khan, M. U. 1982. "Interruption of Shigellosis by Hand Washing." *Transactions of the Royal Society of Tropical Medicine and Hygiene* 76 (2):164–168.

Kielmann, A. A., and C. McCord. 1978. "Weight for Age as an Index of Risk of Death in Children." *Lancet* 1:1247–1250.

Kielmann, A. A., C. DeSweemer, D. Chernichovsky, I. Abroy, N. Masih, C. E. Taylor, R. L. Parker, W. A. Reinke, D. N. Kakar, and R. S. S. Sarma. 1983. *Child and Maternal Health Services in Rural India: The Narangwal Experiment,* Vol 1, *Integrated Nutrition and Child Care.* Baltimore: Johns Hopkins University Press.

Kikuchi, M., N. Fortuna, L. Bambo, and Y. Hayami. 1978. "Polarization of a Laguna Village." IRRI Agricultural Economics Paper 78-01. Los Baños: International Rice Research Institute.

King, E. M. 1990. *Educating Girls and Women: Investing in Development.* Washington, D.C.: World Bank.

King, E. M., and M. A. Hill, eds. 1993. *Women's Education in Developing Countries: Barriers, Benefits, and Policies.* Baltimore: Johns Hopkins University Press.

King, M. H., F. M. King, D. C. Morley, H. J. L. Burgess, and A. P. Burgess. 1972. *Nutrition for Developing Countries.* Oxford: Oxford University Press.

Kirksey, A., G. G. Harrison, O. M. Galal, G. P. McCabe, T. D. Wachs, and A. Rahmanifar. 1992. *The Human Costs of Moderate Malnutrition in an Egyptian*

Village. Human Nutrition Collaborative Research Support Program. Washington, D.C.: USAID, Office of Nutrition.

Klesges, R. C., T. J. Coates, G. Brown, J. Styrgeon-Tillisch, L. Moldenhauer-Klesges, B. Holzer, J. Woolfrey, and J. Vollmer. 1983. "Parental Influences on Children's Eating Behavior and Relative Weight." *Journal of Applied Behavior Analysis* 16:371–378.

Klesges, R. C., J. M. Malott, P. F. Boschee, and J. M. Weber. 1986. "The Effects of Parental Influences on Children's Food Intake, Physical Activity, and Relative Weight." *International Journal of Eating Disorders* 5:335–346.

Knight, J., and S. Grantham-McGregor. 1985. "Using Primary-Schoolchildren to Improve Child-Rearing Practices in Rural Jamaica." *Child: Care, Health, and Development* 11 (2):81–90.

Knodel, J. 1977. "Family Limitation and the Fertility Transaction: Evidence from the Age Patterns of Fertility in Europe and Asia." *Population Studies* No. 31:219–249.

Koenig, M. A., J. F. Phillips, O. M. Campbell, and S. D'Souza. 1990. "Birth Intervals and Childhood Mortality in Rural Bangladesh." *Demography* 27 (2):251–265.

Koenig, M. A., U. Rob, M. A. Khan, J. Chakraborty, and V. Fauveau. 1992. "Contraceptive Use in Matlab, Bangladesh, in 1990: Levels, Trends and Explanations." *Studies in Family Planning* 23 (6):352–362.

Korten, D. C. 1980. "Community Organization and Rural Development: A Learning Process Approach." *Public Administration Review* 40 (5, Special supplement, September–October):480–511.

Koster, F. T., G. Curlin, and K. Azaz. 1981. "Synergistic Impact of Measles and Diarrhoea on Nutrition and Mortality in Bangladesh." *Bulletin of the World Health Organization* 59 (6):901–908.

Kotelchuck, M., and E. H. Newberger. 1983. "Failure to Thrive: A Controlled Study of Familial Characteristics." *Journal of the American Academy of Child Psychiatry* 22 (4):322–328.

Kramer, M. S. 1987. "Determinants of Low Birth Weight: Methodological Assessment and Meta-Analysis." *Bulletin of the World Health Organization* 65 (5):663–737.

Krishnan, T. N. 1985. "Health Statistics in Kerala State India." In *Good Health at Low Cost,* ed. S. B. Halstead, J. A. Walsh, and K. S. Warren. New York: Rockefeller Foundation.

Kuhn, T. 1970. *The Structure of Scientific Revolutions.* Chicago: University of Chicago Press.

Kulin, H., N. Bwibo, D. Mutie, and S. Santner. 1982. "The Effect of Chronic Childhood Malnutrition on Pubertal Growth and Development." *American Journal of Clinical Nutrition* 36 (3):527–536.

Laforgia, G. M. 1986. *Local Organizations for Rural Health in Panama: Community Participation, Bureaucratic Reorientation, and Political Will.* Rural Development Committee Special Series on Rural Local Organization. Ithaca: Cornell University.

Lal, D. 1976. "Agricultural Growth, Real Wages, and the Rural Poor in India." *Economic and Political Weekly* 9 (26):A47–A61.

Lalitha, N. V., and J. Standley. 1988. "Training Workers and Supervisors in

Growth Monitoring: Looking at ICDS." *Indian Journal of Pediatrics* 55 (1, Suppl.):S44–S54.

Lambert, J. 1988. "Pakistan: Update on Breastfeeding." *Mothers and Children* 7 (2):5–6.

Lambert, J., and J. Basford. 1977. "Port Moresby Infant Feeding Survey." *Papua New Guinea Medical Journal* No. 20:175–179.

La Montagne, J., P. L. Engle, and M. F. Zeitlin. 1993. "Maternal Employment and Nutritional Status of 12–18 Month-Old Children in Managua, Nicaragua." Paper presented at the International Nutrition Mini-symposium II: Malnutrition, Growth, and Development, Federation of American Societies for Experimental Biology Annual Meeting, Anaheim, California, 5–9 April. Abstract No. 3256 in *Abstracts of FASEB*.

Lappe, F. M., and J. Collins. 1977. *Food First: Beyond the Myth of Scarcity.* Boston: Houghton Mifflin.

Latham, M. C. 1991. "Growth Monitoring and Promotion." In *Anthropometric Assessment of Nutritional Status,* ed. John H. Himes. New York: Wiley-Liss.

Latham, M. C. 1987. "Strategies for the Control of Malnutrition and the Influence of the Nutritional Sciences." In *Food Policy: Integrating Supply, Distribution, and Consumption,* ed. J. P. Gittinger, J. Leslie, and C. Hoisington. Baltimore: Johns Hopkins University Press.

Latham, M. C. 1984. "Smallness—A Symptom of Deprivation." *Nutrition Foundation of India Bulletin* 5 (3):7–8.

Latham, M. C., L. Bondestam, R. Chorlton, and U. Jonsson. 1988. *Hunger and Society.* Vols. 1, 2 and 3. Cornell University International Nutrition Monograph Series Nos. 17, 18, and 19. Ithaca: Cornell University.

Leaf, M. J. 1983. "The Green Revolution and Cultural Change in a Punjab Village." *Economic Development and Cultural Change* 31:227–270.

Lebshtein, A. K., and A. M. El Bahay. 1976. "The Extent of Breast and Bottle Feeding of Children in Cairo and Its Effects on Their Growth." *Journal of Egypt Public Health Association* No. 51:242–257.

Lechtig, A., and R. E. Klein. 1981. "Prenatal Nutrition and Birth Weight: Is There a Causal Association?" In *Maternal Nutrition in Pregnancy—Eating for Two?* ed. J. Dobbing. London: Academic Press.

Lehman, D., P. Howard, and P. Heywood. 1988. "Nutrition and Morbidity: Acute Lower Respiratory Tract Infections, Diarrhea and Malaria." *Papua New Guinea Medical Journal* No. 31:109–116.

Lele, U. 1989. *Madia Studies: Kenya Case Study.* Washington, D.C.: World Bank.

Lele, U. 1975. *The Design of Rural Development: Lessons from Africa.* Baltimore: Johns Hopkins University Press.

Lerman, C., J. W. Molyneaux, S. Moeljodihardjo, and S. Pandjaitan. 1989. "The Correlation between Family Planning Program Inputs and Contraceptive Use in Indonesia." *Studies in Family Planning* No. 20:26–37.

Leslie, J. 1992. "Women's Lives and Women's Health: Using Social Science Research to Promote Better Health for Women." *Journal of Women's Health* 1 (4):307–318.

Leslie, J. 1989a. "Women's Time: A Factor in the Use of Child Survival Technologies?" *Health Policy and Planning* 4 (1):1–16.

Leslie, J. 1989b. "Women's Work and Child Nutrition in the Third World." In

Women, Work, and Child Welfare in the Third World, ed. J. Leslie and M. Paolisso. Boulder: Westview Press.

Leslie, J. 1988. "Women's Work and Child Nutrition in the Third World." *World Development* 16 (11):1341–1362.

Leslie, J., and G. R. Gupta. 1989. "Utilization of Formal Services for Maternal Nutrition and Health Care in the Third World." International Center for Research on Women, Washington, D.C. Mimeographed.

Leslie, J., and D. T. Jamison. 1990. "Health and Nutrition Considerations in Educational Planning: I—Educational Consequences of Health Problems among School Age Children." *Food and Nutrition Bulletin* 12 (3):191–203.

Leslie, J., M. Lycette, and M. Buvinic. 1988. "Weathering Economic Crises: The Crucial Role of Women in Health." In *Health, Nutrition, and Economic Crises: Approaches to Policy in the Third World,* ed. D. E. Bell and M. R. Reich. Dover, Mass.: Auburn House.

Lettenmeier, C., L. Liskin, C. Church, and J. Harris. 1988. "Mothers' Lives Matter: Maternal Health in the Community." *Population Reports* Series L, No. 7.

Levin, H. M. 1987. "Economic Dimensions of Iodine Deficiency Disorders." In *The Prevention and Control of Iodine Deficiency Disorders,* ed. B. S. Hetzel, J. T. Dunn, and J. B. Stanbury. New York: Elsevier.

Levin, H. M., E. Pollitt, R. Galloway, and J. McGuire. 1990. "Micronutritional Deficiency Disorders." In *Evolving Health Priorities in Developing Countries,* ed. D. T. Jamison and W. H. Mosley. Washington, D.C.: World Bank, Population, Health and Nutrition Division.

LeVine, R. 1987. "Women's Schooling, Patterns of Fertility and Child Survival." *Educational Researcher* 16 (1):21–27.

Levinson, J. 1989. Personal communication and unpublished material about the effectiveness of nutrition education strategies.

Levy, S., B. Iverson, and H. Walberg. 1980. "Nutrition Education Research: An Interdisciplinary Evaluation and Review." *Health Education Quarterly* 7 (2):107–126.

Lindblom, C., and D. Cohen. 1979. *Usable Knowledge: Social Science and Social Problem Solving.* New Haven: Yale University Press.

Lipsitt, L. S., C. Crook, and C. Booth. 1985. "The Transitional Infant: Behavioral Development and Feeding." *American Journal of Clinical Nutrition* 41 (2 supplement):485–496.

Lipton, M. 1983. *Poverty, Undernutrition and Hunger.* World Bank Staff Working Paper No. 597. Washington, D.C.: World Bank.

Lipton, M., and E. de Kadt. 1987. *Agriculture-Health Linkages.* Geneva: WHO.

Lipton, M., and R. Longhurst. 1989. *New Seeds and Poor People.* London: Unwin Hyman.

Liu, K., J. Stamler, A. Dyer, J. McKeever, and P. McKeever. 1978. "Statistical Methods to Assess and Minimize the Role of Intra-Individual Variability in Obscuring the Relationship between Dietary Lipids and Serum Cholesterol." *Journal of Chronic Disease* 31:399–418.

Ljungqvist, B. 1987. *Social Mobilization for Nutrition: The Iringa Experience.* Dar Es Salaam: UNICEF.

Longe, O. G. 1985. "The Role of Women in Production, Processing, and Preservation." Paper presented at the seminar organized by the Institute of African Studies, University of Ibadan, Ibadan, Nigeria, 20–21 June.

Longhurst, R. 1981. *Rapid Rural Appraisal.* IDS Bulletin 12. Sussex, Eng.: Institute for Development Studies.

Loose, E. 1980. "Women's Time Budget in Rural Senegal." Paper presented for the workshop on Sahelian Agriculture, Department of Agricultural Economics, Purdue University, West Lafayette, Ind.

Lopez, C. 1978. "Nutrition and Government Policy in Colombia." In *Nutrition and National Policy,* ed. B. Winikoff. Cambridge: Massachusetts Institute of Technology Press.

Lowbury, E. J. L., H. A. Lilly, and J. P. Bull. 1964. "Disinfection of Hands: Removal of Transient Organisms." *British Medical Journal* No. 5403 (July 25):230–233.

Lozoff, B. 1989. "Nutrition and Behavior." *American Psychologist* 44 (2):231–236.

Lung'aho, M. S., and G. H. Pelto. 1983. "The Weaning Process: A Review of Cross-Cultural Patterns of Infant and Young Child Feeding and Their Determinants." Prepared for WHO, Storrs, Conn. Mimeographed.

Lutter, C., J. Mora, J.-P. Habicht, K. M. Rasmussen, D. S. Robson, S. G. Sellters, C. M. Super, and M. G. Herrera. 1989. "Nutritional Supplementation: Effects on Child Stunting Because of Diarrhea." *American Journal of Clinical Nutrition* 50:1–8.

Lutter, C., J.-P. Habicht, J. A. Rivera, and R. Martorell. 1992. "The Relationship between Energy Intake and Diarrhoeal Disease in Their Effects on Child Growth: Biological Model, Evidence, and Implications for Public Health Policy." *Food and Nutrition Bulletin* 14 (1):36–42.

McAnarney, E. R. 1987. "Young Maternal Age and Adverse Neonatal Outcome." *American Journal of Diseases in Childhood* No. 141:1053–1059.

McCloskey, D. 1985. *The Rhetoric of Economics.* Madison: University of Wisconsin Press.

McCullough, A. L., A. Kirksey, T. D. Wachs, G. P. McCabe, N. S. Bassily, Z. Bishry, O. M. Galal, G. G. Harrison, and N. W. Jerome. 1990. "Vitamin B-6 Status of Egyptian Mothers: Relation of Infant Behavior and Maternal-Infant Interactions." *American Journal of Clinical Nutrition* 51 (6):1067–1074.

MacDonald, M. 1977. *Food, Stamps, and Income Maintenance.* New York: Academic Press.

McFarland, E. L. 1989. "Conclusions." In *Successful Development in Africa: Case Studies of Projects, Programs and Policies.* Washington, D.C.: World Bank.

McGraw, M. B. 1943. *The Neuromuscular Maturation of the Human Infant.* New York: Columbia University Press.

McGuire, J. S., and J. E. Austin. 1987. *Beyond Survival: Children's Growth for National Development.* New York: Assignment Children: UNICEF.

McGuire, J. S., and B. Popkin. 1990. "Helping Women Improve Nutrition in the Developing World: Beating the Zero Sum Game." Technical Paper No. 114. Washington, D.C.: World Bank.

McGuire, J., and B. M. Popkin. 1989. "Beating the Zero-Sum Game: Women and Nutrition in the Third World, Part 1." *Food and Nutrition Bulletin* 11 (4):38–63.

McKay, A., L. Sinisterra, and A. McKay. 1978. "Improving Cognitive Ability in Chronically Deprived Children." *Science* 200 (4339):270–278.

McKenzie, J., and P. Mumford. 1965. "The Evaluation of Nutrition Education Programmes: A Review of the Present Situation." *World Review of Nutrition and Dietetics* 17:91–149.

McMurray, D. N., S. A. Loomis, L. J. Casazza, H. Rey, and R. Miranda. 1981. "Development of Impaired Cell Mediated Immunity in Mild and Moderate Malnutrition." *American Journal of Clinical Nutrition* No. 34:68–77.

McQuail, D. 1989. *Mass Communication Theory.* Newbury Park, Calif.: Sage.

McSweeney, B. G. 1979. "Collection and Analysis of Data on Rural Women's Time Use." *Studies in Family Planning* 10(11–12):379–384.

McSweeney, B. G., and M. Freedman. 1980. "Lack of Time as an Obstacle to Women's Education: The Case of Upper Volta." *Comparative Education Review* 2 (2, Suppl., Part 2):S124–S139.

Magnani, R. J., S. C. Tourkin, and M. J. Hartz. 1984. *Evaluation of the Provincial Water Project in the Philippines.* Washington, D.C.: International Statistical Program Center, Bureau of the Census, U.S. Department of Commerce.

Mahalanabis, D., K. N. Jalan, T. K. Maitra, and S. K. Agarwal. 1976. "Vitamin A Absorption in Ascariasis." *American Journal of Clinical Nutrition* 29 (2):1372–1375.

Mahalanabis, D., T. W. Simpson, M. L. Chakraborty, A. K. Bhattacharjee, and K. L. Mukherjee. 1979. "Malabsorption of Water Miscible Vitamin A in Children with Giardiasis and Ascariasis." *American Journal of Clinical Nutrition* 32 (2):313–318.

Mahmood, T. A., D. M. Campbell, and A. W. Wilson. 1988. "Maternal Height, Shoe Size, and Outcome of Labour in White Primigravidas: A Prospective Anthropometric Study." *British Medical Journal* 297 (6647, August 20–27):515–517.

Malcolm, L. A. 1974. "Ecological Factors Related to Child Growth and Nutritional Status." In *Nutrition and Malnutrition: Identification and Measurement,* ed. A. F. Roche and F. Falkner. New York: Plenum Press.

Manoff International. 1984. *Nutrition Communication and Behavior Change Component: Indonesian Nutrition Development Program, Vol. 4: Household Evaluation; Vol. 5: Kader Evaluation.* Washington, D.C.: Manoff International.

Manoff, R. K. 1987. "Nutrition Education: Lessons Learned." In *Food Policy: Integrating Supply, Distribution, and Consumption,* ed. J. P. Gittinger, J. Leslie, and C. Hoisington. Washington, D.C.: World Bank.

Manoff, R. K. 1985. *Social Marketing, New Imperatives for Public Health.* New York: Praeger.

Marquez, C. B., P. L. Pingali, and F. G. Palis. 1992. "Farmer Health Impact of Long-Term Pesticide Exposure—A Medical and Economic Analysis in the Philippines." Paper presented at a workshop on Measuring the Health and Environmental Effects of Pesticides, Bellagio, Italy, 30 March–3 April.

Marquez, L. 1988. "Growth Monitoring: Ritual or Nutrition Intervention? PRICOR Project, Center for Human Services." Paper presented at the 116th Annual Meeting of the American Public Health Association, Boston.

Marshall, E. 1990. "USDA Admits 'Mistake' in Doctoring Study." *Science* 247 (February):522.

Martin, T. H. 1982. "A Literature Survey Exploring the Impact of Agricultural Development Projects on Nutrition." World Bank, Washington, D.C., Mimeograph.

Martines, J. 1988. "The Interrelationships between Malnutrition and Diarrhea, and Mode of Feeding in Early Infancy among the Urban Poor in South Brazil." Ph.D. diss., London School of Tropical Medicine and Hygiene.

Martines, J., M. Phillips, and R. G. A. Feachem. 1991. *Diarrheal Diseases Health Section Priorities Review.* Washington, D.C.: World Bank.

Martorell, R. 1993. "Enhancing Human Potential in Guatemalan Adults through Improved Nutrition in Early Childhood." *Nutrition Today* (January–February) 28 (1):6–13.

Martorell, R. 1989. "Body Size, Adaptation and Function." *Human Organization* 48 (1):15–20.

Martorell, R. 1985. "Child Growth Retardation: A Discussion of Its Causes and Its Relationship to Health." In *Nutritional Adaptation in Man,* ed. K. Blaxter and J. C. Waterlow. London: John Libbey.

Martorell, R., and G. Arroyave. 1988. "Malnutrition, Work Output and Energy Needs." In *Capacity for Work in the Tropics,* ed. K. J. Collins and D. F. Roberts. Cambridge: Cambridge University Press.

Martorell, R., H. Delgado, V. Valverde, and R. E. Klein. 1981. "Maternal Stature, Fertility, and Infant Mortality." *Human Biology* 53 (3):303–312.

Martorell, R., D. Foote, and C. Kendall. 1986. "Health Education as a Strategy for Improving the Management of Diarrhoea." In *Proceedings of the XIII International Congress of Nutrition,* ed. T. G. Taylor and N. G. Jenkins. London: John Libbey.

Martorell, R., J.-P. Habicht, C. Yarbrough, A. Lechtig, R. E. Klein, and K. A. Western. 1975. "Acute Morbidity and Rural and Physical Growth in Rural Guatemalan Children." *American Journal of Diseases of Children* 129 (2):1296–1301.

Martorell, R., and T. J. Ho. 1984. "Malnutrition, Morbidity, and Mortality." In *Child Survival: Strategies for Research,* ed. H. Mosley and L. Chen. *Population and Development Review* 10 (Supp.):49–68.

Martorell, R., L. K. Khan, and D. G. Schroeder. 1994. "Reversibility of Stunting: Epidemiological Findings in Children from Developing Countries." *European Journal of Clinical Nutrition* 48 (Supplement 1):S45–S57.

Martorell, R., J. Mason, K. Rasmussen, T. J. Ho, and J.-P. Habicht. 1985. "Child Feeding Practices: Knowledge, Research Needs, and Policy Implications." Cornell University, Ithaca, N.Y. Mimeographed.

Martorell, R., and C. O'Gara. 1985. "Breastfeeding, Infant Health, and Socioeconomic Status." *Medical Anthropology* 9 (2):173–181.

Martorell, R., J. Rivera, and H. Kaplowitz. 1990. "Consequences of Stunting in Early Childhood for Adult Body Size in Rural Guatemala." *Annales Nestlé* 48:85–92.

Martorell, R., J. Rivera, H. Kaplowitz, and E. Pollitt. 1992. "Long-Term Consequences of Growth Retardation during Early Childhood." In *Human Growth: Basic and Clinical Aspects,* ed. M. Hernandez and J. Argente. New York: Elsevier Science Publishers B.V.

Martorell, R. and M. Shekar. Forthcoming. "Growth Faltering Rates in Berkeley,

Guatemala, and Tamil Nadu: Implications for Growth Monitoring Programs." *Food and Nutrition Bulletin* 15 (3).

Martorell. R., C. Yarbrough, S. Yarbrough, and R. E. Klein. 1980. "The Impact of Ordinary Illnesses on the Dietary Intakes of Malnourished Children." *American Journal of Clinical Nutrition* 33(2):345–350.

Martorell, R., C. Yarbrough, R. E. Klein, and A. Lechtig. 1979. "Malnutrition, Body Size and Skeletal Maturation: Interrelationships and Implications for Catch-Up Growth." *Human Biology* 51 (3):371–389.

Mason, J. B., J.-P. Habicht, H. Tabatabai, and V. Valverde. 1984. *Nutritional Surveillance*. Geneva: World Health Organization.

Mata, L. 1978. *The Children of Santa Maria Cauque*. Cambridge: Massachusetts Institute of Technology Press.

Mata, L., M. Allen, P. Jimenez, M. Garcia, W. Vargas, M. Rodriquez, and C. Valerin. 1982. "Promotion of Breast-Feeding, Health, and Growth among Hospital-Born Neonates, and among Infants of a Rural Area of Costa Rica." In *Diarrhea and Malnutrition: Interactions, Mechanisms and Interventions*. ed. L. C. Chen and N. S. Scrimshaw. New York: Plenum Press.

Mata, L. J., R. A. Kromal, J. J. Urrutia, and B. Garcia. 1977. "Effect of Infection on Food Intake and the Nutritional State: Perspectives as Viewed from the Village." *American Journal of Clinical Nutrition* 30 (8):1215–1227.

Mateus, A. 1983. *Targeting Food Subsidies for the Needy: The Use of Cost-Benefit Analysis and Institutional Design*. World Bank Staff Working Papers No. 617. Washington, D.C.: World Bank.

Mathew, S. N.d. "Tamil Nadu Integrated Nutrition Project." A presentation in Madras, India.

Mauldin, W. P. 1983. "Population Programs and Fertility Regulation." In *Determinants of Fertility in Developing Countries*. Vol. 2, *Fertility Regulation and Institutional Influences,* ed. R. Bulatao and R. D. Lee. New York: Academic Press.

Mauldin, W. P., and J. Ross. 1991. "Family Planning Programs: Efforts and Results, 1982–89." *Studies in Family Planning* 22 (6): 350–367.

Mauldin, W. P., and S. Segal. 1988. "Prevalence of Contraceptive Use: Trends and Issues." *Studies in Family Planning* 19(6): 335–353.

Maxwell, S., and A. Fernando. 1989. "Cash Crops in Developing Countries: The Issues, the Facts, the Policies." *World Development* 17 (11): 1677–1708.

Meegama, S. A. 1980. *Socio-Economic Determinants of Infant and Child Mortality in Sri Lanka: An Analysis of Post-War Experience*. WFS Scientific Report No. 8. London: World Fertility Survey.

Meehan, R., A. Viveros-Long, J. M. Hernandez, and S. de Heckadon. 1982. *Panama Rural Water*. Project Impact Evaluation Report No. 22. Washington, D.C.: United States Agency for International Development.

Meier, G. M., ed. 1983. *Pricing Policy for Development Management*. EDI Series in Economic Development. Baltimore: Johns Hopkins University Press.

Mellor, J. W. 1978. "Food Price Policies and Income Distribution in Low Income Countries." *Economic Development and Cultural Changes* 21 (1):1–26.

Mellor, J. W., and R. Ahmed. 1988. *Agricultural Price Policy for Developing Countries*. Baltimore: Johns Hopkins University Press.

Mensch, B., H. Lentzner, and S. Preston. 1985. *Socioeconomic Differentials in Child Mortality in Developing Countries*. New York: United Nations.

Merchant, K., and R. Martorell. 1988. "Frequent Reproductive Cycling: Does It Lead to Nutritional Depletion of Mothers?" *Progress in Food and Nutrition Science* No. 12:339–369.

Merchant, K., R. Martorell, T. Gonzalez-Cossio, J. Rivera, and J. D. Haas. 1990. *Maternal Nutritional Depletion: Evidence of Responses in Women to Frequent Reproductive Cycling*. Report No. 3, Maternal Nutrition and Health Care Program. Washington, D.C.: International Center for Research on Women.

Merrick, T. W. 1985. "The Effect of Piped Water on Early Childhood Mortality in Urban Brazil, 1970–1976." *Demography* 22 (1):1–24.

Merson, M. 1988. "WHO's Diarrhoeal Disease Program: An Address by Director." Paper presented at ICORT III, Washington, D.C.

Miller, J. E., J. Trussell, A. R. Pebley, and B. Vaughan. 1992. "Birth Spacing and Child Mortality in Bangladesh and the Philippines." *Demography* 29 (2):305–318.

Millman, S. 1985. "Breastfeeding and Contraception: Why the Inverse Association?" *Studies in Family Planning* No. 16:61–75.

Molla, A. M., A. Molla, S. A. Sarker, and M. M. Rahaman. 1983. "Food Intake during and after Recovery from Diarrhea in Children." In *Diarrhea and Malnutrition: Interactions, Mechanisms and Interventions,* ed. L. C. Chen and N. S. Scrimshaw. New York: Plenum Press.

Montanari, M. 1987. "The Conception of SAM." In *Food Policy in Mexico: The Search for Self-Sufficiency,* ed. J. Austin and G. Esteva. Ithaca: Cornell University Press.

Mora, J. 1989. Personal communication about the socioeconomic and health conditions of the population in the ANEP program evaluated, Dominican Republic.

Mora, J. O., B. de Paredes, M. Wagner, L. de Navarro, J. Suescun, N. Christiansen and M. G. Herrera. 1979. "Nutritional Supplementation and the Outcome of Pregnancy." *American Journal of Clinical Nutrition* 32 (2):455–462.

Mosely, W. H. 1988. "Is There a Middle Way? Categorical Programs for PHC." *Social Science and Medicine* 26 (9):907–909.

Mosley, W. H. 1984. "Child Survival: Research and Policy." In *Child Survival: Strategies for Research,* ed. W. H. Mosley and L. C. Chen. Cambridge, Eng.: Cambridge University Press.

Mosley, W. H., and S. Becker. 1988. "Demographic Models for Child Survival: Implications for Program Strategy." Prepared for the Seminar on Child Survival Programs: Issues for the 1990s by the Institute for International Programs, School of Hygiene and Public Health, Johns Hopkins University.

Msukwa, L., and B. F. Kandoole. 1981. *Water by the People: An Evaluation of the Rural Water Supply Programme in Zomba District*. Zomba: University of Malawi, Centre of Social Research.

Mueller, E. 1979. "Time Use in Rural Botswana." Paper presented at a seminar on the Rural Income Distribution Survey in Gabarone, Botswana, by the Population Studies Center, held at the University of Michigan, Ann Arbor, 26–28 June.

Muhloff, E. 1990. "A Review of Experiences with Early Warning Systems in Ethiopia." Background paper prepared for the Beyond Child Survival project, CFNPP, Ithaca, N.Y. Mimeographed.

Mukarji, D. 1985. "Growth Monitoring—Some Field Problems." In *Growth Monitoring as a Primary Health Care Activity. Proceedings of a Workshop Sponsored by the Foundation for Indonesian Welfare and the Ford Foundation, Held at Yogyakarta, 20–24 August 1984.*

Mull, D. S. 1991. "Traditional Perceptions of Marasmus in Pakistan." *Social Science and Medicine* 32 (2):175–191.

Muller, F. 1983. "Contrasts in Community Participation: Case Studies from Peru." In *Practicing Health for All*, ed. D. Morley, J. Rohde, and G. Williams. Oxford: Oxford Medical Publications.

Munroe, R. H., and R. L. Munroe. 1984. "Infant Experiences and Childhood Cognition: A Longitudinal Study among the Logoli of Kenya." *Ethos* 12 (4):291–306.

Murphy, J. M. 1976. "Psychiatric Labeling in Cross Cultural Perspective." *Science* 191 (5):1019–1028.

Murphy, J., and T. J. Marchant. 1988. *Monitoring and Evaluation in Extension Agencies.* Technical Paper No. 79. Washington, D.C.: World Bank.

Murthy, N. M. 1985. "Growth Monitoring in Tamil Nadu Integrated Nutrition Project." Paper prepared for the Workshop on Growth Monitoring, Yogyakarta.

Musgrove, P. 1989. *Fighting Malnutrition: An Evaluation of Brazilian Food and Nutrition Programs.* Discussion Paper No. 60. Washington, D.C.: World Bank.

Mutahaba, G. 1985. "The Political Economy of Food Policies and Nutritional Improvement in Tanzania." Paper presented at the IFPRI/UNU Workshop on the Political Economy of Nutritional Improvements, Berkeley Springs, W.V.

Mwabu, G. M. 1989. "Nonmonetary Factors in the Household Choice of Medical Factors." *Economic Development and Cultural Change* 37 (2):383–392.

Nabarro, D. 1983. *The Growth Chart—An Attractive Concept, but How Widely Can It Be Applied?* Liverpool: Save the Children Fund.

Nabarro, D., and P. Chinnock. 1988. "Growth Monitoring—Inappropriate Promotion of an Appropriate Technology." *Social Science and Medicine* 26 (9):941–948.

Naeye, R. L. 1981. "Teenaged and Pre-Teenaged Pregnancies: Consequences of the Fetal-Maternal Competition for Nutrients." *Pediatrics* No. 67:146–150.

NAS (National Academy of Sciences). 1989a. *Nutrition and Diarrheal Diseases Control In Developing Countries.* Washington, D.C.: National Academy Press.

NAS (National Academy of Sciences). 1989b. *The Impact of Diet and Physical Activity on Pregnancy and Lactation: Women's Work in the Developing World.* A report prepared by the Subcommittee of Diet, Physical Activity, and Pregnancy Outcome, Committee on International Nutrition Programs, Food and Nutrition Board. Washington, D.C.: National Academy of Sciences, Institute of Medicine.

NAS (National Academy of Sciences). 1982. *Alternative Dietary Practices and Nutritional Abuses in Pregnancy.* Committee on Nutrition of the Mother and Preschool Child, Food and Nutrition Board. Washington, D.C.: National Academy Press.

National Family Planning Coordinating Board (BKKBN), the Universities of Udayana, Brawijaya, and Airlangga, and Community Systems Foundation. 1986. *KB-Gizi—An Indonesian Integrated Family Planning, Nutrition and Health*

Program: The Evaluation of the First Five Years of Program Implementation in West Java and Bali. Ann Arbor: Community Systems Foundation.

National Research Council. 1985. *Nutritional Management of Acute Diarrhea in Infants and Children.* Washington, D.C.: Subcommittee on Nutrition and Diarrheal Diseases Control, Committee on International Nutrition Programs Food and Nutrition Board, Commission on Life Sciences, National Research Council.

Naylor, A. J., and R. A. Wester. 1985. *Lactation Specialist Training for Health Professionals from Developing Nations. Summary Report of Sessions I–IV, August 1983–January 1985.* San Diego: San Diego Lactation Program.

Neumann, C., N. O. Bwibo, and M. Sigman. 1992. *Diet Quantity and Quality: Functional Effects on Rural Kenyan Families.* Human Nutrition Collaborative Research Support Program. Washington, D.C.: USAID, Office of Nutrition.

Neville, M. C., and J. Oliva-Rasbach. 1989. "Is Maternal Milk Production Limiting for Infant Growth during the First Year of Life in Breast-Fed Infants?" In *Human Lactation 3: The Effects of Human Milk on the Recipient Infant,* ed. A. S. Goldman, S. A. Atkinson, and L. A. Hanson. New York: Plenum Press.

Nietschmann, B. 1973. *Between Land and Water: The Subsistence Ecology of the Mistiko Indians, Eastern Nicaragua.* New York: Seminar Press.

Northrup, R., and L. Hendrata. 1988. *Beyond ORT: Linkages to Diarrhea Prevention and Other Primary Health Care Activities.* Washington, D.C.: ICORT III.

Nweke, F. I., and F. E. Winch. 1980. *Bases for Farm Resource Allocation in the Smallholder Cropping Systems of South Eastern Nigeria: A Case Study of Awka and Abakaliki Villages.* Discussion Paper No. 4/80, Agricultural Economics, IITA.

Nygaard, D. F., and P. L. Pellett, eds. 1986. *Dry Area Agriculture: Food Science and Human Nutrition.* Proceedings of a workshop held at the University of Aleppo, Aleppo, Syria, February 21–25. New York: Pergamon Press.

Ochoa, M. 1983. "Targeted Food Stamp Program in Colombia." Paper presented at the International Food Policy Research Institute workshop on Consumer Food Price Subsidies, Washington, D.C.

O'Gara, C. 1989. "Breastfeeding and Maternal Employment in Urban Honduras." In *Women, Work and Child Welfare in the Third World,* ed. J. Leslie and M. Paolisso. Boulder: Westview Press.

Ojo, A., and V. Oronsaye. 1988. "Who Is the Elderly Primigravida in Nigeria?" *International Journal of Gynecology and Obstetrics* No. 26:51–55.

Okeahialam, T. C. 1975. "Non-nutritional Aetiological Factors of Protein-Calorie Malnutrition in Africa." *Environmental Child Health* 21 (1B, February, special issue):20–25.

Olawoye, J. E. 1985. "Factors Affecting the Role of Rural Women in Agricultural Production: A Survey of Rural Women in Oyo State, Nigeria." Paper presented at the Seminar on Nigerian Women and National Development, University of Ibadan, Nigeria, 20–21 June.

Olson, C. M. 1987a. "Pregnancy in Adolescents: A Cause for Nutritional Concern?" *Professional Perspectives* No. 1:1–5.

Olson, C. M. 1987b. "Breastfeeding by Adolescent Mothers: Potential Benefits and Concerns." *Professional Perspectives* No. 2:1–4.

Olson, C. M., and G. L. Kelly. 1989. "The Challenge of Implementing Theory-

Based Intervention Research in Nutrition Education." *Journal of Nutrition Education* 21 (6):280–284.

Olvera-Ezzell, N., T. G. Power, and J. H. Cousins. 1990. "Maternal Socialization of Children's Eating Habits: Strategies Used by Obese Mexican American Mothers." *Child Development* 61 (2):395–400.

Omran, A. R., C. C. Standley, and J. E. Azare. 1976. *Family Formation Patterns and Health: An International Collaborative Study in India, Iran, Lebanon, Philippines, and Turkey.* Geneva: World Health Organization.

Oniang'o, R. 1989. "Community Based Growth Monitoring and Promotion in Embu District, the Republic of Kenya: A Contextual Analysis Focussing on the Mechanisms Contributing to Community Adoption of the Program Activities." Cornell Food and Nutrition Policy Program, Ithaca. Mimeographed.

Orr, E. 1972. *The Use of Protein-Rich Foods for the Relief of Malnutrition in Developing Countries: An Analysis of Experience.* London: Tropical Products Institute.

Otaala, B., R. Myers, and C. Landers. 1988. *Children Caring for Children: New Applications of an Old Idea.* New York: Consultative Group on Early Childhood Care and Development.

Pacey, A. 1982. "Health Planning: Taking Soundings for Development and Health." *World Health Forum* 3 (1):38–47.

Palloni, A., and S. Millman. 1986. "Effects of Interbirth Intervals and Breastfeeding on Infant and Child Mortality." *Population Studies* No. 40:215–236.

Palmer, I. 1979. *The Nemow Case.* New York: Population Council.

Paltiel, L. 1987. "Women and Mental Health: A Post Nairobi Perspective." *World Health Statistical Quarterly* 40 (1):233–266.

Paolisso, M., M. Baksh, and J. C. Thomas. 1989. "Women's Agricultural Work, Child Care, and Infant Diarrhea in Rural Kenya." In *Women, Work, and Child Welfare in the Third World,* ed. J. Leslie and M. Paolisso. Boulder: Westview Press.

Parlato, M. B., and M. N. Favin. 1982. *Primary Health Care: Progress and Problems. An Analysis of 52 AID-Assisted Projects.* Washington, D.C.: APHA.

Partridge, W. L., and A. B. Brown. 1980. *Nutrition Impact of Resettlement, Settlement and Colonization.* Washington, D.C.: USAID.

Paul, S. 1987. "Community Participation in Development Projects: The World Bank Experience." In *Readings in Community Participation* Vol. 1, comp. and intro. by Michael Bamberger. Washington, D.C.: Economic Development Institute.

Pearson, R. 1983. "Thematic Evaluation of UNICEF Support to Growth Monitoring." New York: UNICEF, Evaluation and Research Office.

Pebley, A., and J. DaVanzo. 1988. "Maternal Depletion and Child Survival in Guatemala and Peninsular Malaysia." Paper presented to Population Association of America, New Orleans, April.

Pebley, A., and P. Stupp. 1986. "Reproductive Patterns and Child Mortality in Guatemala." *Demography* 24:43–60.

Peirano, P., I. Fagioli, B. B. Singh, and P. Salzarulo. 1989. "Effect of Early Human Malnutrition on Waking and Sleep Organization." *Early Human Development* 20 (1):67–76.

Pelletier, D. L. 1991a. *Relationships between Child Anthropometry and Mortality in Developing Countries: Implications for Policy, Programs, and Future Research.* CFNPP Monograph No. 12. Ithaca, N.Y.: Cornell Food and Nutrition Policy Program.

Pelletier, D. L. 1991b. *The Uses and Limitations of Information in the Iringa Nutrition Program, Tanzania.* Working Paper No. 5. Ithaca: Cornell Food and Nutrition Policy Program.

Pelletier, D. L., and L. A. H. Msukwa. 1991. "The Use of National Sample Surveys for Nutritional Surveillance: Lessons from Malawi's National Sample Survey of Agriculture." *Social Science and Medicine* 32 (8):887–898.

Pelletier, D. L., and L. A. H. Msukwa. 1990. "The Role of Information Systems in Decision-Making Following Disasters: Lessons from the Mealy Bug Disaster in Northern Malawi." *Human Organization* 49 (3):245–254.

Pelletier, D. L., and R. Shrimpton. 1994. "The Use of Information in the Planning, Management, and Evaluation of Community Nutrition Programs." *Health Policy and Planning* 9 (2).

Perera, P. D. A. 1985. "Health Care Systems of Sri Lanka." In *Good Health at Low Cost,* ed. S. B. Halstead, J. A. Walsh, and K. S. Warren. New York: Rockefeller Foundation.

Phillips, J., R. Simmons, M. Koenig, and J. Chakroborty. 1988. "Determinants of Reproductive Change in a Traditional Setting: Evidence from Matlab, Bangladesh." *Studies in Family Planning* No. 19:313–334.

Pielemeier, N. R. 1982. "The Relationship of Mother's Nutrition Knowledge to Child-Feeding Practices and Child Nutritional Status in Lesotho." Ph.D. diss., Johns Hopkins University.

Pielemeier, N. R., E. M. Jones, and S. J. Munger. 1978. *Use of the Child's Growth Chart as an Educational Tool.* Allison Park, Pa.: Synectics Corporation.

Pillsbury, B., A. Brownlee, and J. Timyan. 1990. *Understanding and Evaluating Traditional Practices: A Guide for Improving Maternal Care.* Washington, D.C.: International Center for Research on Women.

Pines, J. M. 1983. "The Nutrition Consequences of Agricultural Projects: Evidence and Response." In *Papers and Proceedings of a Workshop Held by the UN ACC/SCN.* New York: United Nations.

Pines, J. M. 1982. "National Nutrition Planning: Lessons of Experience." *Food Policy* 7 (4):275–301.

Pinstrup-Andersen, P. 1989. *Government Policy, Food Security and Nutrition in Sub-Sahara Africa.* Pew/Cornell Lecture Series on Food and Nutrition Policy. Ithaca: Cornell Food and Nutrition Policy Program.

Pinstrup-Andersen, P. 1988a. "The Social and Economic Effects of Consumer-Oriented Food Subsidies: A Summary of Current Evidence." In *Food Subsidies in Developing Countries: Costs, Benefits, and Policy Options,* ed. P. Pinstrup-Andersen. Baltimore: Johns Hopkins University Press.

Pinstrup-Andersen, P., ed. 1988b. *Food Subsidies in Developing Countries: Costs, Benefits, and Policy Options.* Baltimore: Johns Hopkins University Press.

Pinstrup-Andersen, P. 1987. "Food Prices and the Poor in Developing Countries." In *Food Policy: Integrating Supply, Distribution, and Consumption,* ed. J. P. Gittinger, J. Leslie, and C. Hoisington. Baltimore: Johns Hopkins University Press.

Pinstrup-Andersen, P. 1985a. "The Impact of Export Crop Production on Human

Nutrition." In *Nutrition and Development* ed. M. Biswas and P. Pinstrup-Andersen. Oxford: Oxford University Press.

Pinstrup-Andersen, P. 1985b. "Food Prices and the Poor in Developing Countries." *European Review of Agricultural Economics* 12:69–81.

Pinstrup-Andersen, P. 1984. *The Nutritional Impact of the Colombian Food and Nutrition Program in the State of Cauca, Colombia.* Washington, D.C.: International Food Policy Research Institute.

Pinstrup-Andersen, P. 1982. *Agricultural Research and Technology in Economic Development.* New York: Longman Group.

Pinstrup-Andersen, P. 1981. *Nutritional Consequences of Agricultural Projects: Conceptual Relationships and Assessment Approaches.* Staff Working Paper No. 456. Washington, D.C.: World Bank.

Pinstrup-Andersen, P. 1971. *The Feasibility of Introducing Opaque-2 Maize for Human Consumption in Colombia.* Technical Bulletin No. 1. Cali, Colombia: Centro Internacional de Agricultura Tropical.

Pinstrup-Andersen, P., and H. Alderman. 1988. "The Effectiveness of Consumer Oriented Food Subsidies in Reaching Rationing and Income Transfer Goals." In *Food Subsidies in Developing Countries: Costs, Benefits, and Policy Options,* ed. P. Pinstrup-Andersen. Baltimore: Johns Hopkins University Press.

Pinstrup-Andersen, P., A. Berg, and M. Forman, eds. 1984. *International Agricultural Research and Human Nutrition.* Washington, D.C.: International Food Policy Research Institute.

Pinstrup-Andersen, P., S. Burger, J.-P. Habicht, and K. Peterson. 1993. "Protein Energy Malnutrition." In *Disease Control Priorities in Developing Countries,* ed. D. T. Jamison, W. H. Mosley, A. R. Measham, and J. L. Bobadilla. New York: Oxford University Press.

Pinstrup-Andersen, P., and P. Hazell. 1985. "The Impact of the Green Revolution and Prospects for the Future." *Food Review International* 1 (1):1–25.

Pinstrup-Andersen, P., and M. Jaramillo. 1989. "The Impact of Drought and Technological Change in Rice Production in Intrayear Fluctuations in Food Consumption: The Case of North Arcot, India." In *Seasonal Variability in Third World Agriculture: The Consequences for Food Security,* ed. D. E. Sahn. Baltimore: Johns Hopkins University Press.

Pitt, M. M. 1983. "Food Preferences and Nutrition in Rural Bangladesh." *Review of Economics and Statistics* 65 (1):105–114.

Pitt, M. M., and M. R. Rosenzweig. 1985. "Health and Nutrient Consumption across and within Farm Households." *Review of Economics and Statistics* 67 (2):212–223.

Pitt, M. M., and M. R. Rosenzweig, and M. N. Hassan. 1990. "Productivity, Health and Inequality in the Intrahousehold Distribution of Food in Low Income Countries." *American Economic Review* 80 (5):1139–1156.

PMPA and Manoff International. 1986. "The Weaning Project: New Strategies to Improve Infant Feeding Practices." PMPA and Manoff International, Washington, D.C. Mimeographed.

Pollitt, E. 1990. *Malnutrition and Infection in the Classroom.* Paris: UNESCO.

Pollitt, E. 1988. "A Critical View of Three Decades of Research on the Effects of Chronic Energy Malnutrition on Behavioral Development." In *Chronic Energy*

Deficiency: Consequences and Related Issues, ed. B. Schurch and N. S. Scrimshaw. Lausanne: International Dietary Energy Consultancy Group.

Pollitt, E. 1984. *Early Childhood Intervention Programs for the Young Child in the Developing World,* Vol. 2, *Child Development Reference Document.* Houston: University of Texas Health Science Center.

Pollitt, E. 1973. "Behavior of Infant in Causation of Nutritional Marasmus." *American Journal of Clinical Nutrition* 26 (3):262–270.

Pollitt, E., and P. Amante, eds. 1984. *Energy Intake and Activity: Current Topics in Nutrition and Disease.* Vol. 2. New York: Alan R. Liss.

Pollitt, E., K. S. Gorman, P. Engle, R. Martorell, and J. Rivera. 1993. "Early Supplementary Feeding and Cognition: Effects over Two Decades." *Monographs of the Society for Research in Child Development, Serial No.* 235 58 (7).

Pollitt, E. and S. Wirtz. 1981. "Mother-Infant Feeding Interaction and Weight Gain in the First Month of Life." *Journal of the American Dietetic Association* 78 (6):596–601.

Polyani, M. 1962. "The Republic of Science: Its Political and Economic Nature." *Minerva* 1 (1):54–73.

Popkin, B. M., and R. M. Doan. 1989. "Women's Roles, Time Allocation and Health." Carolina Population Center, University of North Carolina, Chapel Hill. Mimeographed.

Potter, J. E. 1989. "On the Relationship between Contraceptive Use and Access to Health Care in Developing Countries." Background paper. Washington, D.C.: Working Group on the Health Consequences of Contraceptive Use and Controlled Fertility, Committee on Population, National Academy of Sciences.

Potter, J. E. 1988. "Birth Spacing and Child Survival: A Cautionary Note regarding the Evidence from the WFS." *Population Studies* No. 42:443–450.

Potter, J. E., O. Mojarro, and L. Nunez. 1987. "The Influence of Health Care on Contraceptive Acceptance in Rural Mexico." *Studies in Family Planning* No. 18:144–156.

Powell-Griner, E. 1987. "Risk of Perinatal Death: A Log-Linear Analysis of the Effects of Selected Factors on Pregnancy Outcome." Paper presented to the annual meeting of the Population Association of American, Chicago, May.

Praun, A. 1982. "Nutrition Education: Development or Alienation?" *Human Nutrition: Applied Nutrition* 36A:28–34.

Prentice, A. M., T. J. Cole, F. A. Foord, W. H. Lamb, and R. G. Whitehead. 1987. "Increased Birth Weight after Prenatal Dietary Supplementation of Rural African Women." *American Journal of Clinical Nutrition* 46 (5):912–925.

Preston, S. 1985. "Mortality in Childhood: Lessons from WFS." In *Reproductive Change in Developing Countries: Insights from the World Fertility Survey,* ed. J. Cleland and J. Hobcraft. Oxford: Oxford University Press.

PRICOR. 1989a. "Preliminary Results from Systems Analysis Done by PRICOR in Zaire, Haiti, Philippines, Colombia, and Thailand." Mimeographed.

PRICOR. 1989b. "Operations Research in Growth Monitoring and Promotion." Solution-Development Workshop, K'Palime, Togo, 10–14 April.

PRICOR. 1987. *Adding Nutrition Repletion Education to ORT Program in Egypt.* PRICOR Study Summary. Center for Human Services, Chevy Chase, Md.: Agency for International Development.

PRITECH. 1989. *Summary of Acute Respiratory Infections (ARI) for CDD Technical Advisors.* Arlington, Va.: Management Sciences for Health.

Priyosusilo, A. 1988. "Health in the Balance: The Underfives Weighing Program." *Indian Journal of Pediatrics* No. 55 (Suppl.):S88–S99.

Puffer, R., and C. Serrano. 1973. *Patterns of Mortality in Childhood.* Washington, D.C.: PAHO.

Pyle, D. F. 1981a. *Framework for Evaluation of Health Sector Activities for Private Volunteer Organization Receiving Matching Grants.* Washington, D.C.: USAID Bureau for Peace and Voluntary Cooperation.

Pyle, D. F. 1981b. "From Project to Program: The Study of the Scaling Up/Implementation Process of a Community-Level, Integrated Health, Nutrition, Population Intervention in Maharashtra, India." Ph.D. diss., Massachusetts Institute of Technology.

Rajapurohit, A. 1983. "Recent Trends in Agricultural Growth Rates in Karnatanka." *Indian Journal of Agricultural Economics* 38 (4):589–590.

Rajasekaran, P., P. R. Dutt, and K. A. Pisharoti. 1977. "Impact of Water Supply on the Incidence of Diarrhoea and Shigellosis among Children in Rural Communities in Madurai." *Indian Journal of Medical Research* 66 (2):189–199.

Ramsay, M., and P. R. Zelazo. 1988. "Food Refusal in Failure-to-Thrive Infants: Nasogastric Feeding Combined with Interactive-Behavioral Treatment. *Journal of Pediatric Psychology* 13 (3):329–347.

Rao, C. H. H. 1975. *Technological Change and Distribution of Gains in Indian Agriculture.* Delhi: Macmillan of India.

Rao Gupta, G. 1985. "Role Conflict and Coping Strategies: A Study on Indian Women." Ph.D. diss., Bangladesh University.

Rasmussen, K. M., C. S. Johnson, J. A. Kusin, S. Kardjati, and J.-P. Habicht. 1990. *Role of Compliance with Nutritional Supplementation during Pregnancy: Comparison of Data from Guatemala and Indonesia.* Report No. 18, Maternal Nutrition and Health Care Program. Washington, D.C.: International Center for Research on Women.

Ravallion, M. 1992. *Poverty Comparisons: A Guide to Concepts and Methods.* Living Standards Measurement Survey Working Paper No. 88. Washington, D.C.: World Bank.

Ravindran, S. 1986. *Health Implications of Sex Discrimination in Childhood: A Review Paper and an Annotated Bibliography.* Geneva: WHO.

Reardon, T., T. Tjiombiano, and C. Delgado. 1988. *La substitution des céréales locales par les céréales importées: La consommation alimentaire des menages a Ouagadougou, Burkina Faso.* Ouagadougou and Washington, D.C.: Centre d'Etudes, de Documentation, de Recherches Economiques et Sociales (CEDRES), Ecole Supérieure des Sciences Economiques, with International Food Policy Research Institute.

Reid, J. 1984. "The Role of Maternal and Child Health Clinics in Education and Prevention: A Case Study from Papua New Guinea." *Social Science and Medicine* 19 (3):291–303.

Repetti, R. L., K. A. Matthews, and I. Waldron. 1989. "Employment and Women's Health: Effects of Paid Employment on Women's Mental and Physical Health." *American Psychologist* 44 (11):1394–1401.

Retherford, R. D., M. K. Chioe, S. Thapa, and B. B. Gubhaju. 1989. "To What

Extent Does Breastfeeding Explain Birth-Interval Effects on Early Childhood Mortality?" *Demography* No. 26:439–450.

Reutlinger, S., and M. Selowsky. 1976. *Malnutrition and Poverty: Magnitude and Policy Options.* Baltimore: Johns Hopkins University Press.

Reutlinger, S., and J. van Horst Pellekan. 1986. *Poverty and Hunger: Issues and Options for Food Security in Developing Countries.* Washington, D.C.: World Bank.

Rhoades, R. E. 1985. "Farming Systems Research: Informal Survey Methods for Farming Systems Research." *Human Organization* 44 (3):215–218.

Rhode, J. 1988. "Beyond Survival: Promoting Healthy Growth." *Indian Journal of Pediatrics* 55:S3–S8.

Ricciuti, H. N. 1981. "Adverse Environmental and Nutritional Influences on Mental Development: A Perspective." *Journal of the American Dietetic Association* 79 (2):115–120.

Rifkin, S. B., F. Muller, and W. Bichmann. 1988. "Primary Health Care: On Measuring Participation." *Social Science and Medicine* 26 (9):931–940.

Rifkin, S. B., and G. Walt. 1986. "Why Health Improves: Defining the Issues Concerning 'Comprehensive Primary Health Care' and 'Selective Primary Health Care.'" *Social Science and Medicine* 23 (6):559–566.

Riley, A. P., S. L. Huffman, and A. K. M. Chowdhury. 1989. "Age at Menarche and Postmenarcheal Growth in Rural Bangladeshi Females." *Annals of Human Biology* No. 16:347–359.

Riley, L. W., S. H. Waterman, A. S. G. Farukh, and M. I. Huq. 1987. "Breast-Feeding Children in the Household as a Risk Factor for Cholera in Rural Bangladesh: An Hypothesis." *Tropical and Geographic Medicine* No. 39:9–14.

Rivera, J. A. 1988. "Effect of Supplementary Feeding upon the Recovery from Mild-to-Moderate Wasting in Children." Ph.D. diss., Cornell University.

Roberts, N., ed. 1989. *Agricultural Extension in Africa.* Washington, D.C.: World Bank.

Roche, A. F., S. Guo, and D. L. Yeung. 1989. "Monthly Growth Increments from a Longitudinal Study of Canadian Infants." *American Journal of Human Biology* 1 (3):271–279.

Roche, A. F., and J. H. Himes. 1980. "Incremental Growth Charts." *American Journal of Clinical Nutrition* 33 (3):2041–2052.

Rocissano, L., and Y. Yatchmink. 1983. "Language Skill and Interactive Patterns in Prematurely Born Toddlers." *Child Development* 54 (5):1229–1241.

Rogers, B. L. 1990. "The Internal Dynamics of Households: A Critical Factor in Development Policy." In *Intrahousehold Resource Allocation: Issues and Methods for Development Policy and Planning, Food and Nutrition Bulletin (Supplement),* ed. B. Rogers and N. Schlossman. Tokyo: United Nations University Press.

Rogers, B. L. 1988. "Design and Implementation Considerations for Consumer-Oriented Food Subsidies." In *Food Subsidies In Developing Countries: Costs, Benefits, and Policy Options,* ed. P. Pinstrup-Andersen. Baltimore: Johns Hopkins University Press.

Rogers, B. L., and M. Lowdermilk. 1988. *Food Prices and Food Consumption in Urban Mali.* Report prepared for Nutrition Economics Group, OICD, USDA, and Office of Nutrition, Bureau of Science and Technology, USAID (October). Washington, D.C.: United States Agency for International Development.

Rogers, B., and A. Swindale. 1988. *Determinants of Food Consumption in the Dominican Republic.* Vols. 1 and 2. Report Prepared for Nutrition Economics Group, OICD, USDA, and Office of Nutrition, Bureau of Science and Technology, USAID.

Rogers, E. 1983. *Communication of Innovations.* New York: Longman.

Rohde, J. E. 1988. "Beyond Survival, Promoting Healthy Growth." *Indian Journal of Pediatrics* 55 (1, Suppl.):S3–S8.

Rohde, J. E., and L. Hendrata. 1983. "Development from Below: Transformation from Village-Based Nutrition Projects to a National Family Nutrition Program in Indonesia." In *Practicing Health for All,* ed. D. Morley, J. Rohde, and G. Williams. Oxford: Oxford Medical Publications.

Rohde, J., D. Ismail and R. Sutrinso. 1975. "Mothers as Weight Watchers: The Road to Child Health in the Village." *Journal of Tropical Pediatrics* 21 (6):295–297.

Rohde, J. E., and R. S. Northrup. 1988. "Feeding, Feedback and Sustenance of Primary Health Care." *Indian Journal of Pediatrics* 55 (1, Suppl.):S110–S123.

Rosenzweig, M. 1990. "Economic Analysis of Intra Household Resource Allocation." In *Intrahousehold Resource Allocation: Issues and Methods for Development Policy and Planning, Food and Nutrition Bulletin (Supplement),* ed. B. Rogers and N. Schlossman. Tokyo: United Nations University Press.

Rosenzweig, M. R., and T. P. Schultz. 1984. "Market Opportunities and Intrafamily Resource Distribution: Reply." *American Economic Review* 74 (3):521–523.

Rosenzweig, M. R., and T. P. Schultz. 1982a. "Child Mortality and Fertility in Colombia: Individual and Community Effects." *Health Policy and Education* 2 (3–4):305–348.

Rosenzweig, M. R., and T. P. Schultz. 1982b. "Market Opportunities, Genetic Endowment and Intra-family Resource Distribution: Child Survival in Rural India." *American Economic Review* 72 (4):803–815.

Rosenzweig, M., and K. J. Wolpin. 1988. "Heterogeneity, Intrafamily Distribution, and Child Health." *Journal of Human Resources* 23 (4):437–461.

Rosenzweig, M., and K. J. Wolpin. 1985. "Specific Experience, Household Structure, and Intergenerational Transfers: Farm Family Land and Labor Arrangements in Developing Countries." *Quarterly Journal of Economics* (Supplement C):961–987.

Rosner, B., D. Spielgelman, and W. C. Willet. 1990. "Correction of Logistic Regression Relative Risk Estimates and Confidence Intervals for Measurement Error: The Case of Multiple Covariates Measured with Error." *American Journal of Epidemiology* 132 (4):734–745.

Ross, J. S., and E. Posanai. 1988. "The Activities of the Nutrition Section: Alternatives to Intersectoral Nutrition Planning." *Papua New Guinea Medical Journal* 31 (2):141–145.

Rowland, M. G. M. 1986. "The Weanling's Dilemma: Are We Making Progress?" *Acta Paediatr Scand* (323, Suppl.):33–42.

Rowland, M. G. M., R. Barrel, and R. Whitehead. 1978. "Bacterial Contamination in Traditional Gambian Weaning Foods." *Lancet* 1:136–138.

Rowland, M. G. M., S. G. J. G. Rowland, and T. J. Cole. 1988. "Impact of

Infection on the Growth of Children from 0 to 2 years in an Urban West African Community." *American Journal of Clinical Nutrition* 47 (1):134–138.

Royston, E., and S. Armstrong, eds. 1989. *Preventing Maternal Deaths.* Geneva: WHO.

Rubin, D. S. 1988. *Changing Production Practices in a Sugarcane-Growing Community in Kenya.* Washington, D.C.: International Food Policy Research Institute.

Ruel, M. 1990. "The Role of Maternal Nutrition Knowledge and Formal Education as Determinants of Child's Nutritional Status in Lesotho." Ph.D. diss., Cornell University.

Ruel, M. T., and J.-P. Habicht. 1992. "Growth Charts Only Marginally Improve Maternal Learning from Nutrition Education and Growth Monitoring in Lesotho." *Journal of Nutrition.* 122:1772–1780.

Ruel, M. T., J.-P. Habicht, and C. Olson. 1992. "Impact of a Clinic-Based Growth Monitoring Programme on Maternal Nutrition Knowledge in Lesotho." *International Journal of Epidemiology* 21 (1):59–65.

Ruel, M. T., D. L. Pelletier, J.-P. Habicht, J. B. Mason, C. S. Chobokoane, and A. P. Maruping. 1991. "Comparison of Two Growth Charts in Lesotho: Health Workers' Ability to Understand and Use Them for Action." *American Journal of Public Health* 81 (5):610–616.

Ruel, M. T., D. L. Pelletier, J.-P. Habicht, J. B. Mason, C. S. Chobokoane, and A. P. Maruping. 1990. "Comparison of Mothers' Understanding of Two Child Growth Charts in Lesotho." *Bulletin of the World Health Organization* 68 (4):483–491.

Rush, D. 1982. "Effects of Changes in Protein and Calorie Intake during Pregnancy on the Growth of the Human Fetus." In *Effectiveness and Satisfaction in Antenatal Care,* ed. M. Enkin and I. Chalmers. Philadelphia: J. B. Lippincott.

Rush, D., J. Leighton, N. L. Sloan, J. M. Alvir, D. B. Horvitz, W. B. Seaver, G. C. Garbowski, S. S. Johnson, R. A. Kulka, M. Holt, J. W. Devore, J. T. Lynch, M. B. Woodside, and D. S. Shanklin. 1988a. "Longitudinal Study of Pregnant Women." *National WIC Evaluation: American Journal of Clinical Nutrition* 48 (2, Suppl.):439–483.

Rush, D., J. Leighton, N. L. Sloan, J. M. Alvir, D. B. Horvitz, W. B. Seaver, G. C. Garbowski, S. S. Johnson. R. A. Kulka, M. Holt, J. W. Devore, J. T. Lynch, M. B. Woodside, and D. S. Shanklin. 1988b. "Study of Infants and Children." *National WIC Evaluation: American Journal of Clinical Nutrition* 48 (2, Suppl.):484–511.

Russell, A. 1979. *Report on the Situation of Women in the Target Villages of the* UNICEF *Domestic Water Supply Project in Bahr El Ghazal Province, Sudan.* Khartoum, Sudan: UNICEF.

Russell-Brown, P., P. L. Engle, and J. Townsend. 1994. *The Effects of Early Childbearing on Women's Status in Barbados.* New York: Population Council/ International Center for Research on Women Series.

Rutstein, S. O. 1984a. *Socio-Economic Differentials in Infant and Child Mortality.* WFS Comparative Studies No. 43. London: World Fertility Survey.

Rutstein, S. O. 1984b. *Infant and Child Mortality: Levels, Trends, and Demographic Differentials.* WFS Comparative Studies, No. 43. Voorburg, Netherlands: International Statistics Institute.

Rutter, M. 1990. "Commentary: Some Focus and Process Considerations regarding Effects of Parental Depression on Children." *Developmental Psychology* 26 (1):60–67.

Ryan, J., A. Sheldrake, and S. Yaday. 1974. *Human Nutritional Needs and Crop Breeding Objectives in the Semi-Arid Tropics.* Occasional Paper No. 4. Hyderabad: International Center for Research in the Semi-Arid Tropics.

Sah, R., and J. Stiglitz. 1986. "The Architecture of Economic Systems: Hierarchies and Polyarchies." *American Economic Review* 76 (4):716–727.

Sahba, G. H., and R. Arfaa. 1967. "The Effect of Sanitation on Ascariasis in an Iranian Village." *American Journal of Tropical Medicine and Hygiene* 70 (1):37–39.

Sahn, D. E. 1990. *Malnutrition in Côte d'Ivoire.* Social Dimensions of Adjustment in Sub-Saharan Africa, Working Paper No. 4. Washington, D.C.: World Bank.

Sahn, D. E., and H. Alderman. 1988. "The Effect of Human Capital on Wages, and the Determinants of Labor Supply in a Developing Country." *Journal of Development Economics* 29 (2):157–184.

Sai, F. T. 1978. "Nutrition in Ghana." In *Nutrition and National Policy,* ed. B. Winikoff. Cambridge: Massachusetts Institute of Technology Press.

Samarasinghe, V., S. Kiribamune, and W. Jayatilaka. 1990. *Maternal Nutrition and Health Status of Indian Tamil Female Tea Plantation Workers in Sri Lanka.* Report No. 8, Maternal Nutrition and Health Care Program. Washington, D.C.: International Center for Research on Women.

Sameroff, A. J. 1981. "Longitudinal Studies of Preterm Infants: A Review of Chapters 17–20." In *Preterm Birth and Psychological Development,* ed. S. L. Friedman and M. Sigman. New York: Academic Press.

Sameroff, A. J. 1979. "The Etiology of Cognitive Competence: A Systems Perspective." In *Infants at Risk: Assessment of Cognitive Functioning,* ed. R. Kearsley and I. Sigel. Hillsdale, N.J.: Erlbaum.

Sameroff, A. J., and M. J. Chandler. 1975. "Reproductive Risk and the Continuum of Caretaking Casualty." In *Review of Child Development Research, Vol. 4,* ed. F. D. Horowitz, M. Hetherington, S. Scarr, and A. Siegel. Chicago: University of Chicago Press.

Sameroff, A. J., and R. Seifer. 1983. "Familial Risk and Child Competence." *Child Development* 54 (5):1254–1268.

Sanghvi, T. 1985. *Notes from the Field: AID Supported Oral Rehydration Therapy Activities.* ICORT II. Washington, D.C.: Office of Health, USAID.

Santosham, M. 1987. *Nutritional Aspects of ORT. Symposium Proceedings Cereal-Based Oral Rehydration Therapy: Theory and Practice.* Washington, D.C.: International Child Health Foundation.

Santow, G., and M. Bracher. 1989. "Do Gravidity and Age Affect Pregnancy Outcome?" *Social Biology* No. 36:9–22.

Satorius, N. 1974. "Depressive Illness as a Worldwide Problem." In *Depression in Everyday Practice,* ed. P. Keilholz. Bern: Hans Huber.

Satyanarayana, K., A. Nadamuni Naidu, and B. S. Narasinga Rao. 1979. "Nutritional Deprivation in Childhood and the Body Size, Activity, and Physical Work Capacity of Young Boys." *American Journal of Clinical Nutrition* 32 (9):1769–1775.

Satyanarayana, K., A. Nadamuni Naidu, M. C. Swaminathan, and B. S. Narasinga

Rao. 1981. "Effect of Nutritional Deprivation in Early Childhood on Later Growth—A Community Study without Intervention." *American Journal of Clinical Nutrition* 34 (8):1636–1637.

Satyanarayana, K., A. Nadamuni Naidu, M. C. Swaminathan, and B. S. Narasinga Rao. 1980. "Adolescent Growth Spurt among Rural Indian Boys in Relation to Their Nutritional Status in Early Childhood." *Annals of Human Biology* 7 (4):359–366.

Sazawal, S., and R. E. Black. 1992. "Meta-Analysis of Intervention Trials on Case-Management of Pneumonia in Community Settings." *Lancet* 340:528–533.

Schiller, F. 1955. *Werke in Drei Bänden.* Vol. 2, pp. 74–78. Leipzig: VEB Bibliographisches Institut.

Scholl, E. A. 1985. "An Assessment of Community Health Workers in Nicaragua." *Social Science and Medicine* 20 (3):207–214.

Scholl, T. O., M. L. Hediger, and I. G. Ances. 1990. "Maternal Growth during Pregnancy and Decreased Infant Birth Weight." *American Journal of Clinical Nutrition* 51 (5):790–793.

Scholl, T. O., M. L. Hediger, M. F. Healey, I. G. Ances, and P. Vasilenko III. 1990. "Maternal Growth and Micro-Nutrient Levels during Pregnancy in Adolescence." Abstract of paper prepared for presentation at the 30th annual meeting of the American Society for Clinical Nutrition, Washington, D.C., 3–4 May.

Schroeder, D. G., R. Martorell, J. Rivera, M. Ruel, and J.-P. Habicht. Forthcoming. "Age Differences in the Impact of Nutritional Supplements on Growth." *Journal on Nutrition.*

Schultz, T. P. 1993a. "Investments in the Schooling and Health of Women and Men: Quantities and Returns." Yale University, New Haven, Conn. Mimeographed.

Schultz, T. P. 1993b. "Returns to Women's Education." In *Women's Education in Developing Countries: Barriers, Benefits, and Policies.* Baltimore: Johns Hopkins University Press.

Schultz, T. P. 1990. "Testing the Neoclassical Model of Family Labor Supply and Fertility." *Journal of Human Resources* 25 (4):599–634.

Schultz, T. W. 1975. "The Ability to Deal with Disequilibria." *Journal of Economic Literature* 13:827–846.

Scobie, G. 1983. *Food Subsidies in Egypt: Their Impact on Foreign Exchange and Trade.* IFPRI Research Report No. 40. Washington, D.C.: International Food Policy Research Institute.

Scrimshaw, M. W., and S. C. M. Scrimshaw. 1989. "The Success of Mothers in Maintaining the Health of Their Children: Experiences from a Guatemalan Coastal Plantation." UCLA, School of Public Health. Mimeographed.

Scrimshaw, S., and E. Hurtado. 1987. *Rapid Assessment Procedures for Nutrition and Primary Health Care,* ed. B. G. Valk. UCLA Latin American Center Reference Series 11. Los Angeles: UCLA Publications.

Seckler, D. 1982. "'Small but Healthy': A Basic Hypothesis in the Theory, Measurement, and Policy of Malnutrition." In *Newer Concepts in Nutrition and Their Implications for Policy,* ed. P. V. Sukhatme. Pune, India: Maharashtra Association for the Cultivation of Science Research Institute.

Seeds, J. W. 1986. "Malpresentations." In *Obstetrics: Normal and Problem Pregnancies,* ed. S. G. Gabbe, J. Niebyl, and J. L. Simpson. New York: Livingstone.

Sen, A. 1981. *Poverty and Famines: An Essay on Entitlement and Deprivation.* Oxford: Clarendon Press.

Senauer, B., and N. Young. 1986. "The Impact of Food Stamps on Food Expenditures: Rejection of the Traditional Model." *American Journal of Agricultural Economics* 68 (1):37–43.

Sepúlveda, J., W. Willet, and A. Muñoz. 1988. "Malnutrition and Diarrhea: A Longitudinal Study among Urban Mexican Children." *American Journal of Epidemiology* 127 (2):365–376.

Serdula, M. K., D. Herman, D. F. Williamson, N. J. Binkin, J. M. Aphane, and F. Trowbridge. 1987. "Validity of Clinic-Based Nutritional Surveillance for Prevalence Estimation of Undernutrition." *World Health Organization Bulletin* 65 (4):529–533.

Severin, W. J., and J. W. Tankard. 1988. *Communication Theories: Origins, Methods, Uses.* New York: Longman.

Shah, C. H. 1983. "Food Preference, Poverty, and the Nutrition Gap." *Economic Development and Cultural Change* 32 (1):121–148.

Shekar, M. 1991. *The Tamil Nadu Integrated Nutrition Project: A Review of the Project with Special Emphasis on the Monitoring and Information System.* CFNPP Working Paper No. 14. Ithaca: Cornell Food and Nutrition Policy Program.

Shekar, M., and M. C. Latham. 1992. "Growth Monitoring Can and Does Work! An Example from the Tamil Nadu Integrated Nutrition Project in Rural South India." *Indian Journal of Pediatrics* 59:5–15.

Shiffman, M. A., R. Schneider, J. M. Faigenblum, R. Helms, and A. Turner. 1979. "Field Studies on Water, Sanitation and Health Education in Relation to Health Status in Central America." *Progress in Water Technology* 11 (1):143–150.

Shoemaker, B. 1988. "Primary Health Care Progress and Problems: Three Cases in Southeast Asia." M. P. S. thesis, Cornell University.

Shrimpton, R. 1989. "The Applied Nutrition Education Project of Caritas, the Dominican Republic: A Contextual Analysis Focussing on the Role and Usage of Information for Decision Making." Cornell Food and Nutrition Policy Program, Ithaca. N.Y. Mimeographed.

Sigman, M., C. Neumann, M. Baksh, N. Buribo, and M. A. McDonald. 1989. "Relationship between Nutrition and Development in Kenyan Toddlers." *Journal of Pediatrics* 115 (3):357–364.

Simon, P., M. Manning, and D. Jamison. 1989. "Sex Differences in Iodine Deficiency Disorders: A Review of the Literature." World Bank, Washington, D.C. Mimeographed.

Sims, L. 1983. "The Ebb and Flow of Nutrition as a Public Policy Issue." *Journal of Nutrition Education* 15 (4):132–136.

Sirageldin, I., D. Salkever, and R. Osborn, eds. 1983. *Evaluating Population Programs: International Experience with Cost-Effectiveness Analysis and Cost-Benefit Analysis.* London: Croom Helm.

Sivakumar, B., and V. Reddy. 1975. "Absorption of Vitamin A in Children with Ascariasis." *Journal of Tropical Medicine and Hygiene* 78 (5):111–115.

Slaughter, D. T. 1983. "Early Intervention and Its Effects on Maternal and Child Development." *Monographs of the Society for Research on Child Development* 48 (4):1–91.

Smedman, L., G. Sterky, L. Mellander, and S. Wall. 1987. "Anthropometry and Subsequent Mortality in Groups of Children Aged 6–59 Months in Guinea-Bissau." *American Journal of Clinical Nutrition* 46 (2):369–373.

Soekirman. 1988. "Principles of Institution Building in Nutrition Based on Experience in Indonesia." AGN/SCN, Geneva. Mimeographed.

Soemardjan, S. 1985. "Influence of Culture on Food and Nutrition: The Indonesian Case." In *Nutrition and Development,* ed. M. Biswas and P. Pinstrup-Andersen. Oxford: Oxford University Press.

Solimano, G., and C. Haignere. 1988. "'Free-Market' Politics and Nutrition in Chile: A Grim Future after a Short-Lived Success." In *Hunger and Society,* Vol. 2, ed. M. C. Latham, L. Bondestam, R. Chorlton, and U. Jonsson. Cornell International Nutrition Monograph Series No. 18. Ithaca: Cornell University.

Sommer, A., I. Toswotjo, G. Hussaini, and D. Susarto. 1983. "Increased Mortality in Children with Mild Vitamin A Deficiency." *Lancet* 2:585–588.

Soysa, P. 1987. "Women and Nutrition." *World Review of Nutrition and Dietetics* 52:1–70.

Spencer, D., and D. Byerlee. 1976. "Technical Change, Labor Use, and Small Farmer Development: Evidence from Sierra Leone." *American Journal of Agricultural Economics* 58 (5):874–880.

Sprunt, K., W. Redman, and G. Leidy. 1973. "Antibacterial Effectiveness of Routine Hand Washing." *Pediatrics* 52 (2):264–271.

Spurr, G. B. 1983. "Nutritional Status and Physical Work Capacity." *Yearbook of Physical Anthropology* 26:1–35.

Stansfield, S. K. 1987. "Acute Respiratory Infections in the Developing World: Strategies for Prevention, Treatment and Control." *Pediatric Infectious Diseases Journal* 6 (7):622–629.

Stansfield, S. K., and S. D. Sheppard. 1991. "Acute Respiratory Infection." *Health Sector Priorities Review.* Washington, D.C.: World Bank.

Stanton, B., J. Clemens, B. Wojtyniak, and T. Khair. 1986. "Risk Factors for Developing Mild Nutritional Blindness in Urban Bangladesh." *American Journal of Diseases of Childhood* 140:584–588.

Stephenson, L. A. 1987. "Schistosomiasis." In *The Impact of Helminth Infections on Human Nutrition: Schistosomes and Soil-Transmitted Helminths,* ed. L. S. Stephenson. Philadelphia: Taylor and Francis.

Stevenson, R. 1988. *Communication, Development and the Third World.* New York: Longman.

Stigler, G. 1982. *The Economist as Preacher and Other Essays.* Chicago: University of Chicago Press.

Stinson, W. 1989. *Results of Systems Analyses Studies.* Bethesda, Md.: PRICOR, University Research Corporation.

Stinson, W. 1986. *Women and Health: An Information for Action Issue Paper.* Washington, D.C.: American Public Health Association.

Strauss, J. 1986. "Does Better Nutrition Raise Farm Productivity?" *Journal of Political Economy* 94 (2):297–320.

Subbarao, K. 1989. *Improving Nutrition in India: Policies and Programs and Their Impact.* Discussion Paper No. 49. Washington, D.C.: World Bank.

Suntikitrungruang, C. 1984. "Growth Monitoring: Thailand's Experience." Paper presented at the workshop on Growth Monitoring as a Primary Health Care Activity, Yogyakarta.

Super, C. M., and S. Harkness. 1986. "The Developmental Niche: A Conceptualization of the Interface of Child and Culture." *International Journal of Behavioral Development* 9 (2):545–569.

Super, C. M., M. G. Herrera, and J. O. Mora. 1990. "Long-Term Effects of Food Supplementation and Psychological Intervention on the Physical Growth of Colombian Infants at Risk of Malnutrition." *Child Development* 61 (1):29–49.

Svedberg, P. 1988. *Undernutrition in Sub-Saharan Africa: Is There a Sex Bias?* Seminar Paper No. 421. Stockholm: Institute for International Economic Studies.

Swaminathan, M. C., T. P. Susheela, and B. V. S. Thimmanyamma. 1970. "Field Prophylactic Trial with a Single Annual Oral Massive Dose of Vitamin A." *American Journal of Clinical Nutrition* 23 (1):119.

Swope, M. 1962. "A Review of Nutrition Education Research." In *Nutrition Education Research Project.* New York: Teachers' College, Columbia University.

Taub, B. 1989. "Poverty and Isolation: A Study of Depression in Uruguayan Women." M.A. thesis, University of California at Los Angeles.

Taucher, E. 1982. "Measuring the Health Effects of Family Planning Programs." In *The Role of Surveys in the Analysis of Family Planning Programs,* ed. A. Hermalin and B. Entwisle. Liège: Ordina.

Taussig, M. 1978a. "Nutrition, Development and Foreign Aid: A Case Study of US Directed Health Care in a Colombian Plantation Zone." *International Journal of Health Services* 8 (1): 101–131.

Taussig, M. 1978b. "Peasant Economies and the Development of Capitalist Agriculture in the Cauca Valley, Colombia." *Latin American Perspectives* 5 (3):62–90.

Tayeh, A., and S. Cairncross. 1989. "Aggregation of Dracunculus medinenesis in Communities Using Different Types of Water Sources in Sudan." *Transactions of the Royal Society of Tropical Medicine and Hygiene* 83 (3):431.

Taylor, C., and R. Jolly. 1988. "The Straw Men of Primary Health Care." *Social Science and Medicine* 26 (9):971–977.

Taylor, C. E. 1988. "Child Growth as a Community Surveillance Indicator." *Indian Journal of Pediatrics* 55 (1, Suppl.):S16–S25.

Teitelbaum, J. M. 1977. "Human versus Animal Nutrition: A Development Project among Fulani Cattlekeepers of the Sahel of Senegal." In *Nutrition and Anthropology in Action,* ed. T. K. Fitzgerald. Assen: van Gorcum.

Teller, C. H. 1986a. "Applications of Operations Research in Growth Monitoring/Promotion." Paper presented at the Annual Conference of the National Council for International Health, Washington, D.C., 10–13 June.

Teller, C. H. 1986b. *Operations Research on Growth Monitoring within Primary Health Care: Methodological Advances and Preliminary Findings: Thailand Trip Report, August 14–30.* Washington, D.C.: International Nutrition Unit, Office of International Health.

Teller, C. H., and J. O. Mora. 1988. "Integrating Nutrition in Primary Health Care and Child Survival: Lessons Learned Ten Years since Alma Ata." Paper presented at the 15th Annual International Health Conference, National Council for International Health (NCIH).

Teller, C., V. Yee, and J. O. Mora. 1985. "Growth Monitoring as a Useful Primary Health Care Management Tool." International Nutrition Division, LTS-OIH/DHHS. Paper presented at the 12th Annual International Health Conference of the National Council for International Health, Washington, D.C., 3–5 June.

Teller, C. H., A. Zerfas, and S. Rutstein. 1990. "Growing up beyond Child Survival: Sociodemographic Considerations on Infant/Child Mortality, Chronic Undernutrition and Community/Household Food Insecurity in the Third World." Paper presented at the Third Annual Hunger Research Briefing and Exchange, Brown University, 4–6 April.

Test, K. E., J. B. Mason, P. Bertolin, and R. Sarnoff. 1987. "Trends in Prevalence of Malnutrition in Five African Countries from Clinic Data: 1982 to 1985." Geneva: Administrative Coordinating Committee of the United Nations, Subcommittee on Nutrition.

Thacker, S. B., S. I. Music, R. A. Pollard, G. Berggren, C. Bouloc, T. Nagy, M. Brutus, M. Pamphil, R. O. Ferdinand, and V. R. Joseph. 1980. "Acute Water Shortage and Health Problems in Haiti." *Lancet* 1:471–473.

Thapa, S., R. Short, and M. Potts. 1988. "Breastfeeding, Birth Spacing, and Their Effects on Child Survival." *Nature* 335 (20):679–682.

Thomas, D. 1990. "Intra-Household Resource Allocation: An Inferential Approach." *Journal of Human Resources* 25 (4):635–664.

Thomas, D., J. Strauss, and M. H. Henriques. 1991. "How Does Mother's Education Affect Child Height?" *Journal of Human Resources* 26 (2):183–211.

Thomas, D., J. Strauss, and M. H. Henriques. 1990. "Child Survival, Height for Age, and Household Characteristics in Brazil." *Journal of Development Economics* 33(2):197–234.

Thomas, R. B., S. Paine, and B. P. Brenton. 1989. "Perspectives on Socio-Economic Causes of and Responses to Food Deprivation." *Food and Nutrition Bulletin* 11 (1):41–54.

Thomson, E. C. 1978. "The Symbiosis of Scientist, Planner, and Administrator in Nutrition Program Implementation." In *Nutrition and National Policy*, ed. B. Winikoff. Cambridge: Massachusetts Institute of Technology Press.

Tiffen, M. 1989. *Guidelines for the Incorporation of Health Safeguards into Irrigation Projects through Intersectoral Cooperation with Special Reference to the Vector-Borne Diseases.* PEEM Guidelines Series 1. Joint WHO/FAO/UNEP Panel of Experts on Environmental Management for Vector Control.

Timmer, C. P. 1988a. "Analyzing Rice Market Interventions in Asia: Principles, Issues, Themes and Lessons." In *Evaluating Rice Market Intervention Policies.* Manila: Asian Development Bank.

Timmer, C. P. 1988b. *Food Price Stability and Welfare of the Poor.* Pew/Cornell Lecture Series on Food and Nutrition Policy. Ithaca: Cornell Food and Nutrition Policy Program.

Timmer, C. P. 1986. "Food Price Policy in Indonesia." Graduate School of Business Administration, Harvard University, Cambridge, Mass. Mimeographed.

Timmer, C. P., W. Falcon, and S. Pearson. 1983. *Food Policy Analysis.* Baltimore: Johns Hopkins University Press.

Tinker, I. 1979. *New Technologies for Food Chain Activities: The Imperative of Equity for Women.* Washington, D.C.: USAID, Office of Women in Development.

TINP. 1989. "Tamil Nadu Integrated Nutrition Project: Programme Summary."

Proceedings of Workshop on Managing Successful Nutrition Programes, Seoul, South Korea, 15–18 August.

Tolley, G. S., V. Thomas, and C. M. Wong. 1982. *Agricultural Price Policies and the Developing Countries*. Baltimore: Johns Hopkins University Press for the World Bank.

Tomkins, A. 1981. "Nutritional Status and Severity of Diarrhoea among Preschool Children in Rural Nigeria." *Lancet* 1:860–862.

Tomkins, A., and F. Watson. 1989. *Malnutrition and Infection: A Review*. State of the Art Series, Nutrition Policy Discussion Paper No. 5. Geneva, Switzerland: ACC/SCN.

Trairatvorakul, P. 1984. *The Effects on Income Distribution and Nutrition of Alternative Price Policies in Thailand*. Research Report No. 46. Washington, D.C.: International Food Policy Research Institute.

Tripp, R. 1984. "Nutrition in Agricultural Research at CIMMYT." In *International Agricultural Research and Human Nutrition*, ed. P. Pinstrup-Andersen, A. Berg, and M. Forman. Washington, D.C.: International Food Policy Research Institute.

Tripp, R. 1982. *Cash Cropping, Nutrition and Choice of Technology in Rural Development*. Mexico City: Centro Internacional de Mejoramiento de Maíz y Trigo.

Tripp, R. B. 1981. "Farmers and Traders: Some Economic Determinants of Nutritional Status in Northern Ghana." *Journal of Tropical Pediatrics* 27 (1):15–22.

Trowbridge, F. 1985. *Wasting and Stunting as Factors for Morbidity and Mortality: Proceedings of the XIII International Congress of Nutrition*. London: John Libbey.

Trowbridge, F. L., L. Newton, A. Huong, N. Staehling, and V. Valverde. 1980. *Evaluation of Nutritional Surveillance Indicators*. Pan American Health Organization Bulletin No. 14:238–243.

Tucker, K., and D. Sanjur. 1988. "Maternal Employment and Child Nutrition in Panama." *Social Science and Medicine* 26 (6):605–612.

Tupasis, T. E., M. G. Lucero, D. M. Magdangal, N. V. Mangubat, Ma. E. S. Sunico, C. U. Torres, L. E. de Leon, J. F. Paisdin, L. Baes, and M. C. Javato. 1990. "Etiology of Acute Lower Respiratory Tract Infection in Children from Alabang, Metro Manila." *Reviews of Infectious Diseases* 12 (Supp. 8):S929–S939.

Uauy, R., and M. Miranda. 1983. "Non-Formal Education: An Instrument for Nutrition Intervention." In *Nutrition Intervention: Strategies in National Development*, ed. B. Underwood. Nutrition Foundation Monograph Series. New York: Academic Press.

Underwood, B. A. 1983. "Some Elements of Successful Nutrition Programs." In *Nutrition Intervention: Strategies in National Development*, ed. B. Underwood. Nutrition Foundation Monograph Series. New York: Academic Press.

UNICEF. 1993a. *Child Malnutrition: Progress toward the World Summit for Children Goal*. New York: UNICEF, Statistics and Monitoring Section.

UNICEF. 1993b. *State of the World's Children*. New York: United Nations Children's Fund.

UNICEF. 1993c. "Strategy for Improved Nutrition of Children and Women in Developing Countries." A UNICEF Policy Review.

UNICEF. 1992a. "Towards an Improved Approach to Nutrition Surveillance." Report on a workshop held at UNICEF, New York, October.

UNICEF. 1992b. "Evaluation of Growth Monitoring and Promotion Programmes." Report prepared by the Evaluation Office and Nutrition Cluster, Programme Division of UNICEF, on a workshop held at Nairobi, 7–9 May.

UNICEF. 1989a. "Joint WHO/UNICEF Nutrition Support Program in Iringa, Tanzania: Improving Child Survival and Nutrition." Dar es Salaam: UNICEF.

UNICEF. 1989b. *Iringa: The Child Survival and Development Revolution: JNSP.* New York: UNICEF.

UNICEF. 1987. *A Simple Solution: How Oral Rehydration Is Averting Child Death from Diarrhoeal Dehydration.* UNICEF Special Report. New York: UNICEF.

UNICEF. 1984a. "The Indonesian National Family Nutrition Improvement Programme: Analysis of Programme Experience." New York: Economic and Social Council of UNICEF.

UNICEF. 1984b. "Report on the Botswana Workshop on Clinic-Based Nutritional Surveillance Systems and Integrated Data Bases, Gaborone, Botswana, 10–12 January." *Social Statistics* 7 (1). Ithaca: Cornell Nutritional Surveillance Program.

UNICEF. 1983a. *Report of the Evaluation of Botswana's Nutritional Surveillance System.* Occasional Paper No. 4. Nairobi: Social Statistics Program, Eastern Africa Regional Office. UNICEF.

UNICEF. 1983b. *Evaluation of Botswana's Nutritional Surveillance System.* Supplement Report on the Results of the Evaluation's Field Work No. 5. Nairobi: Social Statistics Program, Eastern Africa Regional Office.

UNICEF. 1981. *Report on the Community Participation Workshop in Agra.* New Delhi: UNICEF. 13–16.

UN-ACC/SCN (United Nations Administrative Committee on Coordination, Subcommittee on Nutrition). 1989. *Update on the Nutrition Situation: Recent Trends in Nutrition in 33 Countries.* New York: United Nations, ACC/SCN.

United Nations. 1979. *The Methodology of Measuring the Impact of Family Planning Programmes on Fertility.* Population Studies No. 66. New York: United Nations Department of International Economic and Social Affairs.

Uribe-Mosquera, T. 1985. "The Political Economy of PAN." Paper presented at the IFPRI/UNU workshop on the Political Economy of Nutritional Improvements, Berkeley Springs, W.V.

USAID (United States Agency for International Development). 1988. *Growth Monitoring and Nutrition Education: Impact Evaluation of an Effective Applied Nutrition Program in the Dominican Republic. CRS/CARITAS, 1983–1986.* Washington, D.C.: USAID, Bureau for Science and Technology, Office of Nutrition.

USDA (United States Department of Agriculture). 1988. "Economic Research Service Food Assistance." *National Food Review* 11 (2):37.

Usoro, E. J. 1972. "Producer Prices and Rural Economic Activity: A Case of Two Itak Villages in the South-Eastern State of Nigeria." *Nigeria Journal of Economics and Social Studies* 14 (2):57–171.

Valenzuela, M. 1990. "Attachment in Chronically Underweight Young Children." *Child Development* 61:1984–1996.

Valenzuela, M. 1988. "Infant-Mother Attachment, Child Development and Quality of Home Care in Young Chronically Undernourished Children." *Nestle Foundation Annual Report,* 75–87. Lausanne: Nestle Foundation.

Valverde, V., H. Delgado, R. Flores, R. Sibrian, and M. Palmieri. 1982. "Uses and Constraints of Schoolchildren's Height Data for Planning Purposes: National Experiences in Central America." *Food and Nutrition* 8 (3):42–48.

Valverde, V., R. Martorell, V. Mejia-Pivaral, H. Delgado, A. Lechtig, C. Teller, and R. E. Klein. 1977. "Relationship between Family Land Availability and Nutritional Status." *Ecology of Food and Nutrition* 6 (1):1–7.

Valverde, V., F. Trowbridge, I. Beghin, B. Pillet, I. Nieves, N. Sloan, T. Farrell, P. R. Payne, J. L. Joy, and R. E. Klein. 1978. "Functional Classification of Undernourished Populations in the Republic of El Salvador: Methodological Development." *Food and Nutrition* 4 (3–4):8–14.

van der Gaag, J., E. Makonnen, and P. Englebert. 1991. "Trends in Social Indicators and Social Sector Financing." Policy Research and External Affairs Working Paper No. 662. Washington, D.C.: World Bank.

van Wijk-Sijbesma, C. 1985. *Participation of Women in Water Supply and Sanitation: Roles and Realities.* UNDP Technical Paper Series No. 22. The Hague: International Reference Centre for Community Water Supply and Sanitation.

Vial, I., E. Muchnik, and J. Kain. 1988. "Evolution of Chile's Main Nutrition Intervention Programs." University of Chile and Catholic University, Santiago, Chile. Mimeographed.

Vial, I., E. Muchnik, and F. S. Mardones. 1989. "Women's Marketwork, Infant Feeding Practices, and Infant Nutrition among Low-Income Women in Santiago, Chile." In *Women, Work, and Child Welfare in the Third World,* ed. J. Leslie and M. Paolisso. Boulder: Westview.

Victora, C. G. 1992. "The Association between Wasting and Stunting: An International Perspective." *Journal of Nutrition* 122:1105–1110.

Victora, C. G., P. Smith, J. Vaughan, L. Nobre, C. Lombardi, A. Teixeir, S. Fuchs, L. Moreira, L. Gigante, and F. Barros. 1987. "Evidence for Protection by Breast-Feeding against Infant Deaths from Infectious Diseases in Brazil." *Lancet* 2:319–322.

Vijayaraghavan, K. A., N. Naidu, N. Pralhad Rao, and S. G. Srikantia. 1975. "A Simple Method to Evaluate the Massive Dose Vitamin A Prophylaxis Program in Preschool Children." *American Journal of Clinical Nutrition* 28 (10):1189–1193.

Vio, F., J. Kain, and E. Gray. 1992. "Nutritional Surveillance: The Case of Chile." *Nutrition Research* 12:321–335.

von Braun, J. 1991. "The Links between Agricultural Growth, Environmental Degradation, and Nutrition and Health." In *Agricultural Sustainability, Growth, and Poverty Alleviation: Issues and Policies,* ed. S. Vosti, T. Reardon, and W. von Urff. Feldafing: Deutsche Stiftung für internationale Entwicklung (DSE) [German Foundation for International Development].

von Braun, J., H. de Haen, and J. Blanken. 1991. *Commercialization of Agriculture under Population Pressure: Effects on Production, Consumption, and Nutrition in Rwanda.* Research Report No. 85. Washington, D.C.: International Food Policy Research Institute.

von Braun, J., D. Hotchkiss, and M. Immink. 1989a. *Nontraditional Export Crops in Guatemala: Effects on Production, Income, and Nutrition.* Research Report No. 73. Washington, D.C.: International Food Policy Research Institute.

von Braun, J., and E. T. Kennedy, eds. Forthcoming. *Agricultural Commercialization, Development, and Nutrition.* Baltimore: Johns Hopkins University Press for the International Food Policy Research Institute.

von Braun, J., and E. Kennedy. 1986. *Commercialization of Subsistence Agriculture: Income and Nutritional Effects in Developing Countries.* Working Papers on Commercialization of Agriculture and Nutrition No. 1. Washington, D.C.: International Food Policy Research Institute.

von Braun, J., E. Kennedy, and H. Bouis. 1988. *Commercialization of Smallholder Agriculture: A Comparative Analysis of the Effects on Household-Level Food Security and Human Nutrition and Implications for Policy.* Washington, D.C.: International Food Policy Research Institute.

von Braun, J., D. Puetz, and P. Webb. 1989b. *Irrigation Technology and Commercialization of Rice in the Gambia: Effects on Income and Nutrition.* Research Report No. 75. Washington, D.C.: International Food Policy Research Institute.

von Braun, J., and P. J. Webb. 1989. "The Impact of New Crop Technology on the Agricultural Division of Labor in a West African Setting." *Economic Development and Cultural Change* 37 (3):513–534.

Wachs, T. D., Z. Bishry, A. Shams, F. Yunis, A. Sobhy, W. Moussa, O. Galal, G. Harrison, N. Jerome, and A. Kirksey. 1988. *Development in Egyptian Toddlers as a Function of Nutrition, Morbidity and Environment.* Symposium presentation at the Sixth International Conference on Infant Studies, Washington, D.C.

Wachs, T. D., and G. E. Gruen. 1982. *Early Experience and Human Development.* New York: Plenum Press.

Wachs, T. D., M. Sigman, Z. Bishry, W. Moussa, N. Jerome, C. Neuman, N. Bwibo, and M. McDonald. 1992. "Caregiver Child Interaction Patterns in Two Cultures in Relation to Nutritional Intake." *International Journal of Behavioral Development* 15 (1):1–18.

Waddington, C. H. 1966. *Principles of Development and Differentiation.* New York: Macmillan.

Wallerstein, N., and E. Bernstein. 1988. "Empowerment Education: Freire's Ideas Adapted to Health Education." *Health Education Quarterly* 15 (4):379–394.

Wandel, M., G. Holmboe-Ottesen, and A. Manu. 1992. "Seasonal Work, Energy Intake and Nutritional Stress: A Case Study from Tanzania." *Nutrition Research* 12 (1):1–16.

Wardlaw, G. M., and A. M. Pike. 1986. "The Effect of Lactation on Peak Adult Shaft and Ultradistal Forearm Bone Mass in Women." *American Journal of Clinical Nutrition* 44 (2):283–286.

Ware, H. 1984. "Effects of Maternal Education, Women's Roles, and Child Care on Child Mortality." In *Child Survival Strategies for Research, Population and Development Review,* Vol. 10 (Supplement), ed. W. H. Mosley and L. C. Chen, pp. 191–214.

Warner, D., J. Briscoe, F. Hafner, and B. Zellmer. 1986. *Malawi Self-Help Rural Water Supply Program: Final Evaluation.* WASH Field Report No. 186. Arlington, Va.: Water and Sanitation for Health Project.

Warren, K. 1988. "The Evaluation of Selective Primary Health Care." *Social Science and Medicine* 26 (9):891–898.

Waterlow, J. C., R. Buzina, W. Keller, J. M. Lane, M. Z. Nichaman, and J. M. Tanner. 1977. "The Presentation and Use of Height and Weight Data for Comparing the Nutritional Status of Groups of Children under the Age of 10 Years." *Bulletin of the World Health Organization* 55 (4):489–498.

WB-IMF (World Bank–International Monetary Fund). 1989. *Strengthening Efforts to Reduce Poverty.* Pamphlet No. 19 of the Development Committee. Washington, D.C.: World Bank–IMF.

WB-IMF (World Bank–International Monetary Fund). 1987. *Protecting the Poor during Periods of Adjustment.* Pamphlet No. 13 of the Development Committee. Washington, D.C.: World Bank–IMF.

Webb, P. 1989. *Intrahousehold Decisionmaking and Resource Control: The Effects of Rice Commercialization in West Africa.* Working Paper on Commercialization of Agriculture No. 3. Washington, D.C.: International Food Policy Research Institute.

Weiss, C. 1977. *Using Social Research in Public Policy Making.* Lexington, Mass.: D.C. Health.

Weissman, M. M., and G. L. Klerman. 1977. "Sex Differences and the Epidemiology of Depression." *Archives of General Psychiatry* 34 (1):989–1111.

Werner, D. 1988. *Empowerment and Health.* Palo Alto, Calif.: Hesperian Foundation.

Werner, D. 1983. *The Village Health Worker—Lackey or Liberator?* Palo Alto, Calif.: Hesperian Foundation.

Werner, E. E. 1988. "A Cross-Cultural Perspective on Infancy: Research and Social Issues." *Journal of Cross-Cultural Psychology* 19 (1):96–113.

Werner, E. E. 1984. *Child Care: Kith, Kin, and Hired Hands.* Baltimore: University Park Press.

West, D. A., and D. W. Price. 1976. "The Effects of Income, Assets, Food Programs, and Household Size on Food Consumption." *American Journal of Agricultural Economics* 58 (3):725–730.

White, G. F., D. J. Bradley, and A. U. White. 1972. *Drawers of Water: Domestic Water Use in East Africa.* Chicago: University of Chicago Press.

Whitehead, F. E. 1973. "Nutrition Education Research." *World Review of Nutrition and Dietetics* 17:91–149.

Whitfield, R. A. 1982. "A Nutritional Analysis of the Food Stamp Program." *American Journal of Public Health* 72 (8):793–799.

Whiting, H., and A. Kristall. N.d. *The Impact of Rural Water Supply Projects on Women.* CARE, New York. Mimeographed.

WHO. 1980. "Disease Prevention and Control in Water Development Schemes." PDO/80.1. Geneva: World Health Organization.

WHO. 1978. "International Conference on Primary Health Care, Alma Ata, USSR, September, 1973." Geneva: WHO.

WHO. 1976. *Methodology of Nutritional Surveillance.* Report of a Joint FAO/UNICEF/WHO Expert Committee, Technical Report Series 593. Geneva: WHO.

WHO/CDD/EPI. 1988. "Improving Infant Feeding Practices to Prevent Diarrhea or Reduce Its Severity: Research Issues." Report of a meeting held at the Johns Hopkins University, Baltimore, April.

WHO, Family Health Division. 1981. "Summary of the Ad Hoc Survey on Infant and Early Childhood Mortality in Sierra Leone." *World Health Statistics Quarterly* No. 34:220–238.

WHO/NRC (World Health Organization and U.S. National Research Council). 1983. "Breast-Feeding and Fertility Regulation: Current Knowledge and Programme Policy Implications." *Bulletin of the World Health Organization* 61:371–382.

WHO/UNICEF. 1989. *Improving Child Survival and Nutrition.* Joint WHO/UNICEF Nutrition Support Program in Iringa, Tanzania. Evaluation Report. Dar Es Salaam: WHO-UNICEF.

WHO-UNICEF. 1978. *Primary Health Care: Joint Report of the Director General of the World Health Organization and of the Executive Director of the United Nations Children's Fund: The Declaration of Alma Ata.* Geneva: WHO-UNICEF.

Williamson-Gray, C. 1982. *Food Consumption Parameters for Brazil and Their Application to Food Policy.* IFPRI Research Report No. 32. Washington, D.C.: International Food Policy Research Institute.

Winikoff, B. 1978. "Program and Policy: Some Specific Questions." In *Nutrition and National Policy,* ed. B. Winikoff. Cambridge: Massachusetts Institute of Technology Press.

Winikoff, B., and M. A. Castle. 1987. "The Maternal Depletion Syndrome: Clinical Diagnosis or Eco-Demographic Condition?" Paper presented at the International Conference for Better Health for Women and Children through Family Planning, Nairobi, Kenya, October.

Wirawan, D. N. 1986. *Survei Perilaku Rumahtangga.* Th. 11985: Propinsi Bali (Seri2: Laporan Utama).

Wisner, B. 1988. "GOBI versus PHC: Some Dangers of Selective Primary Health Care." *Social Science and Medicine* 26 (9):963–969.

Wolfe, B. L., and J. R. Behrman. 1987. "Women's Schooling and Children's Health: Are the Effects Robust with Adult Sibling Control for the Women's Childhood Background?" *Journal of Health Economics* 6 (3):239–254.

Wolfe, B. L., and J. R. Behrman. 1984. "Determinants of Women's Health Status and Health-Care Utilization in a Developing Country: A Latent Variable Approach." *Review of Economics and Statistics* 56 (4):696–703.

Wolff, R. J. 1965. "Meanings of Food." *Tropical Geographic Medicine* 17 (1):45–52.

World Bank. 1993. *World Development Report 1993: Investing in Health.* Washington, D.C.: World Bank.

World Bank. 1992. *Poverty Reduction Handbook.* Washington, D.C.: World Bank.

World Bank. 1988. *Rural Development: World Bank Experience, 1965–1986.* Washington, D.C.: World Bank, Operations Evaluation Department.

World Bank. 1981. *World Development Report, 1981.* Washington, D.C.: World Bank.

Yambi, O., U. Jonsson,and B. Ljungqvist. 1989. *The Role of Government in Promoting Community-Based Nutrition Programs: Experience from Tanzania and Lessons for Africa.* Pew/Cornell Lecture Series on Food and Nutrition. Ithaca: Cornell Food and Nutrition Policy Program, Cornell University.

Yee, V. S-Y. 1984. "Household Level Correlates of Child Nutritional Status in Fiji." M.P.S. thesis, Cornell University.

Yee, V., and A. Zerfas. 1986. *Review of Growth Monitoring: Issues Paper.* Washington, D.C.: LTS/International Nutrition Unit.

Yip, R., K. Scanlon, and F. L. Trowbridge. 1992. "Improving Growth Status of Asian Refugee Children in the United States." *Journal of the American Medical Association* 267:937–940.

Yip, R., and F. L. Trowbridge. 1989. "Limitations of the Current International Growth Reference." Paper presented at the 14th International Congress of Nutrition, Seoul, Korea, 20–25 August. Abstract P4–135:800.

Young, B., and J. Briscoe. 1987. "A Case-Control Study of the Effect of Environmental Sanitation on Diarrhoea Morbidity in Malawi." *Journal of Epidemiology and Community Health* 42 (1):83–88.

Zeitlin, M., and C. Formación. 1981. "Nutrition Education, Study II." In *Nutrition Intervention in Developing Countries: An Overview,* ed. J. Austin and M. Zeitlin. Cambridge, Mass.: Oelgeschlager, Gunn and Hain.

Zeitlin, M. F., G. Griffiths, R. K. Manoff, and T. Cooke. 1984. *Household Evaluation, Nutrition Communication and Behavior Change Component: Indonesian Nutrition Development Program,* Vol. 4. Washington, D.C.: Manoff International.

Zeitlin, M. F., R. Houser, and F. C. Johnson. 1989. "Active Maternal Feeding and Nutritional Status of 8–20 Month Old Mexican Children." Paper presented at the meeting of the Society for Research in Child Development, Kansas City, Mo.

Zeitlin, M., M. Mansour, and M. Boghani. 1990. *Positive Deviance in Nutrition.* Tokyo: United Nations University.

Zeitlin, M., C. Super, M. Beiser, G. Gulden, N. Ahmet, J. Zeitlan, M. Ahmed, and S. Sockalingam. 1990. *A Behavioral Study of Positive Deviance in Young Child Nutrition and Health in Bangladesh.* Washington, D.C.: Office of International Health and USAID.

Zerfas, A. 1986. *Strengthening Community-Based Growth Surveillance in Thailand: Analysis of Phase I Operations Research and Preparations for Phase II.* Thailand trip report, 2–30 October. Rockville, Md.: International Nutrition Unit, Office of International Health.

Zerfas, A. J. 1975. "The Insertion Tape: A New Circumference Tape for Nutritional Assessment." *American Journal of Clinical Nutrition* 28:782.

Zeskind, P. S. 1983. "Cross-Cultural Differences in Maternal Perceptions of Cries of Low-and High-Risk Infants." *Child Development* 54 (5):1119–1128.

Zeskind, P. S., and C. T. Ramey. 1978. "Fetal Malnutrition: An Experimental Study of Its Consequences on Infant Development in Two Caregiving Environments." *Child Development* 49 (4): 1155–1162.

Zinn, F. D., and W. D. Drake. 1988. *Growth Monitoring: Social, Environmental and Institutional Factors Which Influence Successful Implementation.* Ann Arbor: Community Systems Foundation.

Contributors

HAROLD ALDERMAN is a senior economist in the Policy Research Department, Poverty and Human Resources Division of the World Bank. He was formerly a research fellow at the International Food Policy Research Institute.

JERE BEHRMAN is the W. R. Kenan, Jr., professor of economics at the University of Pennsylvania. His research has primarily been on a wide variety of topics related to economic development, in recent years particularly on human resources and household behavior. He has considerable experience in developing countries, has worked with a number of international development-oriented organizations, has been principal investigator on over 40 competitive research grants primarily on development topics, and has authored or co-authored 22 books and over 170 professional articles.

SUSAN BURGER is the director of the Nutrition Unit of Helen Keller International. She formerly held a postdoctoral position at Emory University in the program against micronutrient malnutrition. She has conducted research on the beneficial and detrimental effects of supplementary foods during infancy.

MARIA TERESA CERQUEIRA is presently the regional adviser in Social Participation and Health Education with the Division of Health Systems and Services in the Pan American Health Organization (PAHO). As a nutritionist, she has been a consultant to the Food and Agriculture Organization of the United Nations and the World Bank. She has done extensive research in health and nutrition education dealing with issues of implementation and evaluation of health and nutrition education programs, especially training community workers to facilitate community participation. She has a B.S. from Florida State University (1973), M.S. from the University of Iowa (1975), and is a Ph.D. candidate at Cornell University. She was director for training and research in health and nutrition education with the Ministry of Health in Mexico, head of the Nutrition Education Department of the Nutrition Program, and professor at the Autonomous University in Mexico City.

PATRICE ENGLE is a professor and chair of the Department of Psychology at Cal Poly State University, San Luis Obispo, California. Formerly she was a research associate at UCLA and UC-Davis and psychologist at the Institute of Nutrition of Central America and Panama. Her research has centered on the effects of nutritional deficiencies on children's cognitive development and on the consequences of variations in child caregiving (e.g., maternal work for earnings, food allocation, feeding behavior) for children's health, nutrition, and development.

STEVEN ESREY is a nutritional epidemiologist at McGill University in Montreal. He was formerly a professor at the Johns Hopkins University, School of Hygiene and Public Health in Baltimore. He has conducted extensive research on the social and biological impacts of water and sanitation on children and women in Africa and Latin America. He has also conducted research on food security issues in the Horn of Africa and implemented iron supplementation trials.

JOHN HAAGA is director of the Committee on Population for the National Research Council/National Academy of Sciences. From 1991 to 1993 he was an associate of the Population Council, serving as project director for MCH-Family Planning Extension at the International Center for Diarrheal Disease Research, Bangladesh. He has also worked in the Social Policy Department at RAND and the Nutritional Surveillance Program at Cornell University on studies of family planning, health, and nutrition programs in both poor and rich countries.

SANDRA HUFFMAN, the president of NURTURE, is an adjunct associate professor at Johns Hopkins University, School of Hygiene and Public Health, in the Department of International Health. She founded NURTURE in 1986 while at Johns Hopkins University in an effort to merge academic research with community-level experiences and policy change. She lived and worked in Bangladesh and Colombia for several years. She conducted research on maternal and infant nutrition at the International Center for Diarrheal Diseases in Bangladesh and worked on childhood nutrition intervention programs in Colombia and Peru. She has produced many reports and articles on infant feeding and child nutrition. In addition, she has testified numerous times at congressional hearings on hunger in the United States and in developing countries. She has served as a consultant to UNICEF, the World Health Organization, and the World Bank. In addition, she served on the National Academy of Sciences Committee on International Nutrition Programs.

JOANNE LESLIE, a public health nutritionist, is co-director of the Pacific Institute for Women's Health in Los Angeles and a lecturer in the Community Health Sciences Department at the UCLA School of Public Health. She has previously held research and policy positions at the World Bank and at the International Center for Research on Women in Washington, D.C. Her research has focused on the relationship between health, nutrition, and schooling, and the effects of women's multiple roles on their own health and that of their families.

F. JAMES LEVINSON is a visiting professor, School of Nutrition, Tufts University, and a consultant on international nutrition. He has served as director of the MIT International Nutrition Planning Program and of the Office of Nutrition of USAID. He also is actively involved in the production of food for homeless and elderly persons in the state of Massachusetts.

REYNALDO MARTORELL is the Robert W. Woodruff Professor of International Nutrition at the Emory University School of Public Health. He is chairman of the Advisory Group on Nutrition of the United Nations' Sub-Committee on Nutrition. His current research focuses on the long-term, functional consequences of malnutrition in early childhood.

SABA MEBRAHTU, a sociologist, completed two years of doctoral fieldwork in Nigeria, funded by the Ford Foundation through the International Institute of Tropical Agriculture, Nigeria, and the Dietary Management of Diarrhea Program of the Johns Hopkins University. She has been a visiting scholar at Rutgers University, Women's Studies, and a consultant at the World Health Organization. She is currently at Cornell University in the Population and Development Program, completing her dissertation.

CHRISTINE OLSON is a professor in the Division of Nutritional Sciences at Cornell University. She has conducted numerous research projects focused on nutrition education as an intervention strategy for improving the health of women and children.

DAVID PELLETIER is an associate professor in the Division of Nutritional Sciences, Cornell University, and affiliated with the Cornell Food and Nutrition Policy Program. His research interests are on the uses of information at household, community, and national levels to improve decision making related to nutrition. He also conducts research on the causes and consequences of protein-energy malnutrition, including its effects on child mortality.

PER PINSTRUP-ANDERSEN is director general of the International Food Policy Research Institute. His past positions include professor of food economics at Cornell University, director of the Cornell Food and Nutrition Policy Program, associate professor at the Danish Agricultural University, and economist at the International Center for Tropical Agriculture in Colombia. He has extensive experience in food and nutrition policy and, in addition to research and teaching, has served as a consultant to many government and international agencies.

BEATRICE ROGERS is professor of economics and food policy at the Tufts University School of Nutrition. She has conducted research on food price subsidies, income transfers, and alternative methods of increasing household access to food, in both the United States and developing countries. She has conducted evaluations of health-system-based food supplementation programs in several countries. In addition to food price and income policy, her research deals with intrahousehold resource allocation and its determinants and with methods of measurement.

MARIE RUEL is coordinator of the Human Nutrition Program at the Institute of Nutrition of Central America and Panama/Pan American Health Organization in Guatemala. Her present work involves both basic and applied research in the areas of maternal and child nutrition, growth, micronutrient deficiencies, food and nutrition policies and programs, and nutritional surveillance.

ROGER SHRIMPTON is a nutritionist currently serving with UNICEF in Indonesia as senior program coordinator. He has been a research associate with the Cornell Food and Nutrition Policy Program and with the Brazilian Amazonian Research Institute in Manaus, Amazonas. His research has been related to micronutrients, nutrition and infection interactions, and information systems in nutrition programs.

ADWOA STEEL is a consultant in international health. She was formerly community health adviser at Wellstart International and project director at the Center to Prevent Childhood Malnutrition, both in Washington, D.C. She has worked extensively in Africa on child heath and on ways in which both governments and small communities can address infant and child feeding issues.

Index